Ergonomics
for Therapists

Ergonomics for Therapists

Second Edition

Karen Jacobs, Ed.D., OTR/L, C.P.E., FAOTA
Clinical Associate Professor of Occupational Therapy, Boston University

With 20 contributors

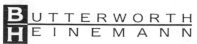

BUTTERWORTH
HEINEMANN

Boston   Oxford   Auckland   Johannesburg   Melbourne   New Delhi

Library of Congress Cataloging-in-Publication Data
Ergonomics for therapists / [edited by] Karen Jacobs. -- 2nd ed.
    p.   cm.
    Includes bibliographical references and index.
    ISBN 0-7506-7051-7
    1. Occupational therapy. 2. Human engineering. 3. Physical therapy.   I. Jacobs, Karen, 1951-   .
RM735.E73   1999
615.8'515--dc21   98-53102
                                                          CIP

British Library Cataloguing-in-Publication Data
A catalogue record for this book is available from the British Library.

The publisher offers special discounts on bulk orders of this book.
For information, please contact

Manager of Special Sales
Butterworth–Heinemann
225 Wildwood Avenue
Woburn, MA 01801-2041
Tel: 781-904-2500
Fax: 781-904-2620

For information on all Butterworth–Heinemann publications available, contact our World Wide Web home page at http://www.bh.com

10 9 8 7 6 5 4 3

Printed in the United States of America

For my parents, Ruth and Lawrence Jacobs,
with much love and admiration

Contents

Contributing Authors

Diane Aja, M.S., OTR
Therapy Coordinator, Work Enhancement and Rehabilitation Center, Fletcher Allen Health Care, Colchester, Vermont

Nancy A. Baker, M.S., OTR/L
Doctoral Candidate in Occupational Therapy, Sargent College of Health and Rehabilitation Sciences, Boston University

Chetwyn C. H. Chan, B.Sc., M.Sc., Ph.D.
Associate Professor, Department of Rehabilitation Sciences, Hong Kong Polytechnic University, Hung Hom, Kowloon

Asnat Bar-Haim Erez, OTR, M.A.
Staff Member, School of Occupational Therapy, Hadassah-Hebrew University, Jerusalem

A. James Giannini, M.D., F.C.P., F.A.P.A., F.R.S.M.
Clinical Professor of Psychiatry, Ohio State University College of Medicine, Columbus; President and Medical Director, Chemical Abuse Centers, Inc., Austintown, Ohio

Juliette N. Giannini
Researcher, Department of History, Poland Seminary, Poland, Ohio

Diane C. Hermenau, M.S., OTR/L
Operations Supervisor for Occupational Therapy, Morton Hospital and Medical Center, Taunton, Massachusetts

Debbie Holmes-Enix, M.P.H., OTR, C.V.E.
Coordinator of Employer Relations and Education and Ergonomics Consultant, Rehabilitation Technology Works, Inc., San Bernardino, California

Karen Jacobs, Ed.D., OTR/L, C.P.E., FAOTA
Clinical Associate Professor of Occupational Therapy, Boston University

Krystal Laflin, P.T.
Therapy Coordinator, Work Enhancement and Rehabilitation Center, Fletcher Allen Health Care, Burlington, Vermont

Paul Chi-Wai Lam, M.Sc.
Assistant Professor, Department of Rehabilitation Sciences, Hong Kong Polytechnic University, Hung Hom, Kowloon

Tatia M. C. Lee, M.Sc., M.Ed., Ph.D.
Assistant Professor, Department of Psychology, Clinical Psychology Program, University of Hong Kong

Karen N. Lindgren, Ph.D.
Neuropsychologist and Research Coordinator, Center for Occupational and Environmental Neurology, Baltimore

Peter Picone, M.S.I.E., C.P.E.
Manager, Commercial Markets Usability Lab, Liberty Mutual Insurance, Danvers, Massachusetts

Valerie J. Berg Rice, Ph.D., C.P.E., OTR/L, FAOTA
Chair of Occupational Therapy, U.S. Army Medical Center and School, San Antonio, Texas; Adjunct Faculty, University of Texas Health Sciences Center, San Antonio

Lynn Shaw, M.Sc., O.T.
Program Manager, Occupational Health and Disability Management, Comcare Health Services, London, Ontario, Canada

Susan Strong, B.Sc., M.Sc., OT(C)
Assistant Clinical Professor and Research Associate, Work Function Unit, School of Rehabilitation Science, McMaster University, Hamilton, Ontario, Canada; Staff Occupational Therapist and Researcher, Hamilton Psychiatric Hospital, Hamilton

Cecilia Tsang-Li, M.Phil.
Associate Professor, Department of Rehabilitation Sciences, Hong Kong Polytechnic University, Hung Hom, Kowloon

Laurie A. Vincello, M.A., P.T.
Physical Therapy Supervisor, The Occupational Health Center of Waltham, Waltham, Massachusetts

Tamar (Patrice L.) Weiss, Ph.D., OT(C)
School of Occupational Therapy, Hadassah-Hebrew University, Jerusalem

Marilyn Wright, M.P.H., OTR
Assistant Professor of Occupational Therapy, School of Allied Health Professions, Loma Linda University, Loma Linda, California

Preface

Ergonomics continues to be a growing service provided by occupational and physical therapists who have advanced knowledge and skills in this area. The second edition of *Ergonomics for Therapists* has been designed as a reference for therapists interested in acquiring knowledge about ergonomics and learning about the tools and techniques used therein. This text is not a substitute for continuing education and advanced academic training in ergonomics and related fields, but it is a complement to lifelong learning and continuing competency.

To provide a framework for understanding ergonomics, the text has been divided into four parts. Part I provides a general overview of ergonomics and a conceptual framework for designing ergonomics services; Part II defines and describes some of the knowledge, tools, and techniques that make up ergonomics; Part III discusses topics worthy of special consideration; and Part IV applies ergonomics to occupational and physical therapy practice.

Appreciation is due to everyone who helped in the completion of this text. Most important, I thank the contributing authors, who eagerly shared their expertise and insights. I am grateful to the editorial staff at Butterworth–Heinemann for their assistance, in particular Leslie Kramer, Assistant Editor in the Medical Division. Finally, I thank my family and friends for their continued support. They are the "wind beneath my wings."

KAREN JACOBS
(kjacobs@bu.edu)

Ergonomics
for Therapists

PART I

Overview and Conceptual Framework

CHAPTER 1
Ergonomics and Therapy: An Introduction

Valerie J. Berg Rice

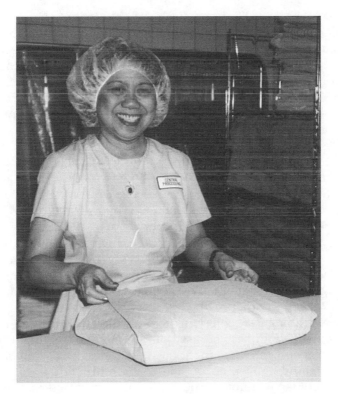

ABSTRACT

This chapter defines ergonomics and provides brief histories of the fields of occupational therapy, physical therapy, and ergonomics. It also describes the relationships between therapists and ergonomists in three areas of practice: (1) workplace analysis, (2) environment and product design and redesign, and (3) research. Principles of therapy and ergonomics are considered in relation to persons with disabilities; persons with temporary injuries, such as work-related musculoskeletal disorders; and persons without disabilities. This chapter also profiles considerations for joint ventures between therapists and ergonomists.

Historical Background

Occupational Therapy

Occupational therapy (OT) is predicated on the belief that eradication of disease alone is insufficient for complete recovery. Before the advent of OT, individuals who had been injured or ill were hospitalized, treated, and discharged, only to find themselves unable to function sufficiently because of physical and mental exhaustion. George Barton, an originator of OT, spent extensive time as a patient in a tuberculosis hospital and recognized the need for additional therapy. Trained as an architect, he formed his own rehabilitation program after leaving the hospital by working with the tools of his profession to strengthen himself physically and mentally. In 1914, he opened Consolation House to provide similar services for others. Other founders of the field of OT held similar beliefs that occupying one's time and doing something of purpose serve both as evaluative tests and as tools for "strength, reserve force, nerve and mental poise, and of the several elements that we take together as character" (Brush 1923). What was important for the founders of OT was that the patient have pursuits that were important to him or her. The purposeful involvement helped reduce weaknesses caused by illness or injury by building on personal strengths, allowing patients to return as productive members of their families and society.

Dr. Adolph Meyer, another of the founders of OT, asked his colleagues at the Chicago Pathological Society in 1893 for their opinions on the types of occupations that could best be used during patient treatment. Gardening and ward and shop work were mentioned, including raffia and basket work, weaving, bookbinding, carpentry, and metal and leather working (Meyer 1921). These crafts were not considered leisure activities; instead, the practice of a craft was an assignment that provided rehabilitation for the patient and could be used as full-time employment to support the patient and patient's family on discharge. Thus, the OT rehabilitation process focused on improving physical and mental functioning, as well as returning the patient to a functional status in society. Indeed, these activities were often used to train patients for specific jobs, and it was with great alarm that therapists first realized their patients did not always enter the craft field for which they had been trained. Questions arose regarding whether time, effort, and funds had been wasted in training. It was noted, however, that with just a few carefully chosen, occupationally based crafts, the habits and skills needed for rehabilitation and employment could be learned and transferred to numerous job opportunities (Report of the Committee on Installations and Advice 1928). Crafts were categorized according to the physical movements (upper and lower extremity, torso, head and neck), balance, and coordination required, as well as according to complexity, pace, stimulation level provided (monotonous or stimulating), the level of problem-solving skills required, initial cost, final product use, level of concentration needed, initiative required, noise created, amount of mental capacity required, and type of patient for which it might be appropriate (Bowman 1928). Thus, the need for simulating the job each patient wanted to return to or undergo new training for was eliminated. The question of whether using a few well-chosen activities for rehabilitation is more effective than individual job simulation has not been clearly answered through outcome research, however. Work hardening, or the simulation of the work environment as a means for recovery of ability, has revived the idea that each job and its commensurate job tasks need to be recreated to provide the best possible rehabilitation and return-to-work program for the industrial worker, but no proof for either argument exists, except anecdotally. The intent is clear, however, that actively engaging the patient in carefully guided physical and mental activities enhances the chances for a more successful return to work.

The fundamental goal of OT is to enhance "the capacity [of the patient] throughout the life span, to perform with satisfaction to self and others those tasks and roles essential to productive living and to the mastery of self and the environment" (Hopkins 1978). OT should also help patients obtain their highest functional performance in all areas of life, including work, recreational activities, and life at home.

Both occupational therapists and ergonomists are trained to be aware of normal human abilities. Therapists must be aware of patients' current physical, cognitive, and psychological limitations and capabilities; their potential abilities and disabilities; and the physiologic and psychological demands of the patients' activities (including work). Therapists must also be aware of the performance competencies and limitations of people without injuries to be able to assess whether a client is functioning within normal range. Maximal functional performance has been the goal of OT since the inception of the profession in 1917 (beginning with the founding of the National Society for the Promotion of Occupational Therapy). The use of purposeful activities (e.g., work simulation) as treatment modalities was integral to the develop-

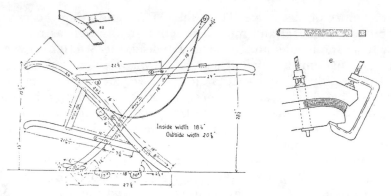

FIGURE 1.1.   Plan of the folding conveying chair. (Reprinted with permission from LJ Haas. A folding conveying chair. Occup Ther Rehabil 1928;7[1]:23.)

ment of the profession, as suggested by its name: *occupational* therapy. It must be noted, however, that work or activity used in a therapeutic manner is not ergonomics, nor is work hardening part of ergonomics.

   The initial articles published in OT literature to use ergonomic principles were published by Haas in the late 1920s and early 1930s. The first article involved what has been termed *ergonomics-for–special populations* (Rice 1998). Haas designed and constructed a weaving frame that could be used for patients who were bedridden (1925). The second article described the combination of the principles of OT (therapeutic activity) with the needs of the hospital (increasing work efficiency): The patients were assigned to build a folding conveying chair for the hospital (Haas 1928) (Figure 1.1). As described in a subsequent article, the building of an adjustable stool that encouraged "good" posture helped hasten recovery, maintain health, and increase productivity through the principles of anatomy (Haas 1930). None of the early articles applied to the general population; instead, they were designs for special patient populations.

Physical Therapy

The early fundamental intention of physical therapy (PT) was "to assess, prevent, and treat movement dysfunction and physical disability, with the overall goal of enhancing human movement and function" (McMillan, as cited by Pinkston 1989). In terms of injury prevention, these goals conform to the objectives delineated by ergonomic engineers, particularly those who design workplaces and equipment for physical safety and effective work performance. For example, as industrial consultants, physical therapists often use knowledge of human motion to evaluate safe and effective working postures. Physical and occupational therapists who work in an industrial environment also evaluate the limitations and capabilities of workers with injuries (functional capacity assessment) and the demands of the work role (workplace analysis) to establish treatment regimens. Assessment and treatment roles are sometimes targeted toward specialty areas, such as back care, strength training, or work hardening. The benefit to companies of having an occupational or physical therapist on an ergonomic team is the increased likelihood of the employee's returning to work earlier, matching worker capabilities with work demands, and preventing injuries. Each of these benefits can translate into increased revenues for a company (Key 1989). A therapist can often provide information about the prognosis of an injury or illness, along with knowledge of the Americans with Disabilities Act.

Ergonomics

Although a concept of ergonomics (also called *human factors*) existed during the Stone Age (humans constructed tools to fit their own hands for hunting and gathering needs), the first documented mention of the field came in 1857, when Wojciech Jastrzebowski published *An Outline of Ergonomics, or The Science of Work Based upon the Truths Drawn from the Science of Nature* (Jastrzebowski 1857):

> Hail, Thou great unbounded idea of work! God, Who, as the Bible teaches us, cursed mankind and subjected him to work, cursed him with a father's heart; for the punishment was also a consolation. He who complains against his work knoweth not life; work is an uplifting force by which all things may be moved. Repose is death, and work is life!

Jastrzebowski felt the ideas of work should be studied and preached with the same rigor applied to more philosophical studies of his time, for he believed that "affections [i.e., beliefs, emotions] are nothing else, but accessories to deeds." According to Jastrzebowski, the study of work, or ergonomics, should involve all aspects of useful work, the four main components of which are physical, aesthetic, rational, and moral (Table 1.1). Jastrzebowski taught that applying each of the four components of work to whatever endeavors one was involved with increased the benefits of those activities exponentially. For example, whereas pure physical work applied to planting might yield a two-for-one harvest, applying aesthetic or sensory forces would increase the yield fourfold. Additional application of intellectual forces would then yield an eightfold gain at harvest time, and so on (Jastrzebowski 1857). His treatise is more complex than this chapter shows; he further subdivided all areas of work. He also sought to identify further areas of study including (1) the animals with which we share work categories, (2) the periods of our lives that are particularly suited to various types of work, (3) the manner of work, and (4) the benefits drawn from work for both the individual and the common good of society. His views are remarkably similar to those of the founders of OT, although the latter applied the theories to individuals who were injured or ill, whereas Jastrzebowski pri-

TABLE 1.1
Jastrzebowski's Divisions of Useful Work

Physical	Aesthetic	Rational	Moral
Kinetic or motor	Emotional or sensory	Intellectual or rational	Spiritual
Labor or toil	Entertainment or pastime	Thinking or reasoning	Devotion or dedication
Breaking stones	Playing with stones	Investigation of a stone's natural properties	Removing stones from the road to remove untidiness and possible suffering for other persons and animals

Source: Adapted from W Jastrzebowski. An Outline of Ergonomics, or The Science of Work Based upon the Truths Drawn from the Science of Nature. Warsaw: Central Institute for Labor Protection, 1997. T Baluk-Ulewiczowa (trans).

marily applied his theories to able-bodied persons with the penultimate objective of bettering humankind.

Ergonomics as a specialty made gains as technological developments emerged during the industrial revolution. Time and motion studies, considered predecessors of ergonomics, focused on evaluation of work methods, workstation design, and equipment design. They were conducted by numerous investigators, including the Gilbreths, Taylor, Muensterberg, and Binet (Christensen 1987).

The field of ergonomics received particular attention during World War II, when the complexity of military equipment frequently surpassed the abilities of the human operators (Damon and Randall 1944): "Man had become the weak link" (Damon et al. 1966). As during World War I, the primary focus was selection and training of personnel; however, even with extensive training, personnel could not always perform as needed (Sanders and McCormick 1987). Because selection and training were not providing an acceptable solution, the focus changed to fitting the task or equipment to the person by using human dimensions, capabilities, and limitations as factors in the design process.

After World War II, the Ergonomics Research Society (the current Ergonomics Society) was founded in England, and the first ergonomics text, *Applied Experimental Psychology: Human Factors in Engineering Design* by Chapanis, Garner, and Morgan, was published (1949). In 1957, the Human Factors Society was formed in the United States, and *Ergonomics*, the journal of the Ergonomics Research Society, began publication. The International Ergonomics Association was formed in 1959 to join ergonomics societies from several countries. Since that time, the field of ergonomics has had tremendous growth, and many areas of specialization have been developed. The interface between humans and computers has given rise to new specializations in ergonomics, and the incident at Three Mile Island accelerated the study of the role of ergonomics in the nuclear power industry. In addition, more attention to product liability has increased the number of ergonomics experts needed in forensics to address design deficiencies, instructions, and warning labels (Sanders and McCormick 1987).

Ergonomics developed from the common interests of a number of professions, particularly engineering, psychology, and medicine. It has remained a multidisciplinary field of study. Ergonomists include professionals with degrees in psychology, engineering, ergonomics, industrial design, education, physiology, medicine, health and rehabilitation sciences, business administration, computer science, and industrial hygiene. However, bachelor's, master's, and doctoral degree programs are now offered specifically in ergonomics/human factors and can be accredited through the Human Factors and Ergonomics Society. Individual certification is also offered through the Board of Certification in Professional Ergonomics (P.O. Box 2811, Bellingham, WA 98227-2811) (see Chapter 14).

Ergonomics Defined

Ergonomics (Greek *ergon* [work] + *nomos* [law]) focuses on the study of work performance with an emphasis on worker safety and productivity. Although several definitions have been proposed, one of the best was provided by Chapanis (1991), who used the terms *ergonomics* and *human factors* interchangeably: "Human factors (ergonomics) is a body of knowledge about human abilities, human limitations, and other human characteristics that are relevant to design. *Human factors engineering* (ergonomics implementation) is the application of human factors information to the design of tools, machines, systems, tasks, jobs, and environments for safe, comfortable, and effective human use."

Considerable debate on the definitions of *ergonomics* and *human factors* has persisted. The controversy has been especially fervent regarding the differentiation of the terms. Proponents of differentiation argue that the term *human factors* was first used in psychology and refers primarily to the interface of humans with technology, whereas *ergonomics* originated in human physiology and biomechanics and therefore refers primarily to physically demanding work (Fraser 1989). The differentiation is capricious at best, and the major human factors and ergonomics texts encourage use of the two terms interchangeably (Gay 1986; Fraser 1989; Kroemer et al. 1994; Meister 1989; Wilson and Corlett 1990). In their introduction, Sanders and McCormick (1987) state that "some people have tried to distinguish between the two, but we believe that any distinctions are arbitrary and that, for all practical purposes, the terms are synonymous."

In this chapter, as well as throughout this book, the two terms are used interchangeably. It is true that *ergonomics* has not been as widely used in the United States and Canada as in other parts of the world. In the United States, the terms *human factors engineering*, *human engineering*, *engineering psychology*, and *human factors* have all been used, although the current term of choice is *human factors*. As noted by Chapanis (1991), "whether we call ourselves human factors engineers or ergonomists is mostly an accident of where we happen to live and where we were trained." *Ergonomics* is quickly becoming the more recognized term among the general public, even in the United States.

Ergonomics focuses on humans and their interactions with the environment. It involves interactions with tools, equipment, consumer products, work methods, jobs, instruction books, facilities, and organizations. Kantowitz and Sorkin (1983) noted that "the first commandment of human factors is 'Honor Thy User.'" Ergonomists design environments and products according to the physical (visual, auditory, tactile, strength, anthropometric), cognitive (learning, information processing, retention), and psychological (cultural influences, behavior, background) characteristics of humans. Accordingly, ergonomics is not solely confined to the workplace. Products and environments should match the abilities, needs, and perceptions of the people who use them. In self-care, ergonomically designed toothbrushes and spigots are found. These spigots conform to users' expectations (i.e., water should emerge when the spigot is turned counterclockwise, and cold water should be controlled by the spigot on the user's right). Bicycles and snow skis are designed with riders and skiers of differing abilities in mind and are designed differently for men and women. Numerous examples of proper and improper ergonomic designs can be found throughout homes and offices. The concept of making the devices and systems "user-friendly" extends beyond the workplace.

To attain the goal of designing user-friendly devices and systems, ergonomists conduct scientific investigations to identify the limitations, capabilities, and responses of humans in a variety of climates and circumstances. This information is used to produce designs that match human characteristics. Part II of this book, Knowledge, Tools, and Techniques, provides examples of how physical and cognitive information can be applied in the workplace. Part III, Special Considerations, demonstrates how human characteristics are applied to specific situations. Ergonomists evaluate equipment, jobs, work methods, and environments to ensure they meet their intended objectives. Chapter 8, on usability testing, describes the procedures for conducting an ergonomic evaluation of rehabilitation equipment.

Ergonomics can be considered a design philosophy that focuses on supplying a product that ensures safety, ease of use, comfort, and efficiency. However, many distinguished human factors practitioners and ergonomists contend that ergonomics is a unitary, scholarly discipline with unique characteristics, just as OT and PT are unique disciplines (Meister 1989, 1997).

Why Use Ergonomics?

Good principles of ergonomics are most noted when they are absent, because their focus is to optimize the relationship between the environment and the person (Kantowitz and Sorkin 1983). When an appropriate ergonomic design is in use, the user should be unaware of environmental design deficiencies and be able to concentrate on the task at hand. For example, in a well-designed office workstation, a worker should not have to hold his or her neck in an awkward posture to use a visual display terminal and should not experience neck and shoulder discomfort. According to Osborne (1982), good ergonomic design in the workplace offers a means to "victory over the oppressive forces that continue to make work less productive, less pleasant, less comfortable and less safe."

In the past, industry focused on work demands, and the needs of workers took second place. Humanistic and economic concerns and litigation, however, have convinced industry that consideration of the worker is good business. The use of sound ergonomic principles has generated many examples of increased worker productivity and safety. One example (Chaney and Teel 1967) demonstrated that less training is required if workers' abilities are considered in the design of equipment. In this example, the detection efficiency of machine parts inspectors was evaluated after either a 4-hour training program or use of a set of visual aids and displays that assisted with the detection of defects. A 32% increase in detected defects was found with the training, a 42% increase was found with the use of appropriate visual aids, and a 71% increase was found when training and visual aids were combined. Although training was useful, a properly designed environment was also needed for superior results.

The Interrelationship between Therapists and Ergonomists

The interrelationship between rehabilitation and ergonomics has received a great deal of attention (Bogner 1994, 1996a, 1996b; Rice 1992, 1998a). Therapists and ergonomists share some common interests, and therapists can contribute to the practice of ergonomics in five principal areas: (1) ergonomics-for-one (individuals who are disabled); (2) ergonomics-for–special populations; (3) prevention of musculoskeletal injuries; (4) equipment design; and (5) the application of the Americans with Disabilities Act (Rice 1998a). These five areas can be simplified into three major practice application arenas, in addition to integrating ergonomic principles into therapeutic clinical practice: (1) workplace analysis aimed at prevention of work-related musculoskeletal trauma; (2) workplace and tool design for individuals with disabilities; and (3) research through the development and use of databases.

Work-Site Analysis

Therapists should be familiar with the field of ergonomics as a whole to understand terminology being used, know how to best describe their own expertise, and recognize when an ergonomist with specialized training should be consulted (Rader Smith 1998; Rice 1998b, 1998c). A review of introductory ergonomics texts (as well as university accreditation requirements for OT, PT, and ergonomics) produced the following observations about the knowledge base of therapists compared with ergonomists (Kantowitz and Sorkin 1983; Konz 1995; Kroemer 1994; Osborne 1982; Sanders and McCormick 1987).

Some areas of ergonomics with which therapists are familiar are sensory nervous system considerations, anthropometry, kinesiology, human development, anatomy and physiology, work capability analysis, and basic research. Areas familiar to occupational therapists (and to physical therapists, depending on their training) include communication, learning, motivation, normal and abnormal psychology (including the effects of stress), job and task analysis, and measure of job satisfaction. Workplace design, seating and posture, and safety may or may not be included in the knowledge of entry-level therapists. Topics in ergonomics with which entry-level therapists also may be unfamiliar include person-machine communication (displays and controls), workstation design, vibration, noise, temperature, illumination, training, inspection and maintenance, error and reliability, signal detection theory, visual displays, legal aspects of product liability, and advanced statistical research. Although therapists may consider themselves educated in safety, for example, they may be unfamiliar with safety as it is taught in ergonomics curriculums. In these classes, safety may include accident losses; Occupational Safety and Health Act; standards, codes, and safety documents; designing, planning, and production errors; hazards; acceleration, falls, and other impacts; pressure and electrical hazards; explosions and explosives; toxic materials; radiation; vibration and noise; and methods of safety analysis (Hammer 1985).

Therapists are well educated in the procedures of problem identification, interviewing, observation, and record review. Their considerable knowledge in anatomy and physiology, neuroanatomy and neurophysiology, kinesiology, anthropometry, and the mechanism and treatment of injuries makes therapists excellent allies for ergonomists. Knowledge of ergonomics allows therapists to apply their expertise by specializing in the field of work-related musculoskeletal ergonomics and injury prevention.

The application of ergonomics for therapists primarily implies workplace consultation directed at preventing musculoskeletal injuries. The goals are to promote safety and to decrease the financial costs associated with lost work time, medical treatment, and retraining. Consultative services can be combined with direct services (client treatment) or can be offered alone. When providing consultative services in addition to direct services, a therapist can offer functional capacity testing, work hardening, and graded return-to-work placements along with workplace evaluations. Ergonomics workplace evaluations may include task analysis, videotaping, measurement and analysis of equipment and workstation, and workspace analysis (Lopez 1998; Sanders 1997). The consultations may be primarily based on physical considerations or may involve psychosocial factors (Haims and Carayon 1998). The last part of this book addresses the ergonomics intervention process from the beginning (program development and marketing) through problem identification, analysis, and implementation to the final product (evaluation and report of results).

Design for Individuals with Disabilities

More than 43 million Americans have physical or mental disabilities. According to the Committee on a National Agenda for the Prevention of Disabilities, one in seven Americans has a disabling condition (Bello 1991; Pope and Tarlov 1991). Vanderheiden (1990) cites Kraus and Stoddard (1989) and uses 12–20% of the total population as an estimate of the number of individuals in the United States who have a disability. As pointed out by Nickerson (1992), an accurate estimate is not necessary to realize that the dilemma is considerable, and ergonomics intervention could do much to enhance quality of life for these populations.

Cannon, an ergonomics consultant in Colorado who has designed equipment for the visually impaired, stated, "No segment of the population suffers more from neglect of human factors requirements in product design than the severely handicapped" (Gay 1986). Opportunities abound within the areas of overlap between ergonomics and health care. For example, modifications and design features of buildings, vehicles, and appliances could improve independent living prospects for those with physical, cognitive, and emotional disabilities (Nickerson 1992).

Many factors contribute to the lapse of information: seeming unavailability of appropriate resources, lack of data, scarcity of ergonomic concept application in health care and rehabilitation, financial expense, lack of public support for funding these areas, and lack of sufficient databases on which to base designs for special populations. The enactment of the Americans with Disabilities Act (1990), it is hoped, will continue to encourage both public and private entities to consider individuals with disabilities in the initial designs of workplaces, accommodations, transportation systems, and communication services. Databases are available on hardware and software for persons with disabilities who use computers (Casali and Williges 1990), and the increase in the geriatric population has increased spending and research on the needs of older Americans. Few data exist, however, on the anthropometric characteristics, capabilities, and limitations of individuals with disabilities and elderly populations in varying climates and conditions. The argument that has prevented the collection of such information is that the capabilities and limitations differ with each disease process and each person. This argument contends that all of the individual differences that exist within an able-bodied population also exist within a disabled population; however, the differences are compounded because of the additional contrasts in residual capabilities of individuals with disabilities. Until the abilities and restrictions of individuals with disabilities and elderly populations are identified, however, suitable products for their use will not be developed on a consistent basis. As noted, the expansion of the older population has resulted in an increased interest and generation of research in geriatrics. A commensurate increase in research for individuals with disabilities has not occurred, however. The resistance, location, and shape of hand and foot controls; workplace design for people who must sit; and seat pan depth and width requirements differ for people with disabilities and vary according to the disabling condition. Therapists have the skills and are in the settings to gather information for a database on various populations with disabilities. Cases of good research exist, however, and one notable exception to the paucity of information is the research conducted by Das (1998) on paraplegic workers. Das has carefully researched anthropometric information used in design guidelines for paraplegics, annotated measurements of his own, and developed isometric strength profiles for male and female paraplegics (Das 1998; Kozey and Das 1992). Another noteworthy epidemiologic research project identified injuries of wheelchair users and design and selection criteria to assist in injury prevention (Gaal et al. 1997).

Technological aids for individuals with disabilities are expensive because small-scale production is not cost-effective. Although this situation may continue for high-level technological equipment, whether assistive equipment designed for individuals with disabilities could also be attractive and useful for the able-bodied population (called *universal design*) is unstudied (Wilkoff and Abed 1994). For example, use of large numerals on telephones; large, well-marked keys on television remote controls; and door levers rather than knobs may be equally desirable for both disabled and able-bodied populations. Only through appropriate usability evaluations will such information become available. Therapists and medical practitioners must become aware of the need for and develop skills in usability testing. Medical and rehabilitation equipment must be designed with the users (medical practitioners, patients, and patients' family members and caregivers) in mind. Appropriate ergonomic design could increase user acceptance, decrease errors, and increase productivity.

Therapists can provide ergonomists and design engineers with valuable information on the functional capabilities and limitations of, environmental effects on, and overall prognosis of individual patients and diagnostic groups. The information is essential to identifying needed accommodations, which is particularly important as industry continues to implement the Americans with Disabilities Act (Kornblau 1998a, 1998b).

Although this text primarily deals with vocational applications, ergonomics applies equally to the interaction of humans and the tools and environments involved in other pursuits. Therefore, therapists and ergonomists might consult in recreational activities, transportation, or home environments both in terms of layout and design (Unsworth 1998).

Research Interests

Therapists and ergonomists often need the same information on human performance. Therapists can and do use ergonomics data in clinical treatment and prevention programs. For example, when treating hospitalized clients, a therapist should be aware of the effects of diurnal variation on muscle strength during muscle strength testing and should also be aware of the effects of sleep deprivation on cognition, perceptual-motor performance, and learning. Therapists use ergonomic data during the evaluation of, goal setting with, and treatment of patients. The same kinds of information are used by ergonomics professionals to recommend design improvements for equipment used by able-bodied individuals and individuals with disabilities (Sanders and McCormick 1987). In addition, therapists can contribute to the body of knowledge on human performance, neurosensory function, and strength testing.

Certainly, national research goals could be established that would cover the common areas between ergonomics and health care and rehabilitation. Some of these goals might include anthropometric and strength (capabilities and limitations) databases to assist with design for special populations, technology use by and design for special populations, epidemiologic investigations of injuries and illnesses common to disabled populations with suggestions for prevention, and compilations of ergonomics-for-one success stories (Rice 1998a).

Conclusion

Common interests and areas of practice can allow ergonomists and therapists to blend their knowledge for the betterment of both disabled and nondisabled populations. Three broad practice areas of common interest are workplace evaluation for the prevention of musculoskeletal evaluations; environment, workspace, and product design; and research.

Ergonomics, in its broadest sense, is the design of products and environments to make the world user-friendly for humans by creating items and places that enhance productivity, are pleasant to use and view, and do not injure the user. Although a more specific definition of *ergonomics* has been identified, it is equally important to recognize what ergonomics is not. Ergonomics is not simply "1) applying checklists and guidelines, 2) using oneself as the model for designing objects, or 3) common sense" (Sanders and McCormick 1987). A "cookbook" approach to ergonomics is an embarrassment to the therapist or ergonomist who uses it and is inherently dangerous. Ergonomics also applies to much more than the prevention of work-related musculoskeletal disorders, although it is in this realm that therapists are most adept.

Ergonomics can be a satisfying area of specialization for therapists. It provides therapists with a growth area of specialization in injury prevention. It also is an area that presents considerable challenge for designing better equipment and environments for the patients therapists serve. Patients, and all persons, deserve to be considered in the design of their equipment and environments. Therapists have the skills, knowledge, and abilities to contribute to the field of ergonomics, and this book provides information and tools to enhance that process.

References

Americans with Disabilities Act of 1990 (July 26, 1990). Public Law Number 101–336.

Bello M (1991). Preventing disability demands new thinking: looking toward a national agenda. News Report XLI(3):2–4.

Bogner MS (1994). Human Error in Medicine: A Frontier for Change. Hillsdale, NJ: Lawrence Erlbaum.

Bogner MS (1996a). Special section preface. Hum Factors 38:551–555.

Bogner MS (1996b). Medical Human Factors. In Proceedings of the Human Factors and Ergonomics Society 40th Annual Meeting. Santa Monica, CA: Human Factors and Ergonomics Society, 752–753.

Bowman M (1928). Report of the round table on crafts for the physically disabled. Arch Occup Ther 2:467–474.

Brush F (1923). Occupational therapy for men in the convalescent period. Arch Occup Ther 2:87–98.

Casali SP, Williges RC (1990). Data bases of accommodative aids for computer users with disabilities. Hum Factors 32:407–422.

Chaney FB, Teel KS (1967). Improving inspector performance through training and visual aids. J Appl Psychol 51:311–315.

Chapanis A (1991). To communicate the human factors message, you have to know what the message is and how to communicate it. Hum Factors Soc Bull 34:1–4.

Chapanis A, Garner WR, Morgan CT (1949). Applied Experimental Psychology. New York: Wiley.

Christensen JM (1987). The Human Factors Profession. In G Salvendy (ed), Handbook of Human Factors. New York: Wiley, 4–15.

Damon A, Randall FE (1944). Physical anthropology in the Army Air Forces. Am J Phys Anthropol 2:293–316.

Damon A, Stoudt HW, McFarland RA (1966). The Human Body in Equipment Design. Cambridge, MA: Harvard University Press.

Das B (1998). Physical Disability Case Study: An Ergonomics Approach to Workstation Design for Paraplegics. In VJB Rice (ed), Ergonomics in Health Care and Rehabilitation. Boston: Butterworth–Heinemann, 123–141.

Fraser TM (1989). The Worker at Work: A Textbook Concerned with Men and Women in the Workplace. New York: Taylor & Francis.

Gaal RP, Rebholtz N, Hotchkiss RD, Pfaelzer PF (1997). Wheelchair rider injuries: causes and consequences for wheelchair design and selection. J Rehabil Res Dev 34(1):58–71.

Gay K (1986). Ergonomics: Making Products and Places Fit People. Hillside, NJ: Enslow.

Haas LJ (1925). Weaving frame for bedside occupational therapy. Arch Occup Ther 4:135–144.

Haas LJ (1928). A folding conveying chair. Arch Occup Ther 7:21–24.

Haas LJ (1930). An adjustable stool chair. Arch Occup Ther 8:367–374.

Haims MC, Carayon P (1998). Psychosocial Factors Case Study: Work Organization and Work-Related Musculoskeletal Disorders. In VJB Rice (ed), Ergonomics in Health Care and Rehabilitation. Boston: Butterworth–Heinemann, 205–230.

Hammer W (1985). Occupational Safety Management and Engineering. Englewood Cliffs, NJ: Prentice-Hall.

Hopkins HL (1978). Current Basis for Theory and Philosophy of Occupational Therapy. In HS Willard, CS Spackman, Occupational Theory. Philadelphia: Lippincott.

Jastrzebowski W (1857). An Outline of Ergonomics, or The Science of Work Based upon the Truths Drawn from the Science of Nature. Warsaw: Central Institute for Labor Protection, 1997. T Baluk-Ulewiczowa (trans).

Kantowitz BH, Sorkin RD (1983). Human Factors: Understanding People-System Relationships. New York: Wiley.

Key GL (1989). Work Capacity Analysis. In RM Scully, MR Barnes (eds), Physical Therapy. New York: Lippincott.

Konz S (1995). Work Design: Industrial Ergonomics. Scottsdale, AZ: Publishing Horizons.

Kornblau BL (1998a). Health Care Ergonomics and the Americans with Disabilities Act: An Introduction. In VJB Rice (ed), Ergonomics in Health Care and Rehabilitation. Boston: Butterworth–Heinemann, 287–294.

Kornblau BL (1998b). The Americans with Disabilities Act: Legal Ramifications of ADA Consultation. In VJB Rice (ed), Ergonomics in Health Care and Rehabilitation. Boston: Butterworth–Heinemann, 295–306.

Kozey J, Das B (1992). An Evaluation of Existing Anthropometric Measurements of Wheelchair Mobile Individuals. Proceedings of the Annual Human Factors Association of Canada Meeting, Hamilton, ON.

Kraus LE, Stoddard S (1989). Chartbook on Disability in the United States: An InfoUse Report. Washington, DC: U.S. Department of Education, National Institute on Disability and Rehabilitation Research.

Kroemer K, Kroemer H, Kroemer-Elbert K (1994). Ergonomics: How to Design for Ease and Efficiency. Englewood Cliffs, NJ: Prentice-Hall.

Lopez MS (1998). Musculoskeletal Ergonomics: An Introduction. In VJB Rice (ed), Ergonomics in Health Care and Rehabilitation. Boston: Butterworth–Heinemann, 155–186.

Meister D (1989). Conceptual Aspects of Human Factors. Baltimore: Johns Hopkins University Press.

Meister D (1997). The Practice of Ergonomics: Reflections on a Profession. Available from the Board of Certification in Professional Ergonomics, P.O. Box 2811, Bellingham, WA 98227-2811.

Meyer A (1921). The philosophy of occupational therapy. Arch Occup Ther 1:1–10.

Nickerson RS (1992). Looking Ahead: Human Factors Challenges in a Changing World. Hillsdale, NJ: Erlbaum.

Osborne DJ (1982). Ergonomics at Work. New York: Wiley.

Pinkston D (1989). Evolution of the Practice of Physical Therapy in the United States. In RM Scully, MR Barnes (eds), Physical Therapy. New York: Lippincott.

Pope AM, Tarlov AR (eds) (1991). Committee on a National Agenda for the Prevention of Disabilities, Division of Health Promotion and Disease Prevention, National Institute of Medicine. Washington, DC: National Academy Press.

Report of the Committee on Installations and Advice (1928). Analysis of crafts. Arch Occup Ther 6:417–421.

Rice VJB (1998a). Ergonomics in Health Care and Rehabilitation. Boston: Butterworth–Heinemann.

Rice VJB (1998b). Defining the Terms. In VJB Rice (ed), Ergonomics in Health Care and Rehabilitation. Boston: Butterworth–Heinemann, 3–14.

Rice VJB (1998c). Ergonomics: A Systems Approach. In VJB Rice (ed), Ergonomics in Health Care and Rehabilitation. Boston: Butterworth–Heinemann, 29–39.

Rice VJB (1992). Defining common ground: human factors engineering and rehabilitation. Rehabil Manage 5:30–32.

Rader Smith E (1998). Evolution of Health Care and Rehabilitation Ergonomics. In VJB Rice (ed), Ergonomics in Health Care and Rehabilitation. Boston: Butterworth–Heinemann, 15–28.

Sanders MS, McCormick EJ (1987). Human Factors in Engineering and Design. New York: McGraw-Hill.

Sanders MJ (1997). Management of Cumulative Trauma Disorders. Boston: Butterworth–Heineman.

Wilson JR, Corlett EN (eds) (1990). Evaluation of Human Work: A Practical Ergonomics Methodology. New York: Taylor & Francis.

Vanderheiden GC (1990). Thirty-something million: should they be exceptions? Hum Factors 32:383–396.

Wilkoff WL, Abed LW (1994). Practicing Universal Design: An Interpretation of the ADA. New York: Van Nostrand Reinhold.

Review Questions

(Answers are found in Appendix D.)

1. Why must therapists and human factors engineers/ergonomists be aware of "normal" human abilities?

2. Ergonomics began as a multidisciplinary field and developed from the common interests of a number of professions, particularly (1) _____, (2) _____, and (3) _____.

3. The first commandment of human factors is "_____," which means   .

4. Why must human factors engineering/ergonomics be well grounded in research? Why is a systems approach, in both research and implementation, important?

5. What are some reasons for the assumed lack of ergonomics research and design for disabled populations?

CHAPTER 2

A Client-Centered Framework for Therapists in Ergonomics

Susan Strong and Lynn Shaw

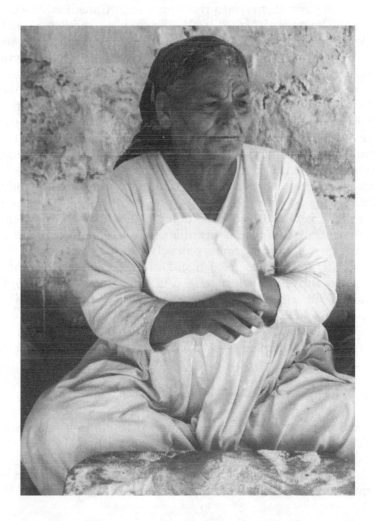

ABSTRACT

This chapter is intended to help the reader (1) understand why and how theoretical frameworks are an integral part of therapists' practice in occupational ergonomics; (2) identify current theoretical approaches being used in this area by therapists; (3) understand and apply client-centered practice concepts to occupational ergonomics; and (4) use the person-environment-occupation (PEO) model as a tool for analysis, intervention planning, and communication within a client-centered framework.

Therapists have been challenged to integrate client-centered values and occupational therapy theory into their practices (Canadian Association of Occupational Therapists [CAOT] 1991; Christiansen and Baum 1991, 1997). Historically, ergonomics has examined the person-machine interface through time and motion studies and anthropomorphic, biomechanical, and kinesiologic measurements. A client-centered practice emphasizes fitting the work to the worker according to the conditions of a particular workplace. The ability of an individual to safely, efficiently, and consistently produce a quality product depends on the complex relationships between the worker, his or her occupation, and his or her work environment. Therapists are beginning to examine ergonomic issues in terms of the interaction of these relationships (Jequier et al. 1989; Webb 1989).

In today's climate of restricted costs and increasing accountability, therapists must focus on effectively achieving clients' goals. The underlying premise of client-centered practice is that time and resources are effectively used by concentrating on the issues that are most important to the client (workers and organizations) and by involving the client throughout the process. The client-centered approach and increased client participation have been associated with more effective results (Greenfield et al. 1985; Henbest and Stewart 1990) and increased client satisfaction (Law and Mills 1998). Organizations are beginning to recognize that happy and satisfied workers perform better (Hallowell et al. 1996; McShane 1998; Shapoff 1996). It follows that a client-centered practice is consistent with good business practices.

Theoretical Framework

A theoretical framework allows the therapist to conceptualize ergonomic issues and guide his or her practice. A framework

- Helps the therapist to understand the ergonomic problem within a greater context—that is, relationships between the worker, workplace, and the work itself. Frameworks enable therapists to *frame* and *name* ergonomic problems.

- Enables a comprehensive assessment that addresses diverse factors and complex contexts that influence productivity in the workplace. The therapist is encouraged not to restrict assessment to the worker with an injury and the biomechanical issues.
- Directs and integrates what the therapist examines, the information-gathering process, and interpretation of findings. It enables the therapist to use critical thinking and a clinical reasoning process. Without a framework, the therapist is left with a collection of tools and a "cookbook" approach to ergonomic practice.
- Helps communicate intervention strategies, how the plans affect outcomes, and the therapist's role in the process.
- Describes the therapist's role, scope, and abilities in relation to other ergonomics practitioners.
- Helps the therapist maintain objectivity throughout the consultative process. Therapists integrate scientific knowledge with knowledge gained from experience in a structural framework.
- Allows the therapist to present a complete plan that identifies areas for enhancement that may or may not be within his or her realm of practice. A framework allows issues to be addressed from a number of perspectives. A therapist is then able to formulate a comprehensive plan that may include recommending actions by other specialists.
- Supports the further development of professional practice.

Ergonomic Approaches

Many different theoretical approaches are used in ergonomics. The approaches presented have been used by therapists within the context of therapeutic practice or occupational ergonomics. Some have roots in other ergonomic applications and have been merged with theories from other disciplines. The six ergonomic approaches discussed in the following sections are (1) occupational biomechanics (Chaffin and Anderson 1991), (2) the functional approach (Isernhagen 1995), (3) the systems approach (Woodson et al. 1992), (4) the Ergonomic Tool Kit approach (Burke 1998), (5) the multidisciplinary approach (Jequier et al. 1989), and (6) the Person-Process-Environment model approach (Webb 1989). These approaches are compared with regard to purpose, theoretical focus, and content in Table 2.1.

Purpose and Application

Biomechanics is a foundation of ergonomics. Chaffin and Anderson (1991) offer a comprehensive overview of occupational biomechanics applied to ergonomics. The objective of occupational ergonomics is to improve work-

TABLE 2.1
Comparison of Ergonomic Approaches

Approach	Purpose/Application	Focus	Content/Components
Occupational biomechanics (Chaffin and Anderson 1991)	Applicant selection/training Hand tool design Workplace and machine control design Seating design Material handling limits	Biomechanics Enhancement of performance Minimization of risk of mechanical trauma	Physical interaction of workers, tools, machines, and materials Kinematics/kinetics Anthropometry Mechanical work capacity evaluations Bioinstrumentation Time/motion studies
Functional (Isernhagen 1995)	Job analysis for functional job descriptions Functional capacity evaluations Injury prevention education Prework screening Ergonomic adaptations Modified work and return-to-work programs Injury management and prevention	Evaluation of human capabilities and job performance requirements Coordination of multiple specialists Comparison of functional abilities of workers with physical demands of job	Assess worker, work, and workplace: 1. Functional components of work 2. Coordination 3. Kinesiologic evaluation of work motions 4. Compare abilities of workers with physical job demands
Systems (Woodson et al. 1992)	Role of ergonomics in systems development	Design of system and machines adapted to workers User satisfaction based on worker comfort and pride of ownership	Reallocation of tasks within jobs and jobs within teams Consider system objectives, functional demands, critical tasks, allocation of functions, grouping of tasks in job descriptions, and teams
Ergonomic Tool Kit (Burke 1998)	Workplace-based ergonomics Workstation design or modification	Client's goals (reducing obstacles to productivity, consistently producing quality products, and	Analysis process: 1. Plan approach and delegate responsibilities

	Change in work process Worker-based programs	removing threats to worker comfort and safety)	2. Assess ergonomic needs 3. Gather background 4. Identify risk factors 5. Explore potential intervention strategies 6. Present report 7. Plan intervention strategies 8. Implement intervention 9. Report on project progress and effectiveness Framework for intervention: 1. Description of restrictions 2. Ergonomic analysis of work (nature of work, task division, work organization, flexibility of work relations, technology, human resources) 3. Intervention protocol Interacting relational systems: 1. Person (sensory, cognitive, physical) 2. Process (tasks, work) 3. Work environment Use with systems approach
Multidisciplinary (Jequier et al. 1989)	Design return-to-work programs for workers with injuries Injury prevention	Vocational rehabilitation and health promotion Incompatibilities between worker's abilities and job requirements Worker and corporate levels (micro-, meso-, and macrolevels)	
Person-Process-Environment (Webb 1989)	Product design Placement and rehabilitation Applicant selection	Vocational rehabilitation Matching task demands with individual's abilities	

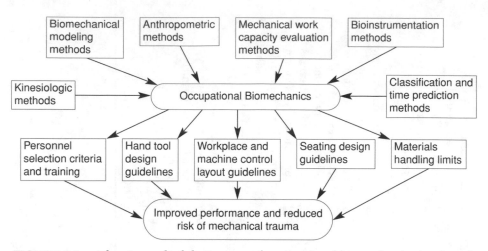

FIGURE 2.1.   The six methodologic areas of occupational biomechanics (top), with some major application areas (bottom). (Reprinted with permission from DB Chaffin, G Anderson. Occupational Biomechanics [2nd ed]. New York: Wiley, 1991;5.)

ers' occupational performance while achieving the organization's productivity goals. Occupational biomechanics is used to guide (1) the selection of job applicants; (2) hand tool design; (3) workplace design and machine control layout; (4) seating design; and (5) appropriate material-handling limits (Figure 2.1). The functional and Person-Process-Environment approaches assist applicant selection. The Person-Process-Environment approach is also applied to product design. Occupational biomechanics, the functional approach, the Ergonomic Tool Kit, and the multidisciplinary approach focus on injury prevention. Work injury management is a primary objective for the functional, multidisciplinary, and Person-Process-Environment approaches. The Person-Process-Environment approach combines with the systems approach (Woodson et al. 1992) to address systems operation and organizational development.

Perspective or Focus

The focus of the ergonomic approach is matching of capabilities of the person to the work demands. The variations among these approaches relate to the context, population, scope, theoretical perspective, and the role of the client. For example, in the Ergonomic Tool Kit approach, the therapist considers the organization's culture, motivational factors, and problems as identified by the facility. The therapist works in concert with the client to define the ergonomic problems and set priorities. Members of the organization are asked for perceptions and suggestions. Management input is sought throughout the process. In contrast, the functional approach involves the coordination of multiple specialists. An important consideration is that some approaches promote injury prevention (Burke 1998; Chaffin and Anderson 1991; Woodson et al. 1992), whereas others are designed for vocational rehabilitation of populations with injuries or disabilities (Isernhagen 1995; Webb 1989) or both (Jequier et al. 1989; Webb 1989; Woodson et al. 1992).

Perhaps the most distinguishing aspect of each approach is the outcomes that are focused on. Occupational biomechanics concentrates on the reduction and minimization of risks related to mechanical trauma in the performance of work tasks. The functional approach used in conjunction with occupational biomechanics examines the abilities of workers in relation to the job demands (Table 2.2). The Ergonomic Tool Kit approach considers the worker's stress level, comfort, and safety. The systems approach examines satisfaction regarding comfort and pride of ownership in relation to the machines and systems used. The Person-Process-Environment and Ergonomic Tool Kit approaches consider the broader work environment. The Person-Process-Environment model (Figure 2.2) specifically examines information processing and decision making at different levels of the organization. Jequier and colleagues (1989) describe micro- (worker), meso (task division, use of technology), and macrolevels (corporate) of intervention (Figure 2.3). The systems approach operates at the mesolevel by examining the production process and allocation of functions between people and machines, and it operates somewhat at the macrolevel by focusing on systems development.

Contents and Components

Components of the ergonomic approaches reviewed in Table 2.1 vary. Some approaches are primarily one-dimensional (Chaffin and Anderson 1991; Woodson et al. 1992), whereas others are multidimensional (Burke 1998; Jequier et al. 1989; Webb 1989). The Ergonomic Tool Kit approach consists of an analytical framework driven by clients to ameliorate risk factors related to workers, the work process, work conditions, and organizational environments (Burke 1998). Similarly, Jequier et al. (1989) offer a broad framework for interaction by sampling barriers to person-work processes. Webb's (1989) approach examines an interacting relational system involving person, process, and work environment. The use of each of these comprehensive frameworks (Burke 1998; Jequier et al. 1989; Webb 1989) can be supplemented by Chaffin and Anderson's (1991) biomechanical techniques, Isernhagen's (1995) job analysis, and Woodson et al.'s (1992) systems perspective.

Client-Centered Practice

Client-centered practice is a collaborative alliance between client and therapist designed to use their combined skills, strengths, and resources to work toward the client's occupational performance goals. "Occupational therapists demonstrate respect for clients, involve clients in decision making, advocate

TABLE 2.2
Three Components of Work Analysis

I. Worker
  A. Gender variables
  B. Age variables
    1. Musculoskeletal system
    2. Cardiorespiratory system
    3. Neurologic-sensory system
  C. Research on combination of age and gender
  D. Anthropometric data
  E. Skill level
  F. Pre-existing conditions
  G. Boeing studies
  H. Conclusion
II. Work
  A. Forces
  B. Angles
  C. Speech
  D. Repetitions
  E. Rest breaks
  F. Rodgers Maximum Voluntary Contraction Chart
  G. Borg Scale
  H. Stress level
  I. Boredom level
  J. Conclusion
III. Work site
  A. Workstation
    1. Work area
    2. Seating
    3. Stand/kneel
  B. Objects of work
    1. Materials to be handled
    2. Objects to be used/manipulated
    3. Controls
    4. Tools
    5. People
  C. Environment
    1. Lighting
    2. Temperature
    3. Noise
    4. Other

Source: Reprinted with permission from SJ Isernhagen. The Comprehensive Guide to Work Injury Management. Gaithersburg, MD: Aspen Publications, 1995;73.

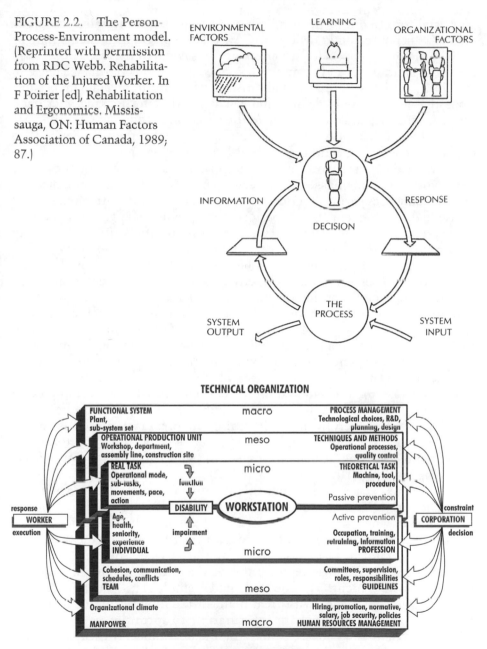

FIGURE 2.2. The Person-Process-Environment model. (Reprinted with permission from RDC Webb. Rehabilitation of the Injured Worker. In F Poirier [ed], Rehabilitation and Ergonomics. Mississauga, ON: Human Factors Association of Canada, 1989; 87.)

FIGURE 2.3. Diagram of the technical and human organization of a corporation (structure and concepts). (R&D = research and development.) (Reprinted with permission from JC Jequier, JM Gauthier, C Lapointe, et al. Model for a Multidisciplinary Approach. In F Poirier [ed], Rehabilitation and Ergonomics. Mississauga, ON: Human Factors Association of Canada, 1989;137–149.)

with and for clients in meeting clients' needs, and otherwise recognize clients' experience and knowledge" (CAOT 1997, p. 49). The clients may be individuals, groups, agencies, governments, or systems such as families, businesses, organizations, and communities. "Occupational performance refers to the ability to choose, organize, and satisfactorily perform meaningful occupations that are culturally defined and age appropriate for looking after one's self, enjoying life, and contributing to the social and economic fabric of community life" (CAOT 1997, p. 30). The goal of client-centered practice is to enhance occupational performance, health, and well-being.

When therapists work in the field of occupational ergonomics, they may work with businesses or other organizations that are not directly experiencing occupational performance problems. Organizations may have individuals with occupational performance problems (e.g., workers with persistent complaints of inability to perform specific work tasks due to back pain). Additionally, various sectors of the organizations may experience occupational performance problems such as decreased productivity due to very hot or very cold work environments, high absenteeism rates, lack of computerization for manual work, or ineffective communication and conflict resolution strategies. Depending on the contractual arrangement, the therapist's consultation may be with the individual, the organization, or with the organization and an external agency (e.g., an insurance agency). Client-centered practice fosters partnerships and encourages collaborative identification of obstacles and options for intervention that are not only person focused but system related. This assists the overall process of managing the changes necessary for individuals to perform safely, efficiently, and effectively while maintaining the organization's goals. Whatever the therapist's role, client-centered practice is "an approach to service which embraces a philosophy of respect for, and partnership with, people receiving services" (Law et al. 1995, p. 253).

To more clearly understand the client-centered model, consider the differences that Chewing and Sleath (1996) highlighted in approaches to intervention when using a client-centered versus a medical model. The client-centered model represents a departure from the medical model's emphasis on clinical status as defined by the service provider. The client defines the priorities together with the service provider, and the emphasis is on self-management. The medical model emphasizes educating clients to encourage compliance with treatment. In the client-centered approach, the client and therapist share information to formulate options from which the client can choose. Unlike the medical model, in which the service provider alone evaluates outcomes, both the client and the provider evaluate outcomes in a client-centered approach.

In *Client-Centered Occupational Therapy*, Law and Mills (1998) review six frameworks of client-centered practice and delineate seven concepts common to all six frameworks. Those concepts and their application to ergonomics are outlined in the following sections.

Respect for Clients and Their Families and the Choices They Make

The frameworks of client-centered practice emphasize that therapists should show respect for the choices clients make and how they go about making those choices. Clients' diverse life experiences and unique backgrounds are considered.

In an ergonomics context, the therapist needs to understand the organizational structure and respect the culture of the organization. Specifically, therapists need to understand the organization's values, attitudes, past ergonomics experiences, and how decisions are made within the organization. Respect extends to the clients' coping styles. It is important to know how the organization has dealt with ergonomic problems and to show respect for how they were managed.

Clients and Families Have the Ultimate Responsibility for Decisions about Daily Occupations and Occupational Therapy Services

The clients are the experts when it comes to knowing their problems and how these problems impact their lives. Although the therapist can leave the situation, the client must continue dealing with these problems. Thus, it makes sense that the client is responsible for making decisions about his or her daily occupation and what services are received. The person receiving services makes the decisions regarding the focus and nature of services.

In the workplace, each level of the organization identifies the ergonomic needs and priorities for services. Therapists can facilitate this process by providing options. At the very start, the therapist needs to clarify expectations about the services that can be provided and about who is responsible for what.

Provision of Information, Physical Comfort, and Emotional Support

To make informed and effective decisions, clients need to feel comfortable and receive adequate information about occupational performance issues. Frameworks emphasize that therapists need to have an open, caring manner and need to carefully listen to clients' descriptions of problems and needs. The issue of comfort arises when clients are placed in unfamiliar settings or situations.

The therapist must pay particular attention to the development and maintenance of relationships with different members of the organization (e.g., union representatives, management, workers, human resources, health and safety representatives). Information needs to be provided in an understandable and useful format. Within the organization, the participants involved in the ergonomics evaluation process have different needs, priorities, and perspectives. Provision of comfort is generally not an issue, as the therapist operates in the client's "home." However, a worker's comfort may involve the presence of a union representative in the evaluation. No matter the setting, the relationship that the therapist has with the client(s) ultimately enables success.

Facilitation of Client Participation in All Aspects of Occupational Therapy Service

Therapy is provided through a collaborative partnership between clients and therapists. Such a partnership requires a power shift from the therapist to the client to enable participation and engagement in mutually satisfying activities.

Different levels of participation in different service-provider interactions can be identified and encouraged. For example, the therapist facilitates the sharing of information and decision making via joint meetings convened with workplace members to analyze information and generate solutions. This can be achieved through one-to-one consultations, group brainstorming, interviews, or some combination of these.

Flexible, Individualized Occupational Therapy

The frameworks identified the importance of attending to the structure of health care delivery systems. Services need to be accessible and coordinated and should avoid unnecessary bureaucracy. Clients must understand the process so that they can participate.

When working in industry, the therapist needs to clearly communicate what he or she has to offer employers or managers and explain how services may or may not help resolve the ergonomic issues under discussion. To be effective, the therapist must be flexible in meeting client needs, respecting the resources and services available uniquely to each organization.

Enabling Clients to Solve Occupational Performance Issues

The therapist is not considered the expert in providing solutions to occupational performance problems. Thus, the therapist facilitates the client's generation and implementation of solutions. In so doing, the client gains skills that he or she can apply in future problem solving.

In industry, the therapist actively solicits suggestions for solutions from various levels of the organization. In particular, the workers and supervisors have access to invaluable information and often can make practical, relevant suggestions. Meetings are held to explore options and changes that could improve product quality and improve productivity by optimizing occupational performance.

Focus on the Person-Environment-Occupation Relationship

The lives and occupational performance difficulties of clients are closely interwoven with their environments and occupations. Environments are multidimensional and vary from one organization to another. Similarly, the skills and abilities required of workers to meet the physical, emotional, and cognitive demands of work vary. Thus, the therapist must be familiar with the relationships among the work processes, the capacities of workers, and the multidimensional factors of the work environment that may contribute to occupational performance issues and their resolution.

Occupational Performance Process Model

Fearing and colleagues developed the occupational performance process model (1997) by integrating primary concepts of occupation and client-centered practice to guide occupational therapy. The model provides a cyclical problem-solving process (Figure 2.4). Rather than assume that clients return to work completely recovered, it concentrates on maintaining or regaining active participation or momentum in daily living. It is flexible and guides rather than dictates practice. The seven stages may be combined or the order altered depending on the client and context. Fearing et al.'s model has been adopted by the Canadian model of occupational performance (Canadian Association of Occupational Therapists 1997).

FIGURE 2.4. The occupational performance (OP) process model. (Reprinted with permission from VG Fearing, M Law, J Clark. An occupational performance process model: fostering client and therapist alliances. Can J Occup Ther 1997;64:7–15.)

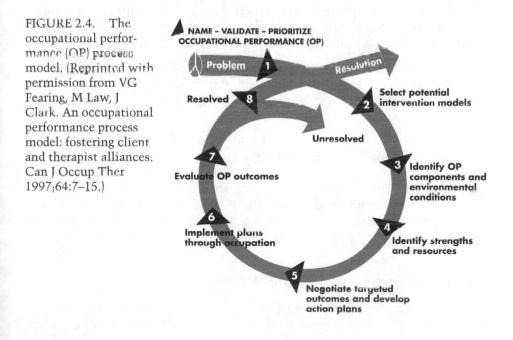

Case Example of the Occupational Performance Process Model

This scenario demonstrates how a therapist can apply the occupational performance process model (Fearing et al. 1997) in the occupational ergonomics process with a client-centered approach. The seven stages of the occupational performance process are used to apply a client-centered approach to ergonomics practice (Table 2.3). An overview of the role of the therapist in ergonomics is presented for each stage. The case example is then applied to each of the seven stages to provide examples of issues that may be identified and resolved with such an approach.

Background

The therapist received a referral from the Centralized Booking Company, a small, private organization of 100 employees that offers a 24-hour booking service for medical, dental, community care, and hospital appointments for national and international clients. The reason for referral was consultation to resolve ergonomic concerns of office workers and to develop and implement a modified duty program to return an employee to his or her preinjury job.

During the initial referral, the following information was relayed:

1. Recently, the company purchased and installed new office equipment to improve worker comfort, reduce time lost because of injuries associated with musculoskeletal strain, and improve productivity. Six months after the office redesign, no improvements have been identified in productivity, lost time injury rates, and absenteeism. Similarly, worker complaints of dissatisfaction associated with the new workstations have continued.

2. An office worker who has been absent from work because of a car accident wants to return to work with a restriction of no shift work. The worker sustained multiple crush injuries to the right hand and a head injury causing permanent figure-ground visual-perceptual problems.

3. Coworkers have forwarded concerns to management regarding fairness of workload. All office workers are required to rotate office duties on a 12-hour basis: 3 days on, 3 days off, 3 nights on, and 3 nights off. Duties include computerized scheduling and booking of appointments for thousands of companies and organizations via a national and international network, invoicing and billing clients while managing telephone inquiries and customer service relations.

Person-Environment-Occupation Model

Derived from environment behavior studies and principles of client-centered practice, the PEO model (Law et al. 1996) is suitable for planning client-

TABLE 2.3
Application of Client-Centered Approach to Ergonomics

Occupational Performance Process	Relation of Occupational Performance Process to Ergonomics	Case Application
1. Name, validate, and prioritize occupational performance issues	The therapist identifies the client or clients (e.g., the worker with an injury, employer, coworkers, union, human resource personnel, health and safety representatives, and other workplace parties) and establishes a relationship with each client. Expectations of the therapist and the outcome of services are negotiated. Interviews with each client are used to define, validate, or clarify the ergonomic issues considered to be priorities. If no ergonomic issues are defined by the clients, the process stops.	The therapist names and clarifies ergonomic issues with clients: 1. A worker with an injury requests modified duties and specific duties not identified or agreed on by the employer. 2. Workers report ongoing unresolved musculoskeletal pain. The workers also have concerns of workload equity related to modified duty programs. They believe each person must rotate and perform duties in the assigned shift. 3. The organization experiences problems with lost time and lowered productivity due to unresolved ergonomic issues, despite purchasing expensive ergonomic workstations. The employer requests external consultation regarding coordination of a return-to-work plan for an individual.
2. Select theoretical approach(es)	The therapist chooses a framework to guide and justify decisions throughout the ergonomic intervention process. Approaches guide selection of measures and application of procedures, which helps maintain objectivity toward and focus on the needs of the client. Approaches are selected that match the organization's management philosophy and decision-making	Examples of potential approaches include the following: 1. A biomechanical approach analyzes the demands of tasks and the physical abilities of the person. 2. The Person-Environment-Occupation model addresses the multiple dynamic interactions of the clients, tasks, and work environment over time. 3. A psychosocial approach examines emotional factors, the social context of the work, the workplace culture, and cognitive demands. 4. Organizational behavior theories assist in understanding political issues (i.e., power and influence in the workplace),

TABLE 2.3
continued

Occupational Performance Process	Relation of Occupational Performance Process to Ergonomics	Case Application
	style. Several approaches may be necessary to deal with issues surrounding the workers, organization, work environment, and work process.	governance (i.e., policies and procedures), communication (i.e., decision-making and conflict resolution processes), and the relationships between individuals and organizations as related to perceptions, values, and beliefs. 5. Health promotion supports positive human resources management and safety in the workplace.
3. Identify occupational performance components and environment	The therapist evaluates work performance and the environment for risk factors by focusing on the ergonomic issues that clients have identified as priorities (e.g., obstacles to productivity, the quality of production, worker comfort, safety, and long-term well-being). Perceptions of contributing ergonomic factors are solicited, clients are interviewed, and work processes are observed. Therapists must also understand ergonomic problems within the context of organizational and legislative systems.	The therapist identifies risk factors such as 1. Environment (e.g., workstation lighting, work surfaces, noise). 2. Absence of ergonomic practices (e.g., use of unsupported awkward postures). 3. Human factors (e.g., the match of worker's abilities and limitations with work demands). 4. Organizational factors (e.g., collective agreements, inadequate workplace policy regarding disability management). 5. Legislative system (e.g., disability-related legislation, health and safety legislation).
4. Identify strengths and resources	The therapist identifies strengths (e.g., attitudes, awareness, experience, problem-solving skills, communication skills, leadership style) and resources (e.g., monetary, personnel, partners, equipment). The therapist uses this information and ideas	1. A worker returning to work identifies the duties he or she can perform and flexibility in organization of tasks. 2. Coworkers suggest improvements in workstation design and work processes to reduce musculoskeletal strains and need for training. The therapist contacts the office equipment supplier to determine the options for training and mechanical adjustments.

from the clients to determine possible solutions.		3. Management identifies human resource issues (e.g., policy development to support collaboration in return-to-work programs). The therapist contacts similar organizations to establish work flow and production benchmarks.
5. Negotiate goals and develop plan of implementation	Directed by the client's needs, the therapist analyzes the gathered information. A report outlines recommended intervention strategies and their rationale. The recommendations are discussed with the clients. The establishment of ergonomic goals and negotiation of the plan and responsibilities may be done individually or in a group depending on the situation.	Ergonomic issues are often interrelated. The therapist must collaborate with all groups involved when developing a plan and delegating responsibilities. For example: 1. The development of modified duty programs to guide work re-entry requires collaboration from all workplace parties. 2. The reduction of lost-time injuries requires the development of an acceptable plan and a commitment to participate in health-promotion programs by everyone in the workplace. 3. The identification of duties the worker can perform requires the collaboration of the worker, the manager, and coworkers.
6. Implement plans through occupation	Implementation involves delegating responsibilities, establishing a time frame for completion, and determining modification strategies for possible difficulties.	The organization, workers, and therapist work together to implement recommendations. For example: 1. The organization identifies who will provide ergonomic training (e.g., the therapist). 2. The organization identifies a team to develop a modified duty and work re-entry policy. 3. The worker desiring to return to work confers with the therapist, management team, and worker representatives to agree on a return-to-work program that accommodates all parties.
7. Evaluate occupational performance outcomes	A time frame is used to evaluate the effectiveness of intervention strategies. The evaluation is used to modify strategies to optimize worker comfort and maximize productivity in a safe environment. Outcomes are evaluated in relation to the initial ergonomic concerns.	A program evaluation of ergonomic recommendations is conducted by measuring outcomes for each initial problem. Data to be surveyed include 1. Length of time until an injured worker successfully rehabilitates. 2. Worker satisfaction with ergonomic changes to workstations. 3. Lost time over the 6-month period after implementation of recommendations.

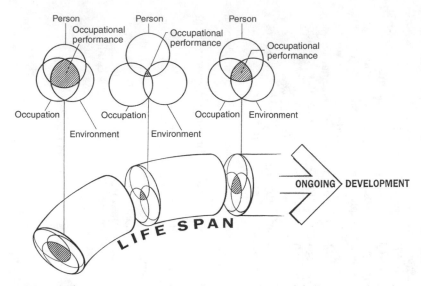

FIGURE 2.5.   The Person-Environment-Occupation model. (Reprinted with permission from M Law, B Cooper, S Strong, et al. The Person-Environment-Occupation model: a transactive approach to occupational performance. Can J Occup Ther 1996; 63:9–46.)

centered interventions on both personal and environmental levels. The *environment* is defined broadly to include cultural, socioeconomic, institutional or structural, and social elements. The model has been used by therapists in various roles in a variety of settings. It has been shown to be a practical tool to conceptualize, communicate, plan, and evaluate occupational performance interventions (Strong et al. 1998).

The model (Figure 2.5) has three components: the person, environment, and occupation, imagined as interrelated spheres that move with respect to each other over time. The spheres represent how a person continuously engages in occupations and interacts with environments. Environments, occupations, and people have enabling or constraining effects on each other; the components shape each other. A cross section taken at any discrete point in time would reveal different interactions.

The greater the degree of overlap between the three components represents increased congruence, or PEO match, resulting in improved occupational performance. Occupational performance is the product of PEO transactions. The aim of interventions is to improve occupational performance and increase the PEO congruence by removing obstacles or providing supports for more harmonious PEO relationships. The model's definitions of person, occupation, environment, and occupational performance are the same as those used by the occupational performance process model (Fearing et al. 1997) and the Canadian model of occupational performance (CAOT 1997).

Application of the Person-Environment-Occupation Model to Ergonomics Practice

To illustrate the PEO model as a practical tool for therapists in ergonomics, the model has been applied to the same three ergonomic problems identified earlier in the case example of the Centralized Booking Company. This model is particularly of value to the therapist in identifying and clarifying barriers to the resolution of ergonomic problems such as worker attitudes, systems issues, organizational issues (e.g., policy, leadership style), and interpersonal relationships within an organization. The PEO model can be used within the occupational performance process (see Table 2.2) by selecting it as a theoretical approach (stage 2) and using it to identify occupational performance components and environmental conditions (stage 3); to identify a client's resources, strengths, and options (stage 4); and to plan, implement, and evaluate outcomes (stages 5–7).

Ergonomic Problem 1

A worker who sustained injuries in a car accident wants to return to work on temporarily modified duties, day shift only. Barriers include the resistance of coworkers and the need to identify the work tasks that will enable the worker to return to work on modified duties.

Analysis and Assessment

The therapist gathers information from the worker regarding his or her current abilities (e.g., physical, cognitive, affective, emotional). Additionally, the therapist gathers data on the actual demands and processes of the working environment from both the worker and a representative from the organization. Analysis of person-occupation, person-environment, and environment-occupation relationships reveals a number of issues.

Person-Occupation Issues
Physical abilities and physical restrictions do not match the physical demands of the job (e.g., pain in hand with prolonged repetitive posture of right hand and visual-perceptual problems working with standard computer screen).

Person-Environment Issues
- Poor match of physical abilities with work expectations (e.g., temporary inability to perform all shifts due to fatigue related to sleep disturbance problems).
- The workplace anticipated a lack of cooperation from coworkers based on experience with other workers with disabilities.

Environment-Occupation Issues

- Lack of formal policy for rehabilitation of workers with injuries and modified duty program
- Workload during modified duty programs perceived as inequitable by coworkers
- Informal workplace expectations that everyone shifts and rotates
- Management wishes to reduce ratings of lost time experience
- Management desires a program to eliminate workplace injuries
- Management wants to improve human relations of staff

Person-Occupation-Environment Interventions

The therapist developed a plan in consultation with all parties, including the workers, coworkers, and management. The therapist takes into consideration the impact of relationships among the workers and the organization (*person*), the work (*occupation*), and the workplace (*environment*). Interventions included the collaborative development of a modified duty program with guidelines acceptable to all parties, increasing the awareness of lost time and reduced workplace productivity.

Once a policy was defined and agreed on, the therapist was able to focus on issues surrounding the worker with an injury. The policy assisted in the acceptance of a plan to return the worker to a modified duty program involving a rotation of duties in the day shift, with a gradual return to all shifts (afternoons followed by night shifts). Subsequently, a plan was developed that involved matching the worker's current abilities with work demands. The development of this plan involved dialogue with the supervisor and the worker and negotiation of what duties matched the worker's abilities under what circumstances. The supervisor, the worker, and the therapist created a plan to gradually increase the worker's duties as endurance and pain control improved. Additionally, the therapist and the worker collaborated to enable the worker to work more efficiently on the computer.

Ergonomic Problem 2

After the corporation-wide installation of new ergonomically designed office equipment, office workers continued to complain of musculoskeletal pain in their necks, shoulders, backs, and wrists.

Analysis and Assessment

The therapist conducted interviews with the staff to ask about the factors they perceived to be contributing to musculoskeletal pain. Additionally, the therapist conducted a review of the office equipment and gathered information associated with the purchase and installation of the new ergonomic office workstations. The following issues were identified.

Person-Occupation Issues

- Pain while performing duties, fears of increasing incapacitation, and reluctance to engage in some duties
- Stress believed to be associated with some work duties in the rotation
- Not all employees have been trained in all work duties within the rotation

Environment-Occupation Issues

- Increased workload demands for each employee
- Rotation of work limited because of absenteeism (i.e., staff experiencing prolonged periods in high-stress duties)
- New equipment installed, but workers received no training on how to manage and adjust new equipment

Person-Occupation-Environment Interventions

The therapist's recommendations included training of staff regarding basic ergonomic principles aimed at skill development in the self-management of their workstations. Training included adjustment and mechanical management of workstations provided to the employees by the vendor and workplace training on basic principles of ergonomics (e.g., methods to prevent workplace strains) provided to employees and management by the therapist. Stretching and exercise programs were included as part of the training package.

Ergonomic Problem 3

The Centralized Booking Company identified that the continuation of lost-time claims, absenteeism, and worker dissatisfaction and discomfort contributed to lost productivity, decreased efficiency, difficulty with staffing, and overall poor staff relations.

Analysis and Assessment

The therapist gathered information regarding claims experience, types of injuries, work flow processes, and so forth to understand and evaluate the workplace injury management program. Additionally, the therapist considered the ergonomic problems within the greater legislative and organizational systems, such as the workplace collective agreements, workplace policy, and health and safety legislation.

Person-Occupation Issues

- Lack of management experience and training in health and safety in office settings
- Management was motivated to return employees to work but lacked successful outcomes in previous cases

- Lack of employee satisfaction with workload and duties

Environment-Occupation Issues

- Time and manpower constraints have limited implementation of work rotation and limit accommodation of workers
- Purchase of ergonomic equipment did not reduce lost-time injuries
- Workplace injury management strategy lacked direction

Person-Occupation-Environment Interventions

The therapist recommended a collaborative approach to identifying a rotation strategy and efficient sequencing of tasks per rotation. This required the therapist, worker representative, and management to design a suitable rotation. The strategy was to develop the skills of the office staff and enable rotation through all tasks, minimizing the length of time on stressful work and allowing recovery time on the most demanding duties. The therapist facilitated a meeting of office staff and a management representative that discussed options for sequencing of tasks and established a trial protocol.

Additionally, a management development and training program was recommended to enhance the skills and knowledge of the management team in injury prevention and management.

Conclusion

The PEO model can be used as a tool in client-therapist alliances to systematically examine complex occupational performance issues. The model focuses on the relationships between the worker, the work environment, and the work itself to create a structure for problem-solving strategies. Therapists clearly articulate solutions and explain how the therapist's services are intended to affect outcome. The PEO model is designed to help facilitate communication with all members of the workplace.

Client-Centered Approach and Ethics

Ethical dilemmas can arise when using a client-centered approach in the ergonomics field. For example, the priorities of key parties may conflict with each other. The workers may believe the most urgent ergonomic issues relate to poor equipment, whereas the employer may identify the workers' unsatisfactory performance and compliance with proper techniques as the problem. The therapist is confronted with the question of which of the clients issues and priorities take precedence. Being client-centered does not mean that the therapist must agree with the client or "take sides." Rather, the therapist focuses on the issues as directed by the client and enters the client's world in a collaborative partnership. The therapist may reclarify and ascertain the priorities and needs of both parties and together negotiate which issues will be addressed and at what time. For the scenario described, an objective evaluation of the concerns of all participants is necessary to identify the extent of all problems. The therapist ensures that all issues are addressed from all perspectives. The goal is to encourage each party to see all points of view.

Funding issues may also pose ethical dilemmas for the therapist. The employer or insurance company may not be able to fund what the client and therapist identify as necessary to resolve the ergonomic problems. The therapist may need to work with clients to identify other options for funding and other methods for arriving at an appropriate solution.

Lack of compliance by the worker or employer in carrying out the agreed-on changes also presents the therapist with a dilemma. The client-centered approach is intended to foster partnerships and actively engage key parties in meaningful plans. In this way, the situation of noncompliance can often be avoided. An effective framework includes the establishment of target dates and identifies an individual responsible for monitoring and re-evaluating changes (e.g., therapist, supervisor, employee). The responsible individual(s) notifies the group if issues are not resolved efficiently and completely.

The therapist may encounter attitudes that have a negative impact on relationships between supervisors and workers. With the client-centered approach, these issues need to be addressed in an objective and respectful manner. Negative attitudes can be identified for workplace parties as barriers to effective solutions. For example, a supervisor may label a worker "unmotivated" or "lazy." Thus, when the worker returns to work on modified duties because of injury, the supervisor may attribute all concerns raised by the worker to laziness. Niemeyer (1991) describes how labeling and stereotyping can bias observers' (i.e., supervisors') beliefs and can delay recovery if the individual accepts the label. The early identification of destructive attitudes allows the therapist to take steps before plans are undermined. For example, the therapist can provide information to counter misinformation and organize sessions to encourage dialogue and provide a forum for parties to be understood.

Conclusion

Ergonomics continues to expand. Organizations are complying with changes in legislation concerning health and safety, human rights, and disability to ensure healthy work environments. A highly competitive marketplace has contributed to the incorporation of ergonomics to maximize productivity and redesign for efficiency. Also, workers are viewed as a valuable resource, and employers are becoming concerned with health promotion and wellness. The practice of ergonomics must continue to develop to meet the changing, complex needs of clients through evidence-based evaluations (see Chapter 13). Using theoretical approaches and frameworks, therapists can think critically about ergonomic issues, create innovative solutions, and further develop the practice of ergonomics.

Approaches direct therapists to consider complex relationships among demands of work (e.g., cognitive, emotional, affective, psychological, physical), the work environment (micro-, meso-, and macrolevels), and the capacities of the client (e.g., worker, organization). Client-centered principles, assisted by the occupational performance process model and the PEO model, have a useful role in ergonomics. A client-centered approach challenges therapists to address the impact of organizational relationships, systems, and attitudes.

References

Burke M (1998). Ergonomics Tool Kit: Practical Applications. Gaithersburg, MD: Aspen Publications.

Canadian Association of Occupational Therapists (1991). Occupational Therapy Guidelines for Client-Centered Practice. Toronto: CAOT Publications ACE.

Canadian Association of Occupational Therapists (1997). Enabling Occupation: An Occupational Therapy Perspective. Ottawa: CAOT Publications ACE.

Chaffin DB, Anderson G (1991). Occupational Biomechanics (2nd ed). New York: Wiley & Sons, 5.

Chewning B, Sleath B (1996). Medication decision-making and management: a client-centered model. Soc Sci Med 42:389–398.

Christiansen C, Baum C (1991). Occupational Therapy: Overcoming Human Performance Deficits. Thorofare, NJ: Slack.

Fearing VG, Law M, Clark J (1997). An occupational performance process model: fostering client and therapist alliances. Can J Occup Ther 64:7–15.

Greenfield S, Kaplan SH, Ware JE (1985). Expanding patient involvement in care: effects on patient outcomes. Ann Intern Med 102:520–528.

Hallowell R, Schlesinger LA, Zornitsky J (1996). Internal service quality, customer and job satisfaction; linkages and implications for management. Hum Res Plan 19:20–31.

Henbest RJ, Stewart M (1990). Patient-centeredness in the consultation. II: Does it really make a difference? Fam Prac 7:28–33.

Isernhagen SJ (1995). The Comprehensive Guide to Work Injury Management. Gaithersburg, MD: Aspen.

Jequier JC, Gauthier JM, Lapointe C, et al. (1989). Model for a Multidisciplinary Approach. In F Poirier (ed), Rehabilitation and Ergonomics. Mississauga, ON: Human Factors Association of Canada, 137–149.

Law M, Baptiste S, Mills J (1995). Client-centered practice: what does it mean and does it make a difference? Can J Occup Ther 62:250–257.

Law M, Cooper B, Strong S, et al. (1996). The Person-Environment-Occupation model: a transactive approach to occupational performance. Can J Occup Ther 63:9–46.

Law M, Mills J (1998). Client-Centered Occupational Therapy. In M Law (ed), Client Centered Occupational Therapy. Thorofare, NJ: Slack, 1–18.

McShane SL (1998). Canadian Organizational Behaviour. Toronto: McGraw-Hill Ryerson.

Niemeyer LO (1991). Social labeling, stereotyping, and observer bias in worker's compensation: the impact of provider-patient interaction on outcome. J Occup Rehabil 1:251–269.

Shapoff SH (1996). Why Corning breathes TQM. Financial Executive 12:22–28.

Strong S, Rigby P, Stewart D, et al. (in press). Application of the person-environment-occupation model: a practical tool. Can J Occup Ther.

Webb RDC (1989). Rehabilitation of the Injured Worker. In F Poirier (ed), Rehabilitation and Ergonomics. Mississauga, ON: Human Factors Association of Canada, 85–94.

Woodson WE, Tillman B, Tillman P (1992). Human Factors Design Handbook: Information and Guidelines for the Design of Systems, Facilities, Equipment, and Products for Human Use. New York: McGraw-Hill.

Review Questions

(Answers are found in Appendix D.)

1. Why does a therapist use a theoretical framework?
   (a) A framework allows the therapist to understand ergonomic problems.
   (b) A framework directs the therapist's observations, data collection, and interpretation of findings.
   (c) A framework lends comprehensiveness to assessments and intervention plans.
   (d) All of the above

2. Theoretical approaches differ with respect to
   (a) history and where they were published
   (b) focus (e.g., matching the capacities of the person with the work demands)
   (c) context, scope, and the extent to which the process is client driven
   (d) none of the above

3. Concepts central to client-centered practice include
   (a) facilitation of client participation in all aspects of service
   (b) flexible, individualized service
   (c) respect for clients and the choices they make
   (d) all of the above

4. The occupational performance process model and the PEO model are
   (a) tools therapists use to facilitate client-centered practice
   (b) intervention models applicable to ergonomics
   (c) flexible and guide rather than dictate practice
   (d) all of the above

5. To be client centered, therapists must
   (a) always agree with the client
   (b) create a collaborative partnership and enter the client's world from
       the client's perspective
   (c) avoid dealing with ethical issues
   (d) rely solely on the client's skills and resources to the exclusion of
       the therapist's skills and resources

PART II

Knowledge, Tools, and Techniques

CHAPTER 3
Anthropometry

Nancy A. Baker

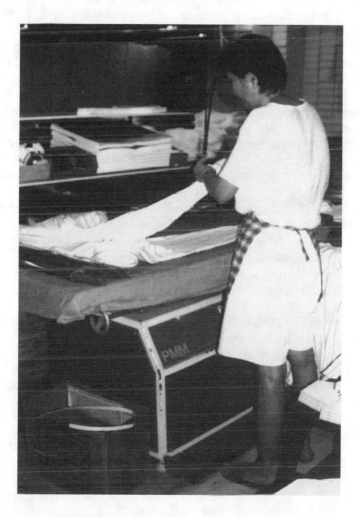

ABSTRACT

Anthropometry, the physical measurement of the human body, provides the therapist with building blocks for understanding the complexities of the human form and how it interfaces with its environment. This chapter reviews the principles and methods of static anthropometry. Discussions of reach, clearance, and posture are included, as well as tables of actual measurements. Methods for the application of these principles to workstation design are also reviewed.

People have always studied and analyzed the human form. Measurements were frequently based on human body parts: A foot was the length of the human foot, and a yard was the length from midline to the fingertip. The Greeks discovered that the proportions of humans were remarkably consistent and that the body could be divided into equal segments, which led to the formulation of the golden section ratio. The golden section ratio was used as a guideline for the design of monuments, sculptures, and paintings. The Greeks believed that the proportions of the human body were especially harmonious and beautiful (Diffrient et al. 1981). These early studies gradually evolved into the modern science of anthropometry. Anthropometry, the measurement of the human body, is the cornerstone of the design of all objects and spaces used by humans. Because ergonomics is concerned with shaping the environment to optimize a worker's ability to perform his or her job, an understanding of anthropometry is essential to the application of ergonomics.

The designer makes many complex choices when creating a work space. In addition to the function of the space, all the parameters of the human form and how it will act within the space must be understood. The designer, therefore, must create a space that is suitable for all potential users, regardless of their physical shape. Often, however, the user is envisioned by the designer to be the same as he or she. Consequently, the designer designs the space to fit his or her own shape and fails to account for the variety of the human form. Such designs are not ergonomically correct and accommodate very few people.

How can a designer understand the population he or she is designing for? He or she could measure everybody who might use this design, but this is often impractical. Alternately, a designer can use anthropometric measurements. Anthropometric measurements provide concrete and scientific information for designing workstations that can fit the largest number of people. Anthropometric measurements give the parameters of human size and shape that allow the designer to fulfill the needs of both comfort and function. Without anthropometry, little science goes into creating a work space, only intuition. Anthropometry provides both the understanding of why a work space fits a worker and the understanding of how a work space may fail the people who work in it. Anthropometry provides important information on how to shape the environment to fit the greatest number of people (the essence of ergonomics). Anthropometric data have been used by NASA to design space capsules (Anthropology Research Project 1978), by biomechanists to estimate lifting limits (Chaffin and Andersson 1991), and by clothing designers to design mittens (Rosenblad-Wallin 1987).

Using anthropometric data for basic ergonomic design is remarkably easy. Many measurements have already been collected and placed in tables. Anthropometric measurements have already been ascertained for those with disabilities, children, and the elderly, as well as a wide variety of ethnic groups. This chapter reviews static anthropometry as it pertains to workstation design, including tables of measurements for persons in the fifth to ninety-fifth percentiles for different populations. The use of link modeling as an alternative for determining body part size is discussed briefly, and a case study that combines all the aspects of anthropometrics provides further information on how to use the data.

Static Anthropometry

Static anthropometry is the science of measuring length, breadths, and widths in the human population. Anthropometrists have reported several universal factors that seem to influence human size and shape. Gender, ethnicity, age, and occupation have all been found to affect anthropometric measurements (Al-Haboubi 1992; Anthropology Research Project 1978; Marras and Kim 1993; Pheasant 1986).

The shape of any stable population changes from generation to generation, a phenomenon termed *secular trend* (Anthropology Research Project 1978; Pheasant 1986). In general, the population has been becoming larger. Although most researchers are cautious in their explanations of this, one theory is that secular trend is due to changes in the environment such as improved diet and the reduction of infectious disease.

Gender Differences

The difference between men and women is more than skin deep. Men generally are larger than women both overall and in limb size. Less of male body weight is composed of fat tissue, and what fat men have tends to accumulate at the abdomen. A woman's fat tends to accumulate at the hips, thighs, and buttocks.

Ethnic Differences

Different ethnic groups do indeed have different anthropometric measurements. A general rule of thumb is that ethnic groups who live primarily in tropical climates have a lower body weight than those who live in colder temperatures (Roberts 1973). Body proportions vary among ethnic groups;

for example, black Africans have proportionally longer lower limbs than Europeans, whereas Asians have proportionally shorter limbs (Pheasant 1986). Differences due to ethnicity, however, tend to diminish as populations migrate and commingle.

Aging

It is easy to see the difference age makes in body size and shape when comparing a child with an adult. Anthropometric changes during adulthood, however, are more subtle. As people pass 30, stature decreases and body weight increases. After age 50 for men and 60 for women, body weight again decreases.

Occupational Differences

The tendency for people of different social classes and occupations to have different anthropometric proportions is poorly understood. Some occupations, such as soldiers or jockeys, are self-selective; a specific size or weight is necessary to perform the job. Why other occupations should be stratified by size is a bit of a mystery. Does the job shape the person or does the correctly sized person select the job?

Persons with Disabilities

Disability is an often overlooked factor that can influence anthropometric measurements. Disability alters not only the size and shape of an individual but also his or her ability to perform activities that may be taken for granted by the general population. Consider a wheelchair user. Not only does he or she have to cope with the disability that placed him or her in the wheelchair, the wheelchair user also has the added anthropometric disadvantages of being both approximately 16 in. lower than most adults and much larger and bulkier because of the wheelchair. Consider, also, the "slightly" disabled. These are individuals who lack full motion or strength because of a mild disability; examples include the frail elderly who cannot rise from a chair because it is too low and the individual with rheumatoid arthritis who cannot open a car door because of weakened hands. A solid understanding of good design principles is vital for designing spaces for these individuals. In a well-designed environment, these individuals may be able to function fully; placed in a poorly designed environment, these individuals may be totally disabled. Thus, designing an environment that supports the independence of those with disabilities is vital. Using anthropometric measurements to design the optimal environment for people with disabilities often provides an optimal environment for all populations.

When designing for people with severe disabilities (particularly those with physical challenges such as kyphosis, axial rotation, or limb discrepancies), however, the use of standard anthropometric measurement and techniques is difficult because of the high degree of statistical variability in this population. Type of disability can markedly affect the distributions of body dimensions. A study of the anthropometrics of a population with severe disabilites reported a need for at least four new linear measurements to capture the spatial requirements of those with physical challenges, as well as five angular measurements to account for the inability of many people with disabilities to assume the "standard" seated posture (Hobson and Molenbroek 1990). Therefore, individual measurements should always be taken for those with physical challenges. The overall "disabled" anthropometric measurements should only be used for those with minimal physical challenges.

Static Anthropometric Measurements

Like most sciences, static anthropometry has conventions. Static anthropometry always looks at human dimensions in one of two planes: (1) sagittal, which divides the body into left and right views, or (2) coronal, which divides the body into front and back views. Static anthropometry also examines two standard postures:

- Standing posture: The person stands erect and looks straight ahead, with his or her arms in a relaxed posture at the side (Figure 3.1).
- Seated posture: The person sits erect and looks straight ahead. The sitting surface is adjusted so that the person's thighs are parallel to the floor and the knees are bent to a 90 degree angle with the feet flat on the floor. The upper arm is relaxed and perpendicular to the horizontal plane, while the forearm is at a right angle to the upper arm and thus also parallel to the floor. Measurements in sitting are made using a horizontal reference point, either the ground or the seat, and a vertical reference point, an imaginary line that touches the back of the uncompressed buttocks and shoulder blades of the subject. Thus, in the standard seated posture, the person is measured with most joints, the ankle, knees, hip, and elbows at 90-degree angles (Figure 3.2).

Some further conventions are as follows:

- Heights are vertical measurements from the floor or seat surface.
- Lengths are horizontal measurements in the sagittal plane.
- Breadths are horizontal measurements in the coronal plane.

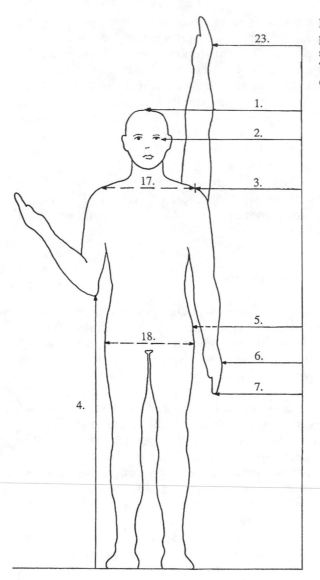

FIGURE 3.1.   Static anthro-pometric dimensions for the standard standing posture. The numbers correspond to data in Tables 3.1–3.4.

The following is a list of the 24 most common measurements. Use Figures 3.1 and 3.2 to help to clarify each measurement.

1. Stature: vertical distance from the floor to the crown of the head
2. Eye height: vertical distance from the floor to the inner corner of the eye
3. Shoulder height: vertical distance from the floor to the acromion of the shoulder

FIGURE 3.2. Static anthropometric dimensions for the
standard sitting posture.
The numbers correspond to
data in Tables 3.1–3.4.

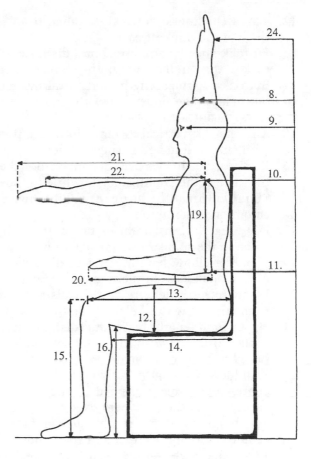

4. Elbow height: vertical distance from the floor to the olecranon
   process of the elbow
5. Hip height: vertical distance from the floor to the greater trochanter
6. Knuckle height: vertical distance from the floor to the knuckle of the
   third metacarpal
7. Fingertip height: vertical distance from the floor to the tip of the third
   digit
8. Sitting height: vertical distance from the seat to the crown of the
   head
9. Sitting eye height: vertical distance from the seat to the inner corner
   of the eye
10. Sitting shoulder height: vertical distance from the sitting surface to
    the acromion of the shoulder
11. Sitting elbow height: vertical distance from the seat to the olecranon
    process of the elbow

12. Thigh thickness: vertical distance from the seat to the top of the thigh at the thickest part
13. Buttock-knee length: horizontal distance from the uncompressed buttock to the patella while in the standard sitting position
14. Buttock-popliteal length: horizontal distance from the uncompressed buttocks to the underside of the knee at the popliteal angle while in the standard sitting position
15. Knee height: vertical distance from the floor to the top of the patella while in the standard sitting position
16. Popliteal height: vertical distance from the floor to the underside of the knee at the popliteal angle while in the standard sitting position
17. Shoulder breadth: horizontal distance across the shoulder from acromion to acromion
18. Hip breadth: horizontal distance at the broadest place on the hips when in the standard sitting position
19. Shoulder-elbow length: vertical distance from the acromion to the olecranon process in the standard sitting position
20. Elbow-fingertip length: vertical distance from the olecranon process to the tip of the third digit while in the standard sitting position
21. Upper limb length: horizontal distance from the acromion to the tip of the third digit with the elbow and wrist extended, and the shoulder flexed to a 90-degree angle
22. Shoulder-grip length: horizontal distance from the acromion to the center of an object gripped in the hand with the elbow and wrist extended and the shoulder flexed to a 90-degree angle.
23. Standing vertical grip reach: vertical distance from the ground to the center of an object gripped in the hand with the shoulder flexed to a 180-degree angle (no excessive stretching)
24. Sitting vertical grip reach: vertical distance from the seat to the center of an object gripped in the hand with the shoulder flexed to a 180-degree angle (no excessive stretching)

These and other measurements have been taken of thousands of people from different populations. The measurements have been compiled to form tables of anthropometric estimates. These tables can be used to determine the best average sizes for aspects of the work space for different ages, genders, and ethnic populations. These tables can also be used to get a sense of the range and complexity of the human form.

These measurements correspond with anthropometric estimates in Tables 3.1–3.4. Table 3.1 provides anthropometric measurements for an American population, Table 3.2 for an elderly British population, Table 3.3 for a Japanese population, and Table 3.4 for a Swedish population. These tables help emphasize the disparity between different ethnic groups and the importance of taking ethnicity into account when designing work spaces. Table 3.5 provides some general estimates for users of wheelchairs and refers to Figures 3.3 and 3.4. Many of these measurements would be similar to a seated population except that the height and breadth of the wheelchair must be taken into consideration. Table 3.6 provides detailed estimates for the hand and refers to Figure 3.5.

Body Segment Links Model

Another method for describing body sizes and shapes in nonstandard postures is to describe the body in terms of segments and links. A simplified example of selected representations of body links (a distance between effective joint centers of location), joint locations, and segment dimensions was developed by Drillis and Contini (1966) and adapted by Roebuck et al. (1975). This model allows the estimation of average body segment lengths and is based on the ratio of the average proportions of different body segments to overall body stature. The average length of any body segment can be determined using this links model, provided the stature is known. These ratios are reasonably correct for white men and are based on 1960s measurements. The ratios would be different, however, for Asians (especially Japanese) or blacks. These proportions have possibly changed over time. For a more realistic, though still somewhat idealized, depiction of body links for the limbs, see the report by Dempster (1955). This report was a major contribution to the study of human factors and biomechanics analysis.

Certain key joint centers of rotation are depicted by open circles in Figure 3.6, although these are highly simplified when compared to the real human body. The height of the head is indicated and the breadths of the chest and feet are depicted with horizontal lines. Because the figure is only shown in a standing posture, some liberties have been taken with regard to combining dimensions of standing and sitting postures, such as the distance from the top of the head to the buttocks, which can only really be applied in the sitting posture.

The primary value of depicting measurements using ratios to a key dimension, such as stature, is that it can be used to compare relative proportions of the average values of anthropometric dimensions from one population to another. When the ratios are similar, dimensions missing from one survey can be estimated from data reported in another. Similar ratios can also be used in a gross approximation method for evaluation and design application. If the heights of individuals working at a site are known, the average sizes of body parts can be estimated. For example, an individual who is 67 in. tall has, on average, a calf height of 19.10 in. (67 in. × the calf segment of 0.285). The proportions can be added to determine an overall length. For example, the average overall arm length from shoulder to fingertip of a 67-in. tall individual would be 29.48 in. ([67 in. × the upper arm link of 0.186] + [67 in. × the forearm link of 0.146] + [67 in. × the hand link segment of 0.108]).

TABLE 3.1
Anthropometric Estimates for American Adults (Refer to Figures 3.1 and 3.2)

No. in Figures	Dimensions	Men			Women		
		2.5th %ile	50th %ile	97.5th %ile	2.5th %ile	50th %ile	97.5th %ile
1.	Stature (in.)	63.58	68.82	74.02	58.70	63.58	68.50
	(cm)	*161.5*	*174.8*	*188.0*	*149.1*	*161.5*	*174.0*
2.	Eye height (in.)	59.61	64.41	69.29	54.68	59.61	64.09
	(cm)	*151.4*	*163.6*	*176.0*	*138.9*	*151.4*	*162.8*
3.	Shoulder height (in.)	51.89	56.61	61.42	47.80	51.89	56.18
	(cm)	*131.8*	*143.8*	*156.0*	*121.4*	*131.8*	*142.7*
4.	Elbow height (in.)	38.58	42.01	45.31	35.20	38.58	41.81
	(cm)	*98.0*	*106.7*	*115.1*	*89.4*	*98.0*	*106.2*
5.	Hip height (in.)	33.31	36.42	39.49	30.39	33.31	36.18
	(cm)	*84.6*	*92.5*	*100.3*	*77.2*	*84.6*	*91.9*
7.	Fingertip height (in.)	23.50	25.79	27.91	21.30	23.50	25.51
	(cm)	*59.7*	*65.5*	*70.9*	*54.1*	*59.7*	*64.8*
8.	Sitting height (in.)	33.11	35.79	38.31	30.79	33.11	35.59
	(cm)	*84.1*	*90.9*	*97.3*	*78.2*	*84.1*	*90.4*
9.	Sitting eye height (in.)	29.09	31.42	33.58	26.81	29.09	31.18
	(cm)	*73.9*	*79.8*	*85.3*	*68.1*	*73.9*	*79.2*

10.	Sitting shoulder height (in.)	21.42	23.39	25.31	19.88	21.46	23.31
	(cm)	54.4	59.4	64.3	50.5	54.5	59.2
11.	Sitting elbow height (in.)	23.66	26.02	28.11	21.57	23.70	25.79
	(cm)	60.1	66.1	71.4	54.8	60.2	65.5
12.	Thigh thickness (in.)	5.71	6.69	7.09	4.02	5.51	7.72
	(cm)	14.5	17.0	18.0	10.2	14.0	19.6
13.	Buttock-knee length (in.)	21.81	23.39	25.71	20.20	22.28	24.41
	(cm)	55.4	59.4	65.3	51.3	56.6	62.0
14.	Buttock-popliteal length (in.)	17.20	18.82	20.12	15.79	17.72	19.80
	(cm)	43.7	47.8	51.1	40.1	45.0	50.3
15.	Knee height (in.)	19.80	21.61	23.50	18.11	19.80	21.6_
	(cm)	50.3	54.9	59.7	46.0	50.3	54.9
16.	Popliteal height (in.)	15.59	17.01	18.50	14.29	15.59	16.89
	(cm)	39.6	43.2	47.0	36.3	39.6	42.9
17.	Shoulder breadth (in.)	15.98	17.72	19.41	14.41	15.98	17.72
	(cm)	40.6	45.0	49.3	36.6	40.6	45.0
18.	Hip breadth (in.)	12.40	13.90	15.79	12.28	14.61	17.72
	(cm)	31.5	35.3	40.1	31.2	37.1	45.0

Source: Adapted from N Diffrient, AR Tilley, JC Bardagly. Humanscale 1/2/3. Cambridge, MA: MIT Press, 1974.

TABLE 3.2
Anthropometric Estimates for British Elderly (Refer to Figures 3.1 and 3.2)

No. in Figures	Dimensions	Men				Women			
		5th %ile	50th %ile	95th %ile	SD	5th %ile	50th %ile	95th %ile	SD
1.	Stature (in.)	59.65	64.57	69.49	3.03	55.12	59.65	64.17	2.76
	(cm)	151.5	164.0	176.5	7.7	140.0	151.5	163.0	7.0
2.	Eye height (in.)	55.51	60.43	65.35	2.99	51.38	55.91	60.43	2.72
	(cm)	141.0	153.5	166.0	7.6	130.5	142.0	153.5	6.9
3.	Shoulder height (in.)	48.23	52.95	57.68	2.83	44.49	48.62	52.76	2.56
	(cm)	122.5	134.5	146.5	7.2	113.0	123.5	134.0	6.5
4.	Elbow height (in.)	36.81	40.35	44.09	2.24	33.86	37.20	40.55	2.05
	(cm)	93.5	102.5	112.0	5.7	86.0	94.5	103.0	5.2
5.	Hip height (in.)	30.91	34.45	37.99	2.17	27.56	30.71	33.86	1.93
	(cm)	78.5	87.5	96.5	5.5	70.0	78.0	86.0	4.9
6.	Knuckle height (in.)	25.20	28.15	30.91	1.77	24.02	26.77	29.33	1.61
	(cm)	64.0	71.5	78.5	4.5	61.0	68.0	74.5	4.1
7.	Fingertip height (in.)	21.65	24.41	27.17	1.65	20.28	23.23	25.98	1.69
	(cm)	55.0	62.0	69.0	4.2	51.5	59.0	66.0	4.3
8.	Sitting height (in.)	30.91	33.46	36.22	1.65	27.95	30.91	34.06	1.89
	(cm)	78.5	85.0	92.0	4.2	71.0	78.5	86.5	4.8
9.	Sitting eye height (in.)	26.57	29.13	31.69	1.57	24.02	26.97	29.72	1.77
	(cm)	67.5	74.0	80.5	4.0	61.0	68.5	75.5	4.5
10.	Sitting shoulder height (in.)	19.49	21.85	24.21	1.46	17.52	20.28	23.03	1.65
	(cm)	49.5	55.5	61.5	3.7	44.5	51.5	58.5	4.2
11.	Sitting elbow height (in.)	6.30	8.46	10.63	1.34	5.91	8.07	10.04	1.26
	(cm)	16.0	21.5	27.0	3.4	15.0	20.5	25.5	3.2
12.	Thigh thickness (in.)	4.72	5.71	6.89	0.67	4.13	5.51	6.69	0.75
	(cm)	12.0	14.5	17.5	1.7	10.5	14.0	17.0	1.9

13.	Buttock-knee length (in.)	20.08	22.24	24.41	1.34	19.29	21.46	23.62	1.34
	(cm)	51.0	56.5	62.0	3.4	49.0	54.5	60.0	3.4
14.	Buttock-popliteal length (in.)	16.14	18.50	20.87	1.42	15.94	18.11	20.28	1.34
	(cm)	41.0	47.0	53.0	3.6	40.5	46.0	51.5	3.4
15.	Knee height (in.)	17.91	20.28	22.44	1.38	16.93	18.90	20.87	1.18
	(cm)	45.5	51.5	57.0	3.5	43.0	48.0	53.0	3.0
16.	Popliteal height (in.)	14.37	16.34	18.50	1.26	12.99	14.96	16.93	1.22
	(cm)	36.5	41.5	47.0	3.2	33.0	38.0	43.0	3.1
17.	Shoulder breadth (in.)	13.19	14.37	15.75	0.79	12.01	13.19	14.57	1.69
	(cm)	33.5	36.5	40.0	2.0	30.5	33.5	37.0	4.3
18.	Hip breadth (in)	11.42	13.39	15.55	1.26	11.22	13.98	16.73	1.69
	(cm)	29.0	34.0	39.5	3.2	28.5	35.5	42.5	4.3
19.	Shoulder-elbow length (in.)	12.01	13.58	14.96	0.87	11.02	12.20	13.58	0.79
	(cm)	30.5	34.5	38.0	2.2	28.0	31.0	34.5	2.0
20.	Elbow-fingertip length (in.)	16.14	17.72	19.09	0.91	14.57	15.94	17.32	0.87
	(cm)	41.0	45.0	48.5	2.3	37.0	40.5	44.0	2.2
21.	Upper limb length (in.)	26.38	28.94	31.50	1.54	23.82	26.18	28.54	1.42
	(cm)	67.0	73.5	80.0	3.9	60.5	66.5	72.5	3.6
22.	Shoulder grip length (in.)	22.44	24.61	26.97	1.38	20.08	22.24	24.41	1.30
	(cm)	57.0	62.5	68.5	3.5	51.0	56.5	62.0	3.3
23.	Vertical grip reach (standing) (in.)	69.68	75.39	81.10	3.46	64.57	69.68	74.80	2.36
	(cm)	177.0	191.5	206.0	8.8	164.0	177.0	190.0	6.0
24.	Vertical grip reach (sitting) (in.)	41.93	46.26	50.39	2.60	38.78	42.72	46.46	2.36
	(cm)	106.5	117.5	128.0	6.6	98.5	108.5	118.0	5.0

Source: Adapted with permission from S Pheasant. Bodyspace: Anthropometry, Ergonomics, and Design. Philadelphia: Taylor & Francis, 1986;110.

TABLE 3.3
Anthropometric Estimates for Japanese Adults (Refer to Figures 3.1 and 3.2)

No. in Figures	Dimensions	Men				Women			
		5th %ile	50th %ile	95th %ile	SD	5th %ile	50th %ile	95th %ile	SD
1.	Stature (in.)	61.42	65.16	68.90	2.28	57.09	60.24	63.39	1.89
	(cm)	156.0	165.5	175.0	5.8	145.0	153.0	161.0	4.8
2.	Eye height (in.)	56.89	60.63	64.37	2.24	53.15	56.10	59.06	1.85
	(cm)	144.5	154.0	163.5	5.7	135.0	142.5	150.0	4.7
3.	Shoulder height (in.)	49.21	52.76	56.30	2.13	42.32	45.08	47.83	1.73
	(cm)	125.0	134.0	143.0	5.4	107.5	114.5	121.5	4.4
4.	Elbow height (in.)	37.99	40.75	43.50	1.69	35.24	37.60	39.96	1.42
	(cm)	96.5	103.5	110.5	4.3	89.5	95.5	101.5	3.6
5.	Hip height (in.)	30.12	32.68	35.24	1.61	27.56	29.72	31.89	1.30
	(cm)	76.5	83.0	89.5	4.1	70.0	75.5	81.0	3.3
6.	Knuckle height (in.)	26.57	29.13	31.69	1.57	25.59	27.76	29.92	1.30
	(cm)	67.5	74.0	80.5	4.0	65.0	70.5	76.0	3.3
7.	Fingertip height (in.)	22.24	24.80	27.36	1.50	21.26	23.62	25.98	1.38
	(cm)	56.5	63.0	69.5	3.8	54.0	60.0	66.0	3.5
8.	Sitting height (in.)	33.46	35.43	37.40	1.22	31.50	33.27	35.04	1.10
	(cm)	85.0	90.0	95.0	3.1	80.0	84.5	89.0	2.8
9.	Sitting eye height (in.)	28.94	30.91	32.87	1.22	27.17	28.94	30.71	1.10
	(cm)	73.5	78.5	83.5	3.1	69.0	73.5	78.0	2.8
10.	Sitting shoulder height (in.)	21.46	23.23	25.00	1.10	20.08	21.85	23.62	1.02
	(cm)	54.5	59.0	63.5	2.8	51.0	55.5	60.0	2.6
11.	Sitting elbow height (in.)	8.66	10.24	11.81	0.91	8.46	9.84	11.22	0.79
	(cm)	22.0	26.0	30.0	2.3	21.5	25.0	28.5	2.0
12.	Thigh thickness (in.)	4.33	5.31	6.30	0.55	4.13	5.12	6.10	0.55
	(cm)	11.0	13.5	16.0	1.4	10.5	13.0	15.5	1.4

	5th	50th	95th	SD	5th	50th	95th	SD
13. Buttock-knee length (in.)	19.69	21.65	23.62	1.14	19.09	20.87	22.64	1.02
(cm)	50.0	55.0	60.0	2.9	48.5	53.0	57.5	2.6
14. Buttock-popliteal length (in.)	16.14	18.50	20.08	1.22	15.94	17.72	19.49	1.02
(cm)	41.0	47.0	51.0	3.1	40.5	45.0	49.5	2.6
15. Knee height (in.)	17.72	19.29	20.87	0.91	16.54	17.72	18.90	0.71
(cm)	45.0	49.0	53.0	2.3	42.0	45.0	48.0	1.8
16. Popliteal height (in.)	14.17	15.75	17.32	0.94	12.80	14.17	15.55	0.83
(cm)	36.0	40.0	44.0	2.4	32.5	36.0	39.5	2.1
17. Shoulder breadth (in.)	13.78	14.96	16.14	0.71	12.40	13.39	14.37	0.59
(cm)	35.0	38.0	41.0	1.8	31.5	34.0	36.5	1.5
18. Hip breadth (in.)	11.02	12.01	12.99	0.55	10.63	12.01	13.39	0.79
(cm)	28.0	30.5	33.0	1.4	27.0	30.5	34.0	2.0
19. Shoulder-elbow length (in.)	11.61	12.99	14.37	0.83	10.63	11.81	12.99	0.55
(cm)	29.5	33.0	36.5	2.1	27.0	30.0	33.0	1.4
20. Elbow-fingertip length (in.)	15.94	17.32	18.70	0.79	14.57	15.75	16.93	0.67
(cm)	40.5	44.0	47.5	2.0	37.0	40.0	43.0	1.7
21. Upper limb length (in.)	26.18	28.15	30.12	1.14	23.82	25.39	26.97	0.98
(cm)	66.5	71.5	76.5	2.9	60.5	64.5	68.5	2.5
22. Shoulder grip length (in.)	22.24	24.02	25.79	1.02	20.28	21.65	23.03	0.87
(cm)	56.5	61.0	65.5	2.6	51.5	55.0	58.5	2.2
23. Vertical grip reach (standing) (in.)	71.06	76.38	81.69	3.27	66.14	70.67	75.20	2.72
(cm)	180.5	194.0	207.5	8.3	168.0	179.5	191.0	6.9
24. Vertical grip reach (sitting) (in.)	43.50	46.65	49.80	1.93	40.55	43.11	45.67	1.61
(cm)	110.5	118.5	126.5	4.9	103.0	109.5	116.0	4.1
25. Forward grip reach (in.)	24.80	27.17	29.53	1.46	22.44	24.41	26.38	1.22
(cm)	63.0	69.0	75.0	3.7	57.0	62.0	67.0	3.1

Source: Adapted with permission from S Pheasant. Bodyspace: Anthropometry, Ergonomics, and Design. Philadelphia: Taylor & Francis, 1986;117.

TABLE 3.4
Anthropometric Estimates for Swedish Adults (Refer to Figures 3.1 and 3.2)

No. in Figures	Dimensions	Men				Women			
		5th %ile	50th %ile	95th %ile	SD	5th %ile	50th %ile	95th %ile	SD
1.	Stature (in.)	64.17	68.50	72.83	2.68	60.63	64.57	68.50	2.44
	(cm)	163.0	174.0	185.0	6.8	154.0	164.0	174.0	6.2*
2.	Eye height (in.)	59.84	64.17	68.50	2.68	56.50	60.43	64.37	2.44
	(cm)	152.0	163.0	174.0	6.8	143.5	153.5	163.5	6.2*
3.	Shoulder height (in.)	52.95	56.89	60.83	2.44	49.41	53.35	57.28	2.36
	(cm)	134.5	144.5	154.5	6.2	125.5	135.5	145.5	6.0*
4.	Elbow height (in.)	40.16	43.31	46.46	1.93	35.63	40.35	45.08	2.87
	(cm)	102.0	110.0	118.0	4.9	90.5	102.5	114.5	7.3*
5.	Hip height (in.)	32.09	35.04	37.99	1.77	29.33	32.68	36.02	2.05
	(cm)	81.5	89.0	96.5	4.5	74.5	83.0	91.5	5.2*
6.	Knuckle height (in.)	28.35	29.92	31.50	0.98	26.57	28.94	31.30	1.42
	(cm)	72.0	76.0	80.0	2.5	67.5	73.5	79.5	3.6
7.	Fingertip height (in.)	23.43	25.79	28.15	1.46	22.44	25.00	27.56	1.50
	(cm)	59.5	65.5	71.5	3.7	57.0	63.5	70.0	3.8
8.	Sitting height (in.)	32.68	35.43	38.19	1.69	31.69	33.86	36.02	1.30
	(cm)	83.0	90.0	97.0	4.3	80.5	86.0	91.5	3.3*
9.	Sitting eye height (in.)	28.15	30.91	33.66	1.65	27.76	29.72	31.69	1.18
	(cm)	71.5	78.5	85.5	4.2	70.5	75.5	80.5	3.0*
10.	Sitting shoulder height (in.)	21.46	23.62	25.79	1.34	20.67	22.64	24.61	1.18
	(cm)	54.5	60.0	65.5	3.4	52.5	57.5	62.5	3.0*
11.	Sitting elbow height (in.)	6.89	8.86	10.83	1.22	6.50	8.46	10.43	1.22
	(cm)	17.5	22.5	27.5	3.1	16.5	21.5	26.5	3.1*
12.	Thigh thickness (in.)	4.72	5.98	7.09	0.71	5.12	6.10	7.09	0.63
	(cm)	12.0	15.2	18.0	1.8	13.0	15.5	18.0	1.6*

13.	Buttock-knee length (in.)	21.46	23.43	25.39	1.18	20.67	23.03	25.39	1.38
	(cm)	*54.5*	*59.5*	*64.5*	*3.0*	*52.5*	*58.5*	*64.5*	*3.5**
14.	Buttock-popliteal length (in.)	16.93	18.90	20.37	1.18	16.93	19.09	21.26	1.30
	(cm)	*43.0*	*48.0*	*53.0*	*3.0*	*43.0*	*48.5*	*54.0*	*3.3**
15.	Knee height (in.)	18.90	20.87	22.83	1.18	17.91	19.69	21.46	1.10
	(cm)	*48.0*	*53.0*	*58.0*	*3.0*	*45.5*	*50.0*	*54.5*	*2.8**
16.	Popliteal height (in.)	15.16	16.93	18.70	1.06	13.78	15.75	17.72	1.14
	(cm)	*38.5*	*43.0*	*47.5*	*2.7*	*35.0*	*40.0*	*45.0*	*2.9*
17.	Shoulder breadth (in.)	14.37	15.75	17.13	0.79	12.80	13.73	14.76	0.59
	(cm)	*36.5*	*40.0*	*43.5*	*2.0*	*32.5*	*35.0*	*37.5*	*1.5*(w)*
18.	Hip breadth (in.)	12.20	14.17	16.14	1.14	27.17	29.72	32.28	1.50
	(cm)	*31.0*	*36.0*	*41.0*	*2.9*	*69.0*	*75.5*	*82.0*	*3.8*
19.	Shoulder-elbow length (in.)	12.99	14.37	15.75	0.79	12.01	13.19	14.37	0.67
	(cm)	*33.0*	*36.5*	*40.0*	*2.0*	*30.5*	*33.5*	*36.5*	*1.7*
20.	Elbow-fingertip length (in.)	17.32	18.70	20.08	0.79	6.30	6.89	7.48	0.39
	(cm)	*44.0*	*47.5*	*51.0*	*2.0*	*16.0*	*17.5*	*19.0*	*1.0*(w)*
21.	Upper limb length (in.)	28.35	30.71	33.07	1.38	25.98	27.76	29.53	1.10
	(cm)	*72.0*	*78.0*	*84.0*	*3.5*	*66.0*	*70.5*	*75.0*	*2.8*(w)*
22.	Shoulder grip length (in.)	24.21	26.18	28.15	1.22	21.85	23.43	25.00	0.94
	(cm)	*61.5*	*66.5*	*71.5*	*3.1*	*55.5*	*59.5*	*63.5*	*2.4*
23.	Vertical grip reach (standing) (in.)	75.98	81.10	86.22	3.07	71.85	76.38	80.91	2.76
	(cm)	*193.0*	*206.0*	*219.0*	*7.8*	*182.5*	*194.0*	*205.5*	*7.0*
24.	Vertical grip reach (sitting) (in.)	45.47	49.02	52.76	2.28	42.91	46.26	49.61	2.09
	(cm)	*115.5*	*124.5*	*134.0*	*5.8*	*109.0*	*117.5*	*126.0*	*5.3*

w = women only; m = men only.
Note: All other measurements are estimates based on E coefficients. See Pheasant (1986) for further details of this method.
*Dimensions are quoted directly from the source.
Source: Adapted with permission from S Pheasant. Bodyspace: Anthropometry, Ergonomics, and Design. Philadelphia: Taylor & Francis, 1986;114.

TABLE 3.5
Anthropometric Estimates for Wheelchair Users (Refer to Figures 3.3 and 3.4)

No. in Figures	Dimensions (Seated in Wheelchair)	Small Woman	Avg. Woman/ Small Man	Avg. Adult	Large Woman/ Avg. Man	Large Man
1.	Stature* (in.)	58.3	63.2/63.2	65.8	68.1/68.4	73.6
	(cm)	148.1	160.5/169.5	167.1	173.0/173.7	186.9
2.	Top of head height (in.)	47.8	51.5	53.1	54.3	55.8
	(cm)	121.4	130.8	134.9	137.9	141.7
3.	Eye height (in.)	42.8	46.3	47.7	48.6	51.1
	(cm)	108.7	117.6	121.2	123.4	129.8
4.	Shoulder height (in.)	35.8	38.6	39.8	40.4	42.8
	(cm)	90.9	98.0	101.1	102.6	108.7
5.	Knuckle height (in.)	14.6	16.0	16.0	16.0	16.5
	(cm)	37.1	40.6	40.6	40.6	41.9
6.	Thigh height (in.)	23.5	24.5	25.0	25.5	26.5
	(cm)	59.7	62.2	63.5	64.8	67.3
7.	Toe height (in.)	8.8	6.5	6.2	5.8	8.5
	(cm)	22.4	16.5	15.7	14.7	21.6
8.	Easy forward reach (in.)	18.5	20.2	20.8	21.3	22.3
	(cm)	47.0	51.3	52.8	54.1	56.6
9.	Maximum forward reach (in.)	31.3	34.2	35.3	36.3	38.3
	(cm)	79.5	86.9	89.7	92.2	97.3
10.	Floor to high forward reach (in.)	45.5	51.5	53.5	55.5	59.2
	(cm)	115.6	130.8	135.9	141.0	150.4
11.	Easy side reach (in.)	16.2	17.3	18.6	19.9	22.5
	(cm)	41.1	43.9	47.2	50.5	57.2
12.	Maximum side reach (in.)	22.2	23.8	25.3	26.9	30.1
	(cm)	56.4	60.5	64.3	68.3	76.5
13.	Floor to high side reach (in.)	53.0	59.3	62.0	64.6	71.2
	(cm)	134.6	150.6	157.5	164.1	180.8

*Stature refers to the height of the individual if standing.
Source: Adapted from N Diffrient, AR Tilley, JC Bardagly. Humanscale 1/2/3. Cambridge, MA: MIT Press, 1974.

FIGURE 3.3. Static anthropometric dimensions for wheelchair users (side view). The numbers correspond to data in Table 3.5.

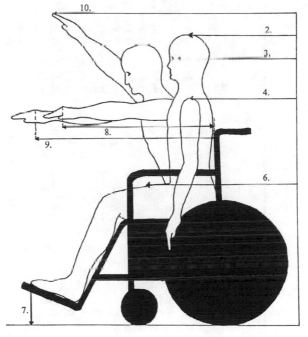

FIGURE 3.4. Static anthropometric dimensions for the wheelchair users (front view). The numbers correspond to data in Table 3.5.

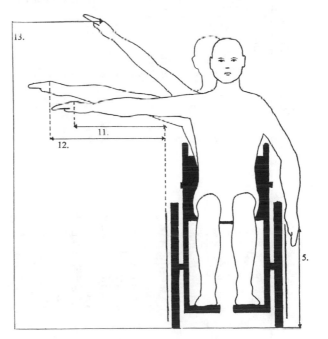

TABLE 3.6
Anthropometric Estimates for the Hand (Refer to Figure 3.5)

# in Figures	Dimensions	Men				Women			
		5th %ile	50th %ile	95th %ile	SD	5th %ile	50th %ile	95th %ile	SD
1.	Hand length (in.)	6.81	7.44	8.07	0.39	6.26	6.85	7.44	0.04
	(cm)	17.3	18.9	20.5	1.0	15.9	17.4	18.9	0.9
2.	Palm length (in.)	3.86	4.21	4.57	0.24	3.50	3.82	4.13	0.20
	(cm)	9.8	10.7	11.6	0.6	8.9	9.7	10.5	0.5
3.	Thumb length (in.)	1.73	2.01	2.28	0.16	1.57	1.85	2.09	0.16
	(cm)	4.4	5.1	5.8	0.4	4.0	4.7	5.3	0.4
4.	Index finger length (in.)	2.52	2.83	3.11	0.20	2.36	2.64	2.91	0.20
	(cm)	6.4	7.2	7.9	0.5	6.0	6.7	7.4	0.5
5.	Middle finger length (in.)	2.99	3.27	3.54	0.20	2.72	3.03	3.31	0.20
	(cm)	7.6	8.3	9.0	0.5	6.9	7.7	8.4	0.5
6.	Ring finger length (in.)	2.56	2.83	3.15	0.16	2.32	2.60	2.87	0.16
	(cm)	6.5	7.2	8.0	0.4	5.9	6.6	7.3	0.4
7.	Little finger length (in.)	1.89	2.17	2.48	0.16	1.69	1.97	2.24	0.16
	(cm)	4.8	5.5	6.3	0.4	4.3	5.0	5.7	0.4
8.	Thumb breadth (IPJ) (in.)	0.79	0.91	1.02	0.08	0.67	0.75	0.83	0.08
	(cm)	2.0	2.3	2.6	0.2	1.7	1.9	2.1	0.2
9.	Thumb thickness (IPJ) (in.)	0.75	0.87	0.94	0.08	0.59	0.71	0.79	0.08
	(cm)	1.9	2.2	2.4	0.2	1.5	1.8	2.0	0.2
10.	Index finger breadth (PIPJ) (in.)	0.75	0.83	0.91	0.04	0.63	0.71	0.79	0.04
	(cm)	1.9	2.1	2.3	0.1	1.6	1.8	2.0	0.1
11.	Index finger thickness (in.)	0.67	0.75	0.83	0.04	0.55	0.63	0.71	0.04
	(cm)	1.7	1.9	2.1	0.1	1.4	1.6	1.8	0.1
12.	Hand breadth (metacarpal) (in.)	3.07	3.43	3.74	0.20	2.72	2.99	3.27	0.16
	(cm)	7.8	8.7	9.5	0.5	6.9	7.6	8.3	0.4

13.	Hand breadth (across thumb)	(in.)	3.82	4.13	4.49	0.20	3.31	3.62	3.90	0.20
		(cm)	*9.7*	*10.5*	*11.4*	*0.5*	*8.4*	*9.2*	*9.9*	*0.5*
14.	Hand breadth (minimum)	(in.)[a]	2.80	3.19	3.35	0.24	2.48	2.80	3.11	0.20
		(cm)	*7.1*	*8.1*	*8.5*	*0.6*	*6.3*	*7.1*	*7.9*	*0.5*
15.	Hand thickness (metacarpal)	(in.)	1.06	1.30	1.50	0.12	0.94	1.10	1.30	0.12
		(cm)	*2.7*	*3.3*	*3.8*	*0.3*	*2.4*	*2.8*	*3.3*	*0.3*
16.	Hand thickness (including thumb)	(in.)	1.73	2.01	2.28	0.16	1.57	1.77	1.97	0.12
		(cm)	*4.4*	*5.1*	*5.8*	*0.4*	*4.0*	*4.5*	*5.0*	*0.3*
17.	Maximum grip diameter	(in.)[b]	1.77	2.05	2.32	0.16	1.69	1.89	2.09	0.12
		(cm)	*4.5*	*5.2*	*5.9*	*0.4*	*4.3*	*4.8*	*5.3*	*0.3*
18.	Maximum spread (in.)		7.01	8.11	9.21	0.67	6.50	7.48	8.46	0.59
		(cm)	*17.8*	*20.6*	*23.4*	*1.7*	*16.5*	*19.0*	*21.5*	*1.5*
19.	Maximum functional spread (in.)[c]		4.80	5.59	6.38	0.47	4.29	5.00	5.71	0.43
		(cm)	*12.2*	*14.2*	*16.2*	*1.2*	*10.9*	*12.7*	*14.5*	*1.1*
20.	Minimum square access (in.)[d]		2.20	2.60	2.99	0.24	1.97	2.28	2.64	0.20
		(cm)	*5.6*	*6.6*	*7.5*	*0.6*	*5.0*	*5.8*	*6.7*	*0.5*

IPJ = interphalangeal joint (i.e., the articulation between the two segments of the thumb); PIPJ = proximal interphalangeal joint (i.e., the finger articulation nearest the hand).

[a] As for hand breadth (metacarpal), except that the palm is contracted to make it as narrow as possible.
[b] Measured by sliding the hand down a graduated cone until the thumb and middle finger just touch.
[c] Measured by gripping a flat wooden wedge with the tip end segments of the thumb and ring fingers.
[d] The side of the smallest equal aperture through which the hand will pass.
Source: Adapted with permission from S Pheasant. Bodyspace: Anthropometry, Ergonomics, and Design. Philadelphia: Taylor & Francis, 1986;126.

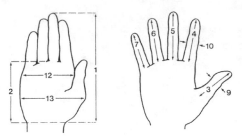

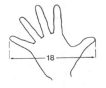

FIGURE 3.5.   Static anthropometric dimensions for the hand. The numbers correspond to data in Table 3.6. (Reprinted with permission from S Pheasant. Bodyspace: Anthropometry, Ergonomics, and Design. Philadelphia: Taylor & Francis, 1986;127.)

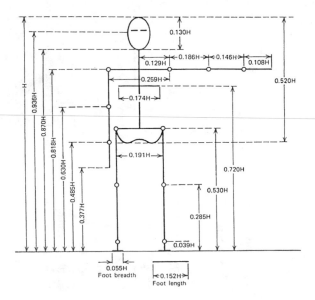

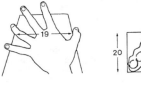

FIGURE 3.6.   The segment links model. (H = height of standing subject [stature].) (Reprinted with permission from JA Roebuck, KHE Kroemer, WG Thompson. Engineering Anthropometry Methods. New York: Wiley, 1975;176.)

This method provides a general estimate of body segment sizes for specific heights that may not be mentioned in the tables.

These estimates must be used with caution, however; a set of values calculated by the preceding method can only define the set of averages, never the set of dimensions, for any particular individual. It is not at all unusual for a real person to have a ninetieth percentile sitting height, a tenth percentile arm length, and a twentieth percentile foot length. Weight and fat distribution, as well as posture, diet, breathing, and muscular training, can create changes at various times. If more accurate estimates of segment lengths are desired for a specific person, a variety of estimation equations as well as different combinations of actual anthropometric measurements of that individual should be used (Pheasant 1986, 1996; Roebuck 1995).

Limitations of the Static Anthropometric Estimates

All the information described is useful for understanding the shape of humans. However, as with any averages, these measurements have some limitations. Remember: Anthropometric data offer a guide, not an absolute.

Accuracy

Measuring the human form is a tricky business. Not only is the body composed of round, soft outlines that are prone to compression, but people also tend to slouch. Measurement methods may vary from study to study depending on the researchers. Sometimes, because of the time and expense of anthropometric research, estimates are made using mathematical equations based on stature (similar to the segment links model). Although these provide a very reasonable estimate, they may not be totally accurate (Pheasant 1996). Fortunately, unless form-fitting spaces are being designed (such as a space capsule [NASA does its own measurements]), exact measurements are not always necessary.

Clothing

One of the greatest flaws in anthropometric measurements, at least for workstation design, is that all the measurements are taken of unclothed, unshod persons. Fortunately, most clothing adds only minimal bulk, unless it is protective equipment or bulky outdoors clothing. If workers are likely to be wearing bulky clothing, adjust the measurements accordingly. As a rule of thumb, use the following:

- Shoes: Add approximately 1.0–1.5 in. (2.5–3.8 cm) for men and 1–3 in. (4.5–7.6 cm) for women to all measurements involving leg height (these heights do not reflect extremes in fashion). Shoes add approximately 2 lb (0.9 kg) to male weight and 1.1 lb (0.5 kg) to female weight (Diffrient et al. 1974).

- Overcoat: Add 4 in. (10 cm) to elbow-to-elbow measurements and 1.0–1.5 in. (2.5–3.8 cm) to floor-to-shoulder heights (Diffrient et al. 1974). Reach is shortened and movements are slowed by a bulky overcoat.
- Safety helmet: Add 4 in. (10 cm) to stature (Diffrient et al. 1974).

Population

As mentioned, different populations have different sizes. Estimates should correspond with the population that will use the design. For example, if the population is predominantly Asian, using the information from an occidental group will provide measurements that are too large. Unfortunately, not all populations have anthropometric estimates that designers can use. Even the segment links model is sized to white men and must be used with caution.

Averages

All the measurements are averages of a large population. Variations exist for all the measurements when applied to the individual level. Using the average (fiftieth percentile) creates workstations that are too large or small for most people. Even using the fifth and ninety-fifth percentile, as recommended by ergonomic texts, misses 10% of the population. Data from the ninety-ninth and first percentiles exclude fewer people but have a greater potential for error. The data may not be reliable because the population used for the measurement is very small.

Although anthropometric data may have flaws, they still provide valuable insights into the overall size and shape of the population. They provide a solid foundation of information that can be used to create a workstation that will fit the largest number of people comfortably. The estimates provided in the tables should be used as a stepping-stone to understanding human form when improving or designing the work environment. Use of these estimates should help prevent the mistake of designing for only a few members of a population.

Uses of Anthropometric Data

The next sections of the chapter build on the static anthropometric estimates and review concepts such as reach and clearance. These concepts are vital to understanding how to construct a workstation. As with all measurements, these are averages. Always consider the overall population and the purpose of the workstation before using any measurement.

Reach

Reach is often defined as a sphere around the worker that can be touched by the worker at all points without moving the body from the starting point. The shoulder is the axis or center of the sphere, and the length of the arm is equal to the radius. In some cases, when reach is limited to what is available from elbow to fingertips (as when working on a table), the elbow is the axis, and the forearm/hand is the radius. When designing to accommodate reach, consider the smallest user, the fifth percentile female. If she can reach an object, all larger individuals can reach it too. (All reaching data are from Diffrient et al. 1974.)

Vertical Reach

Operating buttons on a control panel and getting objects off high shelves are examples of activities that occur during vertical reach.

- The highest any button or control should be from the ground is 71 in. (177 cm), if the person is able to stand directly against the control panel.
- The highest button from a seated position (with the knees up against the controls) should be 21 in. (51 cm) above the person's shoulder height.
- If the person must grasp the object, not just press a button, the heights must be reduced further by the length of the fingers (2.8 in. [7 cm]). If the person must be able to view and reach to the back of a 24-in (60-cm) shelf, the highest that shelf should be is 56 in. (140 cm) from the ground.

Horizontal Reach

Horizontal height is usually defined by a table top or counter; the worker manipulates objects on its surface. Four zones need to be considered (Figure 3.7):

1. *Normal work distance* is the arc made by the forearm when the body is as close to the table as is comfortable and the elbow is held at the side. This is the area where most precision work is performed. This distance for a small woman is a radius of approximately 8 in. (20 cm).

2. *Extended working distance* is the area made by the arc of the forearm when the elbow is actually resting at the edge of the table. This area is also a good work area, but is better for storing frequently used tools, supplies, and heavy objects. This distance is a radius of approximately 16 in. (40 cm).

3. *Maximum work distance* is established when the body leans forward as the person leans into the work. This area is best for infrequently used supplies and tools. It is also the area that is considered for the placement of push-buttons and other controls. This distance is a radius of approximately 19 in. (48 cm).

4. *Most efficient work space* is defined by a 10-in. (25-cm) square directly in front of the worker and about a hand's span from the edge of the

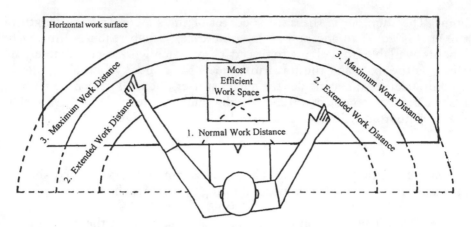

FIGURE 3.7.   The four zones of horizontal reach.

table. This is the area where most people prefer to work, as it places material at the most comfortable distance from the body.

These reaches are optimal when conditions are perfect. Reach distances can be constrained by the following:

- Balance: Greater reach can be achieved by leaning forward and backward. However, this may not be possible if the worker is in a precarious situation or on slippery surfaces. It also increases fatigue for repetitive reaching.
- Clothing: Bulky clothing such as coats and other protective suits reduces reach.
- Overall joint mobility: Persons with decreased motion, such as a person with arthritis or in a wheelchair, may not be able to reach far objects easily.
- Blocking by other surfaces: If a person must reach over or around other objects, reach is decreased.
- Job requirements: Reach can be constrained by needs for precision or strength.

"Visual" Reach (Seeing over Objects)

In the consideration of any work space, visual contact with important objects is necessary. Workers must be able to see what they are doing, as well as lights, controls, and alarms (Figure 3.8). Some rules for visual reach are as follows:

- Objects should not block the normal line of sight.
- The most relaxed line of sight when the head is erect is not actually on the horizontal plane: Relaxed sight occurs about 10–15 degrees below the horizontal. Thus, work that requires continuous

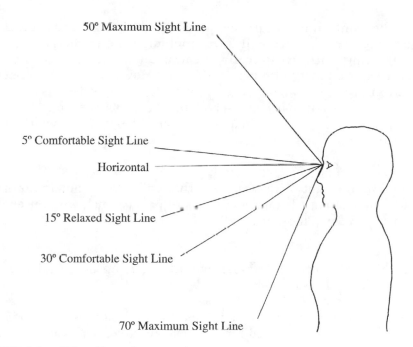

50° Maximum Sight Line

5° Comfortable Sight Line

Horizontal

15° Relaxed Sight Line

30° Comfortable Sight Line

70° Maximum Sight Line

FIGURE 3.8. "Visual" reach.

visual contact, such as work at a computer, should be placed 10–15 degrees below the horizontal eye line (Grandjean 1988).

- The eye can comfortably rotate about 15 degrees above and below this imaginary angle. Thus, controls that need to be read frequently should be placed between 30 degrees below the horizontal and 5 degrees above the horizontal (Grandjean 1988).
- The maximum the eyes can rotate without moving the head is between 70 degrees below the horizontal and 50 degrees above the horizontal. Objects that need occasional viewing or objects that flash on and interact with the peripheral vision are best placed in this area (Diffrient et al. 1974). This area does increase, of course, when the head is moved.
- Displays, particularly those that need to be read, should be large enough to be read at a distance. Grandjean (1988) recommends that characters 19.6 in. (50 cm) away be at least 0.12 in. (0.3 cm) high, whereas those that are 27.5 in. (70 cm) away be at least 0.17 in. (0.43 cm). Sharpness and contrast also play important roles in the ability of a worker to read a display.

Clearance

Clearance is the space needed to allow free passage of a person or a body segment. Clearance can be as narrow as a hatchway into a submarine or as wide as a doorway in a civic center that allows many people to pass in and out at the same time. Clearance, as with any design, must take into account the uses the area will have, including the traffic patterns and clothing being worn. Historically, clearance has been designed for the biggest user, the ninety-fifth percentile man. However, in today's society, clearance must take into account the wheelchair user, because a wheelchair requires considerably larger spaces in which to maneuver.

The following are some general clearance heights and widths based on a large man or, when appropriate, a user of a wheelchair.

Height

The minimum height of a passageway that will allow a ninety-ninth percentile man wearing a helmet and shoes to pass through without ducking is 77 in. (195.5 cm) (Pheasant 1986).

Width

The minimum width of a passageway depends on potential use. (All widths are from Pheasant 1986.)

- The clearance required for one person to walk alone is 25.5 in. (65 cm).
- The clearance required for two persons to walk abreast is 53.1 in. (135 cm).
- The clearance required for one person in a wheelchair is 42 in. (106.7 cm).
- The clearance required for a person in a wheelchair to complete a 360-degree turn is a 74-in. (188-cm) square.

Table Work

Working at a table requires elbow room. (All table work measurements are from Diffrient et al. 1981.)

- The ninety-fifth percentile man requires a 41.8-in. (106.2-cm) diameter circle with his body as the center to prevent him from banging his elbows into objects and other people when he is working.
- If he must swing an object, he requires a 76.7-in. (194.8-cm) diameter circle to not hit others.

Hand Clearance

Sliding the hand in and out of small spaces can be very important for certain tasks.

- The smallest aperture a ninety-fifth percentile man can slide his hand into is a square with each side measuring 5.1 in. (7.6 cm). If the opening is at least 2.3 in. (3.8 cm) thick and 4.6 in. (11.4 cm) wide, the hand can slide in. However, he cannot grasp and remove anything in this size, only press buttons.

- If hand access to a place is to be prevented, for example with hand guards, the opening must be less than 2 in. (5.0 cm) square or no thicker than 1.5 in. (2.3 cm) and no wider than 3.3 in. (8.3 cm) (Pheasant 1986).
- Seated work requires leg room. Any area designated for seated work should have enough space for a large person to comfortably place his or her legs under the space. Generally, work space designated for seated work should not have drawers or thick countertops, as this reduces knee space (all leg space estimates are from Grandjean 1988)
- The space should be at least 27.2 in. (68 cm) wide and 27.6 in. (69 cm) high.
- When they sit, most people like to lean back and stretch their legs under the space; therefore the depth of the space should accommodate this at least at floor level. The space should be 24 in. (60 cm) at knee level and 32 in. (80 cm) at floor level.

Posture

Essentially the orientation of body parts in space, posture is believed to have a profound effect on the health and well-being of the worker. Working in one unchanging position, or static posture, has been associated with the development of musculoskeletal disorders (Bernard 1996). Postures that position the body or body parts so that muscles must work strongly against gravity, such as holding the arms out at shoulder height or working with the torso bent, often cause discomfort in the worker. Anthropometric data is commonly used to place the body in the best posture for the job. But what is the best posture? In general, maintaining the limbs and torso as close to the neutral posture as possible is considered to place the least strain on the body. When a person is standing, the neutral posture can be achieved by having the head upright over the torso, the torso upright with the center of gravity over the hips, the knees slightly bent, and the arms in a relaxed position at the sides. Working positions that allow the worker to maintain or return to this posture frequently are considered to put the least amount of stress on the body. For sitting, the posture is similar, except it is shaped by the chair on which the worker is sitting.

One question is often considered: Is it better to sit or stand on the job? Both have good points. Whether a person should sit or stand on the job depends on the requirements of the task.

Advantages of Standing to Work
(Diffrient et al. 1981)

- Increases mobility
- Allows the worker to cover a larger work area
- Makes large control motions possible
- Allows the worker to exert body weight as force
- Saves space

Advantages of Sitting to Work
(Diffrient et al. 1981)

- Minimizes operator fatigue
- Increases operator stability
- Provides support to exert force
- Permits the use of pedals
- Accommodates a wide range of operator sizes

Sitting Posture

The position in which an individual sits can place a great deal of stress on the lower back. The so-called correct sitting posture in which the individual is positioned at 90-degree hip flexion, 90-degree knee flexion, and 90-degree elbow flexion, with ramrod-straight back and erect head, is a myth that may have caused some harm. Research on discal pressure during sitting suggests that this position places greater pressure on the lower back than sitting in a relaxed posture in the chair (Chaffin and Andersson 1991). Observations of workers suggest the posture most often selected is one that allows them to lean back in the chair at about an angle of 105 degrees (Grandjean et al. 1983). This position allows the back to be supported by the chair, taking some of the weight off the spinal disks and musculature. The best chair allows the worker to recline slightly.

The following rules should be kept in mind to help decrease the effects posture may have on the body:

- Position should be changed frequently. Prolonged static postures place a great deal of stress on the worker.
- Positions that cause forward inclination of the head should be avoided. The torque caused by the weight of the head (approximately 8 lb) increases dramatically the further from midline the head is placed. Make sure visual work is high enough to keep the head balanced over the spine.
- Upper arms should be kept next to the body, and raising arms overhead should be avoided. As with the neck, the torque on the shoulders increases as the arms move toward 90-degree angles.
- Body parts should be kept aligned, and twisting and asymmetry should be avoided. Asymmetry tends to place muscles in positions of weakness.
- Neutral postures should be maintained and extremes of range avoided. This is especially true for the wrist and hands, which can wind up in some very awkward postures.
- A back support should always be provided, preferably one that can be inclined to greater than 90 degrees.
- Body parts should be placed in the positions of greatest strength.

Precision and Strength

Anthropometrics directly affect a worker's ability to do work that requires precision or strength. As with posture, an understanding of anthropometrics can help correctly position workers to perform such tasks.

Precision

Precision is strongly influenced by the need to see work; the smaller the work, the closer it must be held to the eyes. Precision is enhanced by the worker's ability to hold the work close to the body and to support his or her arms or hands while working. In general, precise work should be positioned about 2–4 in. (5–10 cm) above elbow height (Grandjean 1988). This does not necessarily refer to work-surface height. The actual surface may be lower or higher than this for tools, and job demands may require the worker to position the job above or below the work surface. For example, when considering how to position the work for a welder, the therapist must take into account the height of the welding wand, and position the work low enough so that the hand holding the wand is 2–4 in. (5–10 cm) above elbow height.

Strength

Strength is directly influenced by posture and therefore anthropometries. All muscles have an optimal muscle-tension length at which they are strongest (Chaffin and Andersson 1991). When the body part is positioned at this optimal length, greater strength is achieved. Strength alone, however, is not all that is necessary for a job. Some tasks are more dependent on leverage, body equilibrium, and friction. Pulling often requires the use of body weight to counter balance the task. In general, however, jobs that require strength should be performed with the object 6–16 in. (15–40 cm) lower than the elbow (Grandjean 1988).

After the basics of anthropometry are understood, the question becomes how to integrate the information into actual design. The following is a hypothetical case study that uses anthropometric estimates to help determine equipment for a group of office workers. After applying anthropometric estimates for designing a workstation, a therapist must allow a range of real individuals to test arrangements and equipment.

Case Study

A large company is considering redesigning their data-entry department to improve the configuration of each workstation. The company has three shifts of 50 data-entry personnel. All workstations are used by at least three employees during these three shifts, and sometimes floaters (temporary employees) also use the workstations. The therapist hired to consult about the purchase of equipment has ascertained the following information:

1. The population of the company is predominantly female (90%).
2. The primary ethnicity is white (75%). An equal mix of ethnicities occurs in the remaining 25%.
3. The company states they are willing to replace the chairs and provide some additional small equipment. No budget is provided for completely redesigning all the capital equipment.
4. Each workstation has a standard 30-in. desk and a 4-in.–high computer with a 16-in.–tall monitor on top of it. This configuration places the top of the monitor 50 in. from the floor. The keyboard is placed on the 30-in. desk. Each station has a computer wrist rest. The chairs are adjustable up and down from 17.5 to 22.5 in.
5. Most of the data entry is numeric; thus, the employees use the number pad. The mouse and the alphanumeric part of the keyboard are seldom used.

The therapist realizes she is unable to design each workstation to fit individuals. Instead, she concentrates on making the workstation fit the greatest variety of workers by using the static anthropometric tables to determine the optimal sizes for the greatest number of people.

Using the static measurements for American adults (see Table 3.1), the therapist creates a table to help estimate the variety of sizes likely to occur within this population (Table 3.7). He or she makes the following recommendations based on the table:

1. Purchase adjustable chairs. A review of available models suggests that most chairs adjust between 16 and 21 in. These meet the height requirements of taller men and women, although footrests for shorter men and women will need to be available. The chairs should have adjustable arm rest heights from 7 to 9.5 in. The arm rests should also be adjustable in and out to allow for hip breadth. The seat pan should be no more than 18-in. deep and the back of the chair should adjust forward so that the seat pan depth can be reduced by 4 in.

2. Provide all desks with adjustable keyboard holders. The holders should be adjustable from between 2 and 7 in. below the desk height (because no chair is going lower than 16 in., the measurement of the elbow height from the ground is adjusted to a 16-in. height for 2.5 percentile females). A keyboard holder with space for a mouse is recommended.

3. The monitor should be removed from the computer and placed on an adjustable monitor holder that raises from desk level to 9 in. above the desk.

These three recommendations provide enough versatility to meet the needs of 95% of the workers. The therapist also provides education on how to adjust the workstation to meet individual needs.

TABLE 3.7
Case Study Using Static Anthropometric Estimates to Help Determine Equipment
Requirements for Office Workers

Anthropometric Segment	Smallest Estimate: Women in 2.5th %ile	Largest Estimate: Men in 97.5th %ile	Corresponding Workstation Measurement
Popliteal height	14.3 in.	18.5 in.	Chair seat height
Sitting elbow height	12.57 in.	28.11 in.	Keyboard height
Hip breadth	12.3 in.	17.7 in. (97.5th %ile woman)	Seat pan width
Buttock popliteal length	15.8 in.	20.1 in.	Seat pan depth (subtract 2 in. for actual seat pan depth)
Elbow height from chair (sitting elbow height minus popliteal height)	21.57 in. – 14.3 in. = 7.3 in.	28.11 in. – 18.5 in. = 9.6 in.	Armrest height
Eye height (popliteal height plus sitting eye height)	14.3 in. + 26.8 in. – 41.1 in.	18.5 in. + 33.6 in. = 52.1 in.	Top of monitor height

Summary

This chapter has reviewed the uses of static anthropometric tables for designing workstations for large populations. Static anthropometric and segment links modeling provide the essentials for understanding the variability of the human form. They can greatly reduce time and effort while greatly increasing the accuracy of design by providing the designer with information concerning the broadest ranges of a population, including individuals with disabilities. These estimates can provide the designer with information about clearance, reach, and posture that is essential to good design. Although these methods do have limitations, such as high variability, lack of measurements with clothes, and missing a percentage of the population, they do provide the best estimates of human size now available. Taken as a whole, static anthropometric measurements are invaluable tools for the therapist and ergonomist.

Acknowledgments

I would like to thank David Lee, who helped draft many of the illustrations in this chapter. I also would like to acknowledge the support of a traineeship from the National Center for Medical Rehabilitation Research of the

National Institute of Child and Development of the National Institute of Health (#5T3207462-04).

References

Al-Haboubi MH (1992). Anthropometry for a mix of different populations. Appl Ergonomics 23:191–196.

Anthropology Research Project (1978). Anthropometric Source Book. Vol I: Anthropometry for Designers (NASA Reference Publication 1024). Springfield, VA: National Technical Information Service.

Bernard BP (ed) (1997). Musculoskeletal Disorders and Workplace Factors. DHHS (NIOSH) Publication No. 97-141. Washington, DC: U.S. Department of Health and Human Services.

Chaffin DB, Andersson GBJ (1991). Occupational Biomechanics (2nd ed). New York: Wiley.

Dempster WT (1955). Space Requirements of the Seated Operator. Geometrical, Kinematic, and Mechanical Aspects of the Body with Special Reference to the Limbs. Dayton, OH: Wright Air Development Center, USAF. WADC TR 33–159.

Diffrient N, Tilley AR, Bardagly JC (1974). Humanscale 1/2/3. Cambridge, MA: MIT Press.

Diffrient N, Tilley AR, Harman D (1981). Humanscale 7/8/9. Cambridge, MA: MIT Press.

Drillis R, Contini R (1966). Body Segment Parameters. Report No. 1166-03 of the Office of Vocational Rehabilitation, Department of Health, Education and Welfare. New York: New York University School of Education and Science.

Grandjean E (1988). Fitting the Task to the Man (4th ed). New York: Taylor & Francis.

Grandjean E, Hünting W, Pidermann (1983). VDT workstation design: preferred settings and their effects. Hum Factors 25:161–175.

Hobson DA, Molenbroek JFM (1990). Anthropometry and design for the disabled: experiences with seating design for the cerebral palsy population. Appl Ergonomics 21:43–54.

Marras WS, Kim JY (1993). Anthropometry of industrial populations. Ergonomics 36:371–378.

Pheasant S (1986). Bodyspace: Anthropometry, Ergonomics, and Design. Philadelphia: Taylor & Francis.

Pheasant S (1996). Bodyspace: Anthropometry, Ergonomics, and the Design of Work (2nd ed). Philadelphia: Taylor & Francis.

Roberts DF (1973). Climate and Human Variability. An Addison-Wesley Module in Anthropology. Number 34. Reading, MA: Addison-Wesley.

Roebuck JA (1995). Anthropometric Methods: Designing to Fit the Human Body. Santa Monica, CA: Human Factors and Ergonomics Society.

Roebuck JA, Kroemer KHE, Thomson WG (1975). Engineering Anthropometry Methods. New York: Wiley.

Rosenblad-Wallin E (1987). An anthropometric study as the basis for sizing anatomically designed mittens. Appl Ergonomics 18:329–333.

Review Questions

(Answers are found in Appendix D.)

1. Which factor does not influence the size and shape of the human form?
   (a) Gender
   (b) Ethnicity
   (c) Education
   (d) Occupation
   (e) Clothing

2. The horizontal distance from the acromion to the tip of the third digit, with the elbow and wrist extended and the shoulder flexed to 90 degrees, is the
   (a) shoulder grip length
   (b) fingertip height
   (c) popliteal height
   (d) upper limb length
   (e) sitting vertical grip reach

3. On average, a Japanese woman in the fiftieth percentile would require a chair seat how many inches from the ground?
   (a) 12.80
   (h) 14.17
   (c) 15.59
   (d) 16.54
   (e) 17.72

4. Using the body segment links model, calculate the average elbow height in inches of an individual who is 5 ft 9 in. tall.
   (a) 24.84
   (b) 26.01
   (c) 42.01
   (d) 43.47
   (e) 49.68

5. Using anthropometric estimates, an accurate prediction of the exact size and shape of any individual is possible.
   (a) True
   (b) False

CHAPTER 4
Basic Biomechanics

Laurie A. Vincello

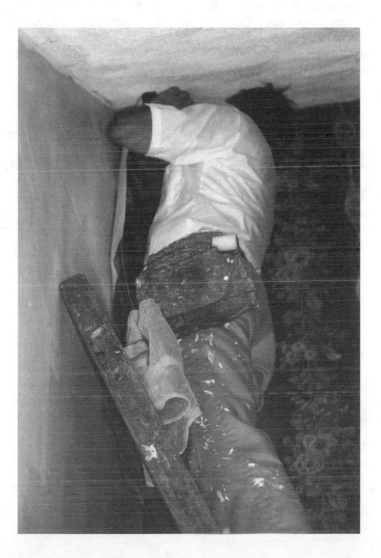

ABSTRACT

This chapter provides an overview of the principles of biomechanics. The biomechanical model uses the laws of physics to explain motion of the body segments and the forces that act on them. The chapter explains how to use functional units in analysis. It then uses the model to solve basic problems that involve the upper extremities, the trunk, and hand grip. Information in this chapter is useful for increasing understanding of person-machine systems and helping in the design of rehabilitation programs.

An understanding of biomechanics is necessary to appreciate the laws that govern movement of the human body. The biomechanical model can be used to estimate the forces that act on different component structures and sometimes to predict the maximum allowable magnitude for a load held in various postures, the appropriate size of tools, and the least stressful configuration of the workplace (Chaffin and Anderson 1984). The application of these principles maximizes performance, conserves energy, and prevents skeletal disorders in industry. Person and machine systems are designed with biomechanics in mind (Grandjean 1988). "Biomechanics uses laws of physics and engineering concepts to describe motion undergone by the various body part segments and the forces acting on these body parts during normal daily activities" (Frankel and Nordin 1980, p. ix). This chapter provides only a brief overview of the field of biomechanics. Many texts offer methods for multidimensional and dynamic analysis that are not discussed here.

Two areas of biomechanics exist: statics and dynamics. Statics is the study of a body at rest or equilibrium. Dynamics is the study of moving bodies. Dynamics involves kinematics, which examines the relationship between displacement, velocity, and acceleration in transitional or rotational motion, and kinetics, which involves moving bodies and the forces on them that produce motion (LeVeau 1992).

Anatomy

An understanding of the composition and function of the tissues involved in body mechanics is important in biomechanics. The following sections provide a review of tissues and structures.

Bone

The important mechanical properties of bone in biomechanics are strength and stiffness. Loading the bone causes temporary deformation unless the load is excessive and goes beyond the elastic stage into the plastic phase, which leads to failure. Bone is subjected to many types of loading, including tension, compression, bending, shear, torsion, or any combination of forces.

Tension occurs when equal and opposite forces are applied inward from the surface of the structure. The structure lengthens and narrows as tension is applied. Compression force exists when equal and opposite loads are applied toward the surface of the structure. In this case, the structure shortens and widens. Shear force is applied parallel to the structure and deforms the structure in an angular manner. Bending is a combination of tension and compression. The loads are applied to cause the structure to bend around an axis. Therefore, tension occurs on the convex side and compression on the concave side of the structure. Torsion occurs when the forces applied cause the structure to twist around an axis. Living bone seldom experiences a load in only one mode; it is most often subjected to a combination of these loads (Nordin and Frankel 1989). When a structure has been injured and is healing, the maximum loads the structure can withstand may be altered. The therapist may need to modify a task or progressively increase the intensity of a task to match the ability of the structure to withstand the load.

Tendons and Ligaments

Tendons transmit tensile loads from muscle to bone, causing joint movement. Ligaments provide stability; they guide motion and prevent excessive motion. According to physiologic studies (Nordin and Frankel 1989), in normal conditions, these structures are subjected to a stress magnitude of only one-third of the maximum stress they can withstand. If the maximum stress value of a structure is exceeded, complete, rapid failure occurs with loss of load-bearing ability. In normal circumstances, these structures undergo deformation and recovery. Residual strain occurs when a tendon or ligament is subjected to repeated stretch with insufficient recovery time (Chaffin 1984). The tendon or ligament may elongate 1–2% of its noload length. This leads to weakening, inflammation, and decreased function. Could residual strain be responsible for many of the lumbosacral strain injuries seen in clinics? Perhaps the client's hamstring, paraspinal, or hip flexor muscles were too short to allow sufficient motion for the bending task. If the muscles had sufficient length, could the individual perform that repetitive task without injury? Additional research is needed in this area.

Skeletal Muscle

Muscles provide strength and protection to the skeleton by distributing loads and absorbing shock. They perform both static (to maintain posture)

TABLE 4.1
Mathematical Relationships

Space: length is measured in meters, area in square meters, and volume in liters
Time: measured in seconds
Matter: that which occupies space
Mass: the quantity of an object; measured in kilograms
Vector: a line that has quantity and direction; it indicates displacement
Displacement: indicates the difference between the initial position and the ending position
Acceleration: the final velocity minus the initial velocity divided by time: $\dfrac{V_f - V_i}{t}$
Weight: measured in newtons and equal to mass multiplied by gravity: $W = (m)(a)$
Force: that which causes movement; force is measured in newtons and can be compressive (directed toward the surface), tensile (directed away from the surface), or shear or tangential (directed parallel to the surface)
Stress: found within the material the forces are acting on; measured in newtons per meter squared (N/m^2) and determined by multiplying the force by the specific quantity of the tissue
Friction: determined by the normal force multiplied by the coefficient of friction for a particular material
Lifting work: defined as weight (mass × gravity) multiplied by height multiplied by number of repetitions: $Lw = (m)(a)(h)(r)$
Gravity: a constant defined as the rate of acceleration in proportion to the square root of the distance traveled; the earth's gravity equals 9.8 m/sec^2 (for the purposes of this chapter, it is rounded to 10 m/sec^2)

Source: Reprinted from SL Roberts, SA Falkenburg. Biomechanics: Problem Solving for Functional Activity. St. Louis: Mosby–Year Book, 1992.

and dynamic (for locomotion and positioning) work. The maximum amount of contractile tension is achieved when the muscle is halfway between its shortest and longest lengths. This position is called the *resting length*. The ability of the muscle to produce contractile tension decreases as the muscle shortens or lengthens beyond the resting length. In a concentric contraction, the greater the external load, the slower the velocity of movement will be. When the external load reaches the maximum force that a muscle can exert, the velocity becomes zero; this is called an *isometric contraction*, and the muscle is in biomechanical equilibrium. When the external load exceeds the maximum muscular force, the contraction is eccentric; the greater the external load, the faster the velocity of movement will be. In the force-velocity relationship, the slower the muscle contracts, the greater the internal muscular tension, and the faster the muscle contracts, the less the internal muscular tension (Nordin and Frankel 1989) (Table 4.1).

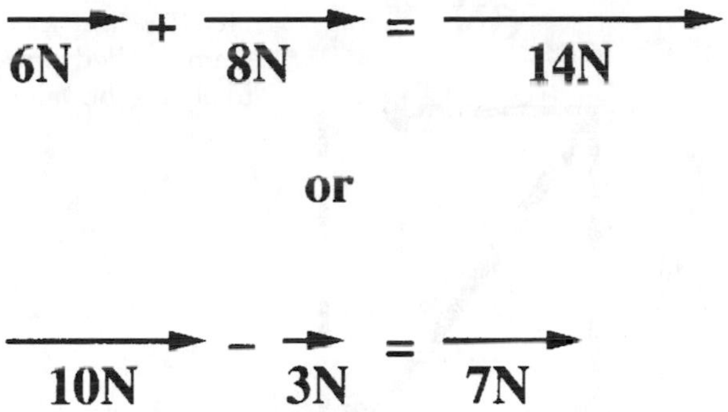

FIGURE 4.1. Linear vec-
tors. Simple mathematics is
used to obtain the value of
the resultant vector.

$$\overrightarrow{\text{6N}} + \overrightarrow{\text{8N}} = \overrightarrow{\text{14N}}$$

or

$$\overrightarrow{\text{10N}} - \overrightarrow{\text{3N}} = \overrightarrow{\text{7N}}$$

Principles of Physics

Vectors

Linear vectors lie in the same line of application as one another. Added together, these vectors equal a single vector called the *resultant vector* (Figure 4.1).

Concurrent vectors are two vectors that act on the same body part in different directions. Two-dimensional models are used to examine them. Concurrent vectors can be resolved by the parallelogram method or by mathematics into the resultant vector (Figure 4.2).

The parallelogram method involves drawing the concurrent vectors, represented by 3 N and 4 N in Figure 4.2, that originate from the same point. Lines are then drawn parallel to the concurrent vectors, starting at the end points of the vectors, illustrated by the dashed lines in Figure 4.2. The resultant vector (C) is drawn from the original starting point and ends at the intersection of the two lines that were drawn parallel to the concurrent vectors. The value of C in newtons is its length in the drawing.

The Pythagorean theorem is used to calculate the length of the resultant vector C. The theorem states that in a right triangle the sum of the squared sides equals the hypotenuse squared:

$$a^2 + b^2 = c^2$$

In Figure 4.2,

$$3^2 + 4^2 = c^2$$
$$9 + 16 = c^2$$
$$25 = c^2$$
$$\sqrt{25} = c^2$$
$$5 - c$$

The value of vector C is 5 N.

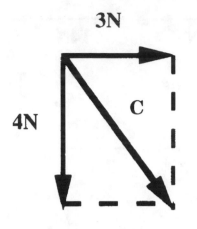

FIGURE 4.2. Concurrent vectors. The parallelogram method or the Pythagorean theorem is used to obtain the value of the resultant vector, C.

Circular Relationships

Circular relationships occur when movement takes place around a fixed axis such as a joint. The force that travels around the axis is called the *moment*. The distance from the axis to a location perpendicular to the point of application of the force is called the *moment arm*. An example of a circular relationship is that between the elbow joint and a force at the middle of the forearm (Figure 4.3).

The length of the moment arm at the range of motion depicted in Figure 4.3 is represented by d. The length of the moment arm changes from instant to instant throughout the range of motion. The length of d is longest

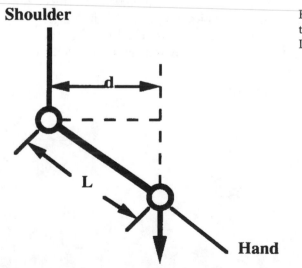

FIGURE 4.3. Circular relationship. (d = moment arm; L = lever arm.)

when the elbow is at 90 degrees of flexion and shortest when the elbow is in full extension.

In Figure 4.3, L represents the lever arm, which is the distance along a body part from the axis to the point of application of the force. L remains constant throughout the range of motion. The lever is the rigid body that moves around an axis. In the example, the lever arm is the bones of the forearm.

Equilibrium occurs when forces in one direction equal forces in the opposite direction. Figure 4.4 shows a seesaw arrangement. The goal is to keep the seesaw level, in equilibrium; the sum of the forces equals zero $(\Sigma F = 0)$.

In this problem, the force (X) required to keep the seesaw from moving must be calculated. The forces to the left of the fulcrum equal the force (5 N) multiplied by the lever arm (10 m).

Therefore,

$$F = (5\,N) \times (10\,m)$$

The forces to the right of the fulcrum equal the force (X) multiplied by the length of the lever arm (5 m), so

$$F = (X) \times (5\,m)$$
$$(5\,N)(10\,M) - (X\,N)(5\,m) = 0$$
$$(5\,N)(10\,M) = (X\,N)(5\,m)$$
$$50\,Nm = 5X\,Nm$$
$$\frac{50\,Nm}{5m} = X\,N$$
$$10 = X$$

The force required by X to keep this seesaw from tipping is 10 N.

Figure 4.4 shows an example of a first-class lever, in which the axis lies between the two forces. An example in the human body is the triceps brachii muscle. A second-class lever is that in which the resistance is

FIGURE 4.4.   A state of equilibrium. The forces on each side of the fulcrum are equal.

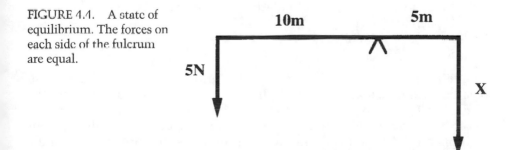

between the effort force and the axis. An example of such a lever is a wheel-barrow or the gastrocnemius and soleus muscles when a person raises him- or herself up onto his or her toes while standing. A third-class lever is that in which the effort force is located between the axis and the resistance. An example of this type of lever is the biceps brachii muscle and most of the musculoskeletal levers. The best mechanical advantage exists when the effort arm, the distance from the axis to the effort, is longer than the resistance arm, the distance from the axis to the resistance. This condition exists in a second-class lever. Because most levers in the human body are third-class levers, the body is not efficient and requires muscular effort several times greater than the weight of the object lifted. Therapists advise clients to keep the load close to the body to reduce the length of the resistance arm. Tools and properly arranged workstations can minimize the effects of the body's third-class levers (Yates and Lindberg 1970).

In addition to levers, two other musculoskeletal arrangements provide movement. The first is similar to a wheel-and-axle arrangement. An example in the human body is medial rotation of the humerus around the longitudinal axis of the humerus. The other type is a pulley arrangement, an example of which is the pulling of the patella between the condyles of the femur during knee extension (White and Panjabi 1990).

Center of Gravity

The center of gravity of an object is defined as the point within the body where the total mass of the body is concentrated. If a body rests on its center of gravity, it is in equilibrium (White and Panjabi 1990). The center of gravity of a human body resting in an erect posture is just anterior to the first sacral vertebra. That location is approximately at the level of 55% of the height of a person. Therapists are taught that increasing the base of support increases the stability of clients. The goal is to lower the center of gravity and to keep it positioned over the base of support. When the center of gravity falls outside the base of support, equilibrium is lost. The center of gravity does not always remain within the body. In a quadruped stance, the center of gravity falls outside the body just anterior to the pelvic region, but because the center of gravity is within the base of support, this is a stable stance (Rasch and Burke 1978). Each body segment has a center of gravity, and its location is used when calculating the forces acting on that body segment (Appendix 4.1).

Torque

Torque is the amount of force required to produce a rotation around an axis. It is expressed as mass multiplied by acceleration multiplied by the moment arm [F = (m)(a)(moment arm)]. The units for torque are newton-meters or foot-pounds. External torque is the weight of the body segment multiplied by the moment arm. Internal torque is that produced around a joint by muscles, tendons, and other soft tissues. Internal torque is equal to the force of the muscular contraction multiplied by the moment arm. The values of both external and internal torque change throughout the range of motion because of the change in the length of the moment arm.

Biomechanical Relationships

Trunk

Back pain has three causes: (1) abnormal strain on a normal back; (2) normal stress on an abnormal back; and (3) normal stress on a normal back unprepared for stress. Abnormal strain on a normal back becomes painful during a prolonged lift. Muscle fatigue puts stress on the ligaments, which eventually fail, forcing the joints to take the load. Pain arises from muscular ischemia, excessive strain on the ligaments, or capsular stretch. Normal strain on an abnormal back occurs when a structural abnormality exists, such as scoliosis, tight hamstrings, or tight or weak lumbar spinal muscles. These conditions cause a shift in the center of gravity and therefore a reduction in the efficiency of the lift. Normal stress on an unprepared back occurs with improper anticipation of the weight of a load to be lifted or with a fatigued back, both of which cause improper positioning (Caillet 1988).

The biomechanical functional unit of the trunk is the vertebral column. It provides the framework on which the body and the extremities move. From cervical to lumbar regions, the structures become larger, and the direction of the articular surfaces changes. The parts of the vertebrae are as follows: The body is the main load bearing section; the pedicles form the neural arch; the four facets on each vertebra have different orientations and direct the movement at that level; and the spinous and transverse processes provide muscle attachments (White and Panjabi 1990). Eighty-five percent to 95% of all disc herniations occur at L4-5 and L5-S1 in equal frequency. In the next problem, the L5-S1 disc represents lumbar stress during lifting because it incurs the largest moment during lifting owing to the long moment arm relative to a load in the hands (Chaffin and Anderson 1984).

Figure 4.5 shows the solution to a basic lifting problem. A person is holding a box that weighs 15 kg. The center of gravity of the box is 0.2 m ventral to the center of motion of the L5-S1 disc. The force of the weight of the upper body passes 0.02 m dorsal to the transverse axis of motion of the L5-S1 disc. First, determine the weight of the upper body. The head, neck, trunk, and arms are approximately 68.8% of the total body weight (Dempster 1955) or 66.1% of the total body weight (Roberts and Falkenberg 1992). See Appendix 4.2 for proportional percentages of body segments to total body weight. The weight of the upper body in this example is 40 kg.

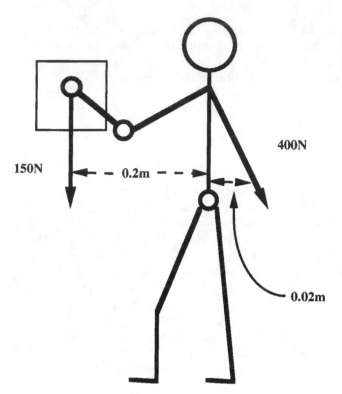

FIGURE 4.5.   Lifting. The box weighs 15 kg. Its center of gravity is 0.2 m ventral to L5-S1 disc. Upper body weighs 40 kg and passes 0.02 m dorsal to L5-S1 disc.

The amount of force (F) the erector spinae muscles must exert if the moment arm is 0.04 m must be determined.

The therapist first calculates the forces exerted by the box and upper body by multiplying mass by acceleration (F = [m][a]). Acceleration in this example is equal to the force of gravity (10 m/s^2) because the person is stationary. The force exerted by the box equals 15 kg × 10 m/s^2 = 150 N. The force exerted by the upper body equals 40 kg × 10 m/s^2 = 400 N. The sum of the forces must equal zero to maintain the lift. The sum of the forces is found by multiplying the force by the length of the moment arm:

$$(150\,\text{M} \times 0.2\,\text{m}) - (400\,\text{N} \times 0.02\,\text{m}) - (\text{F} \times 0.04\,\text{m}) = 0$$
$$(150\,\text{N} \times 0.2\,\text{m}) - (400\,\text{N} \times 0.02\,\text{m}) = \text{F} \times 0.04\,\text{m}$$
$$\frac{30\,\text{Nm} - 8\,\text{Nm}}{0.04\,\text{m}} = \text{F}$$
$$550\,\text{N} = \text{F}$$

Therefore, the erector spinae muscles must exert a force of 550 N to maintain this lift. If the box were held farther from the body, the moment arm for the box would be larger, and the force exerted by the erector spinae muscles would be greater. This is why clients are taught to keep the load close during a lift or carry. The goal is to keep the moment arm as short as possible and therefore the muscular effort as small as possible. The formula $\Sigma F = 0$ is used again to calculate the reaction force on the L5-S1 disc. The forces of gravity of the box, upper body, and erector spinae muscles all pull downward; the reaction force on the L5-S1 disc must be upward of equal magnitude. The reaction force on the disc is represented by D, as follows:

$$0 = D - 150\,N - 400\,N - 550\,N$$
$$D = 150\,N + 400\,N + 550\,N$$
$$D = 1,100\,N$$

The reaction force on the L5-S1 disc equals 1,100 N.

Controversy exists regarding the proper lifting technique. Research by Wiktorin and Nordin (1986) demonstrated that compressive forces on the disc do not lead to rupture, and the authors advocated the squat and lift technique. Other research indicates that when an object is too large to straddle, stooping over the object to lift it produces less compressive force than the squat and lift technique. However, the shear forces are greater in the stooped posture, so maintaining an erect torso is preferred. Unfortunately, the best lordotic posture has not yet been determined and requires more research (Chaffin and Anderson 1984).

Upper Extremity

Five functional units reside in the upper extremity: (1) the shoulder girdle, (2) the shoulder joint, (3) the elbow, (4) the radioulnar joint, and (5) the wrist and hand. These units are designed for either stability or mobility.

Shoulder Girdle

The shoulder girdle complex is designed for mobility. It consists of the clavicle and the scapula and their articulations. The sternoclavicular joint has little stability. It is the site of the most movement and acts as an axis for rotation of the shoulder girdle. It also absorbs lateral shock. The acromioclavicular joint is weak and absorbs the stress of impacts on the shoulder. The muscles of the shoulder girdle provide stability because the bony and ligamentous arrangements are weak. A lack of upper body strength is a factor in a number of injuries (White and Panjabi 1990).

Shoulder Joint

The shoulder joint consists of the glenoid fossa and the head of the humerus. It is a multiaxial joint designed for mobility; at any given time less than one-half of the head of the humerus is in the socket. The rotator cuff muscles and the labrum offer stability.

The muscles that cross the shoulder joint provide a range of movement. The infraspinatus and teres minor muscles insert on the posterior aspect of the humerus. They are arranged in a wheel-and-axle mechanism to cause lateral rotation of the humerus around a longitudinal axis. The subscapularis muscle inserts on the anterior aspect of the head of the humerus. It also functions in a wheel-and-axle manner, causing medial rotation of the humerus around a longitudinal axis. The supraspinatus muscle inserts on the distal aspect of the head of the humerus above the anterior posterior axis of rotation of the shoulder joint. It is a first-class lever mechanism that pulls the head of the humerus medially to allow for abduction of the humerus. The latissimus dorsi and teres major muscles originate on the posterior trunk and insert on the anterior aspect of the humerus. They are arranged in a wheel-and-axle formation to cause medial rotation and extension of the humerus (White and Panjabi 1990).

Elbow Joint

The elbow joint consists of the distal end of the humerus, the proximal end of the ulna, and the proximal end of the radius. The humeral-ulnar arrangement is designed for stability, but the humeral-radial joint is weak. Continual excessive stress at the humeral-radioulnar area is common and leads to injury.

The main elbow flexors are the biceps, brachialis, and brachioradialis muscles. Elbow extension is achieved by the action of the triceps brachii muscle. The other muscles act as stabilizers because their lines of force pass so closely to the elbow joint that they generate only small rotary torques (White and Panjabi 1990).

Radioulnar Joint

The radioulnar joint consists of proximal, distal, and middle joints. It lacks bony stability, so the ligaments provide stability. The movements are supination and pronation around a longitudinal axis. The biceps brachii muscle has a wheel-and-axle arrangement that causes supination. The supinator muscle provides stability and assists in supination. The pronator teres and pronator quadratus muscles provide stability in adduction to cause pronation (White and Panjabi 1990).

The muscular effort required by the biceps muscle to maintain different angles of the elbow joint is calculated in the following example. A person has a 1-kg weight around the wrist. The length of the forearm is 0.3 m. The center of gravity of the forearm is 0.172 m below the elbow joint. (See Appendix 4.1 for the center of gravity locations for each body segment.) The arm weighs 1.58 kg. First, the value of the muscular effort required with the forearm at a 90-degree angle relative to the upper arm should be calculated. The values used for center of gravity and arm weight are for the average man based on anthropometric measurements (Figure 4.6).

The force exerted by the forearm itself is calculated with the formula $F = (m)(a)$: $F = (1.58 \text{ kg}) \times (10 \text{ m/s})$. Therefore, $F = 15.8 \text{ N}$. The force exerted by the weight at the wrist is $F = (1 \text{ kg}) \times (10 \text{ m/s}) = 10 \text{ N}$. The formula $\Sigma F = 0$

FIGURE 4.6. Elbow 90 degrees, 1-kg weight at the wrist.

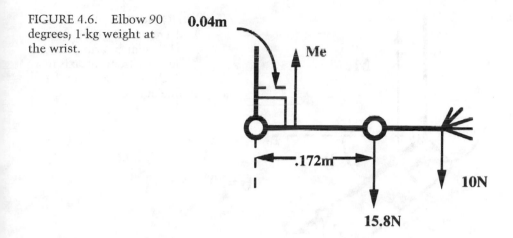

is used to calculate the muscular effort (Me) required by the biceps to keep the forearm at a 90-degree angle:

$$0 = (Me \times 0.04\,m) - (0.172\,m \times 15.8\,N) - (0.3\,m \times 10\,N)$$
$$(Me \times 0.04\,m) = (0.172m \times 15.8N) + (0.3m \times 10N)$$
$$Me = \frac{[(0.172m \times 15.8N) + (0.3m \times 10N)]}{0.04m}$$
$$Me = 142.9\,N$$

The biceps exerts a force of 142.9 N in an upward direction to maintain this position.

The muscular effort required with the forearm 30 degrees below horizontal is diagrammed in Figure 4.7. All other values remain unchanged.

To calculate the length of the moment arm, one uses the formula cos 30 degrees = X/0.04. (Table A4.1 provides trigonometric functions; see Appendix 4.3 to determine the proper trigonometric function.)

$$X = 0.8660 \times 0.04$$
$$X = 0.035\,m$$

The sum of the forces is zero, this time using the new value for the length of the moment arm:

$$0 = (Me \times 0.035) - (0.172 \times 15.8) - (0.3 \times 10)$$
$$Me \times 0.035 = (0.172 \times 15.8) + (0.3 \times 10)$$
$$Me = \frac{[(0.172 \times 15.8) + (0.3 \times 10)]}{0.035}$$
$$Me = 163.36\,N$$

The biceps must exert an upward force of 163.36 N to maintain the forearm 30 degrees below horizontal. This example demonstrates how the muscular

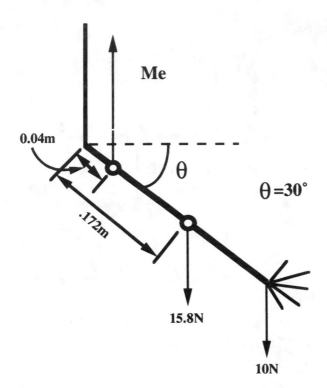

FIGURE 4.7.   Elbow 30 degrees below horizontal. The moment arm is the distance from the axis to a line perpendicular to the line of force.

effort changes with the range of motion. The shorter the moment arm, as in Figure 4.7, the greater the muscular effort required to lift the same load. This is why carrying a heavy load at waist level is possible, whereas placing the same load on a shelf higher than the waist is difficult or even impossible.

Wrist joint

The wrist joint consists of the distal ends of the radius and ulna and the carpal bones. The movements are flexion, extension, radial deviation, and ulnar deviation. The bony arrangements lack stability, so stability is provided by the ligaments and the tendons (White and Panjabi 1990).

Hand

Problems can arise in the workplace if the wrong type of grip is used. A great difference exists between the forces required by the flexor digitorum profundus muscles in partial-hand grip and in whole-hand grip. The forces required by the flexor digitorum profundus muscle to maintain the grip are calculated in the following example: The object grasped is 0.085 m in diameter, and maintaining the grip requires 3 kg of pressure. In both types of grasp, the thumb is abducted to 70 degrees. In the partial-hand grip, the force is applied at an 80-degree angle to the tendon, and contact is made at the distal pha-

FIGURE 4.8.   Whole-
hand grip. Most of hand
is in contact with object.

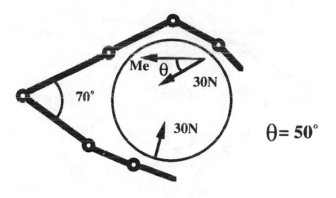

$\theta = 50°$

langes. In the whole-hand grip, the force is applied at a 50-degree angle. The
tendons are 0.005 m from the axis of motion of the finger joints.

The formula used to calculate the muscular effort required is as follows (Figure 4.8; see Table A4.1):

$$\cos 50 \text{ degrees} = \frac{30 \text{ N}}{Me}$$

$$Me = \frac{30 \text{ N}}{\cos 50 \text{ degrees}}$$

$$Me = \frac{30}{0.6428}$$

$$Me = 46.7 \text{ N}$$

In the whole-hand grip, a force of 46.7 N is required to grasp this object.

The same formula is used to calculate the muscular effort in partial-
hand grip (Figure 4.9; see Table A4.1):

$$\cos 80 \text{ degrees} = \frac{30 \text{ N}}{Me}$$

$$Me = \frac{30 \text{ N}}{\cos 80 \text{ degrees}}$$

$$Me = \frac{30}{0.1736}$$

$$Me = 172.8 \text{ N}$$

A partial-hand grip requires a force of 172.8 N instead of the 46.7 N required
by a whole-hand grip. Therefore, using the partial-hand grip requires almost
four times the force required when using a whole-hand grip. This is important in the evaluation of factors that contribute to carpal tunnel problems
(Roberts and Falkenburg 1992).

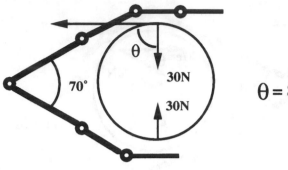

FIGURE 4.9.   Partial-hand grip. Contact is at thumb and distal phalanges.

$\theta = 80°$

Discussion

Therapists should not apply biomechanics principles in isolation. A therapist should use caution and common sense when using biomechanics in the design of workstations. Discussion has taken place among health professionals about the effects of minimizing the amount of movement and force a client should exert. The concern is that applying the stresses in such limited motions, although deemed optimal, ignores the fact that the body was designed for movement. A workstation or rotating work schedules on assembly lines that involve a variety of movements and postures may be most advisable.

Conclusion

Biomechanics describes the actions of the human body. Study of biomechanics led to design criteria for seating for aircraft pilots and office workers; the establishment of permissible control forces and locations in aircraft and the cabs of industrial cranes and in turning lathes and other machines; limits for loads to be lifted and carried in various postures; and design guides for hand tools (Shackel 1976). The human body has limits, and guidelines should be followed. Guidelines can be obtained from the National Institute for Occupational Safety and Health.

Compared to the breadth of information available and the research being conducted, this chapter is a brief discussion of biomechanics. The examples in this chapter are for illustrative purposes only and do not necessarily reflect actual situations. The information is meant to expose therapists to the field of biomechanics to enhance their knowledge of person-machine interactions and to aid them in designing rehabilitation programs. To make computations for a specific client, the therapist should consult a book that focuses on problem-solving methods.

Acknowledgments

I give special thanks to my husband, David, for his support and understanding; and to my children, Stephanie and Timothy, for their love and patience.

References

Caillet R (1988). Low Back Pain Syndrome. Philadelphia: Davis.

Chaffin DB, Anderson G (1984). Occupational Biomechanics. New York: Wiley.

Dempster WT (1955). Space Requirements of the Seated Operator. WADCTR 55-159. Wright-Patterson Air Force Base, OH: Acrospace Medical Research Laboratory.

Frankel VH, Nordin M (1980). Basic Biomechanics of the Skeletal System. Philadelphia: Lea & Febiger.

Grandjean E (1988). Fitting the Task to the Man: A Textbook of Occupational Biomechanics. London: Taylor & Francis.

LeVeau BF (1992). Williams and Lissner's Biomechanics of Human Motion (3rd ed). Philadelphia: Saunders.

Nordin M, Frankel VH (1989). Basic Biomechanics of the Musculoskeletal Systems. Philadelphia: Lea & Febiger.

Rasch PJ, Burke RK (1978). Kinesiology and Applied Anatomy. Philadelphia: Lea & Febiger.

Roberts SL, Falkenburg SA (1992). Biomechanics: Problem Solving for Functional Activity. St. Louis: Mosby–Year Book.

Shackel B (1976). Applied Ergonomics Handbook. Vol. 3. Guilford, UK: IPC.

White AA III, Panjabi MM (1990). Clinical Biomechanics of the Spine. Philadelphia: Lippincott.

Wiktorin CH, Nordin M (1986). Introduction to Problem Solving in Biomechanics. Philadelphia: Lea & Febiger.

Yates JA, Lundberg AC (1970). Moving and Lifting Patients: Principles and Techniques. Minneapolis: Sister Kenny Institute.

Suggested Reading

Fritjof C (1984). The Tao of Physics. New York: Bantam.

Fung YC (1990). Biomechanics—Motion, Flow, Stress and Growth. New York: Springer-Verlag.

Fung YCB (1967). Elasticity of soft tissues in simple elongation. Am J Physiol 213: 1532–1544.

Hall SJ (1991). Basic Biomechanics. St. Louis: Mosby–Year Book.

Holder LI (1984). College Algebra and Trigonometry (3rd ed). Belmont, CA: Wadsworth.

Review Questions

(Answers are found in Appendix D.)

1. What is a vector?
   (a) An arrow
   (b) A line that indicates quantity and direction
   (c) A parallelogram

2. What is equilibrium?
   (a) A condition occurring when the sum of the forces equals zero
   (b) The midpoint
   (c) A concentric contraction

3. What is the most common class of levers in the human body?
   (a) First class
   (b) Second class
   (c) Third class

4. When do you have the best mechanical advantage?
   (a) When the effort arm is longer than the resistance arm
   (b) When the resistance arm is equal to the effort arm
   (c) When the resistance arm is longer than the effort arm

5. When is the least amount of muscular effort required in a lift?
   (a) When the moment arm is shortest
   (b) When the moment arm is longest
   (c) When the moment arm is zero

Appendix 4.1

TABLE A4.1
Trigonometric Functions

Degrees	Sines	Cosines	Tangents	Cotangents	
0	.0000	1.0000	.0000		90
1	.0175	.9998	.0175	57.290	89
2	.0349	.9994	.0349	28.636	88
3	.0523	.9986	.0524	19.081	87
4	.0698	.9976	.0699	14.301	86
5	.0872	.9962	.0875	11.430	85
6	.1045	.9945	.1051	9.5144	84
7	.1219	.9925	.1228	8.1443	83
8	.1392	.9903	.1405	7.1154	82
9	.1564	.9877	.1584	6.3138	81
10	.1736	.9848	.1763	5.6713	80
11	.1908	.9816	.1944	5.1446	79
12	.2079	.9781	.2126	4.7046	78
13	.2250	.9744	.2309	4.3315	77
14	.2419	.9703	.2493	4.0108	76
15	.2588	.9659	.2679	3.7321	75
16	.2756	.9613	.2867	3.4874	74
17	.2924	.9563	.3057	3.2709	73
18	.3090	.9511	.3249	3.0777	72
19	.3256	.9455	.3443	2.9042	71
20	.3420	.9397	.3640	2.7475	70
21	.3584	.9336	.3839	2.6051	69
22	.3746	.9272	.4040	2.4751	68
23	.3907	.9205	.4245	2.3559	67
24	.4067	.9135	.4452	2.2460	66
25	.4226	.9063	.4663	2.1445	65
26	.4384	.8988	.4877	2.0503	64
27	.4540	.8910	.5095	1.9626	63
28	.4695	.8829	.5317	1.8807	62
29	.4848	.8746	.5543	1.8040	61
30	.5000	.8660	.5774	1.7321	60
31	.5150	.8572	.6009	1.6643	59
32	.5299	.8480	.6249	1.6003	58
33	.5446	.8387	.6494	1.5399	57
34	.5592	.8290	.6745	1.4826	56
35	.5736	.8192	.7002	1.4281	55
36	.5878	.8090	.7265	1.3765	54
37	.6018	.7986	.7536	1.3270	53
38	.6157	.7880	.7813	1.2799	52
39	.6293	.7771	.8098	1.2349	51
	Cosines	Sines	Cotangents	Tangents	Degrees

TABLE A4.1
Continued

Degrees	Sines	Cosines	Tangents	Cotangents	
40	.6428	.7660	.8391	1.1918	50
41	.6561	.7547	.8693	1.1504	49
42	.6691	.7431	.9004	1.1106	48
43	.6820	.7314	.9325	1.0724	47
44	.6947	.7193	.9657	1.0355	46
45	.7071	.7071	1.0000	1.0000	45
	Cosines	Sines	Cotangents	Tangents	Degrees

Degrees: For angles above 45 degrees, be sure to see the headings that appear at the bottom of the columns.

Source: Reprinted with permission from SL Roberts, SA Falkenburg. Biomechanics: Problem Solving for Functional Activity. St. Louis: Mosby–Year Book, 1992.

Appendix 4.2

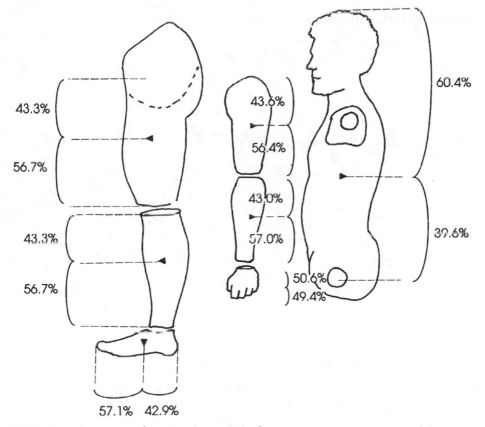

FIGURE A4.1. Center of gravity for each body segment as a percentage of distance from the end of the body segment. (Reprinted with permission from SL Roberts, SA Falkenburg. Biomechanics: Problem Solving for Functional Activity. St. Louis: Mosby–Year Book, 1992.)

Appendix 4.3*

Trigonometric Functions

For a right triangle:

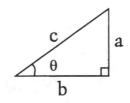

$$Sin = \frac{a}{c} \qquad\qquad CSC = \frac{c}{a}$$

$$COS = \frac{b}{c} \qquad\qquad SEC = \frac{c}{b}$$

$$tan = \frac{a}{b} \qquad\qquad cot = \frac{b}{a}$$

Supplementary Angles

A line intersected by another line forms two angles, which when added together equal 180 degrees. Therefore, A + B = 180 degrees:

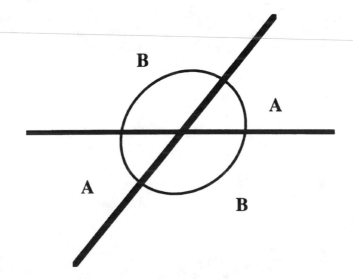

*Source: LI Holder. College Algebra and Trigonometry (3rd ed). Belmont, CA: Wadsworth, 1984.

Alternate Angles

When two parallel lines are intersected by a third line, the angles on opposite sides of the intersecting lines are equal. Therefore, angles A are equal, and angles B are equal:

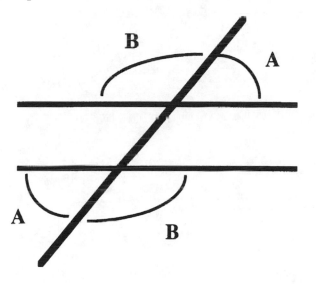

Pythagorean Theorem

In a right triangle, the sum of the squared sides equals the hypotenuse squared:

$$a^2 + b^2 = c^2$$

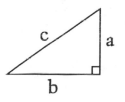

CHAPTER 5
Cognitive Workload and the Organization of Mental Space

A. James Giannini and Juliette N. Giannini

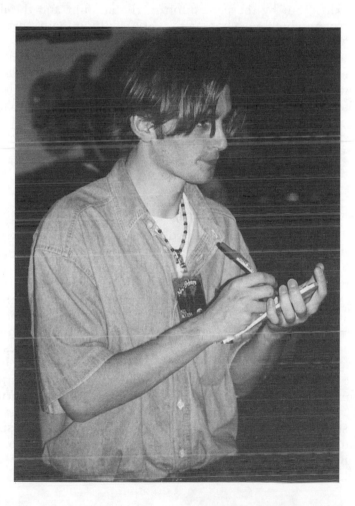

ABSTRACT

Worker efficiency declines when the worker believes that the workload exceeds his or her abilities. Cognitive workload has been studied
since the Middle Ages. Many approaches to reducing the workload
use the model of mental space. A number of variables, including
inherited abilities, environmental factors, personality type, and status level, determine the parameters of this space. By modifying the
worker's mental space, the occupational therapist can produce a comfortable fit for the worker and the job.

Cognitive workload is a subjective term operantly defined as a worker's
perception of work performance and work difficulty. It is measured not by
actual workload but by the perception of the amount and the difficulty.
The intensity at which one chooses to work is a function of this cognitive
workload (Gamberale 1988).

In evaluating a worker and his or her job, the therapist evaluates not
merely the physical or intellectual performance. The worker's subjective
perception of the workload must be integrated into any job analysis
because the individual's perception of work tolerance may not correspond
with the capacity of work measured (Fiori 1991; Luczah 1991). The mental
space may be overcrowded or chaotic and in need of organization (Giannini
et al. 1997).

History

The first studies of cognitive workload were developed by Medieval guilds
and Medieval and Renaissance universities for apprentices to improve performance and decrease subsequent job-related stress. In the guilds, nonliter-
ate masters used diagrams, models, and symbols to reduce the trepidation
associated with task performance in high-status jobs such as cathedral and
castle building (Giannini 1993).

These techniques were later applied in nonsystematic fashion to university students and scholars by a variety of Medieval academics. In these
cases, irrational ordering methods were used. The most popular was the
peripatetic method. Concepts were taught while professors led students on
walks. During the lecture, each concept was linked to some feature of the
landscape. These features, such as trees or fountains, helped fix the concept in a student's mind. Other methods were also popular. Instrumental
music could be used to reduce internally perceived stress for laboring
scholars. Bible reading by professional readers reduced the sense of time

pressure for workers (Wright 1962). Another favorite technique was to present the work in pieces so that workers would not be overwhelmed by the enormity of their tasks. In such ways, the perception of work demand was diminished by reorganizing the worker's mental space.

These techniques were eventually subjected to critical analysis by the academician Marsilio Ficino (1433–1499), who modified and combined these in a comprehensive program. In the sixteenth century, Bartholomew Aneau (c. 1520–1584) limited these studies to visual tasks and thus ran the study of cognitive workload into an intellectual dead-end.

Twentieth-century researchers avoided this dead-end by placing these studies into biopsychophysiologic categories. Initial studies dealt with general psychophysiologic problems of subjective force and cognitive workload. Early results of this work suggested that subjective intensity increased with the perceived load (Hermansen and Saltin 1956; Winscott 1965).

Measurement

A variety of techniques have been developed to measure elements of cognitive workload. Somatic perception of the task can be measured by the Somatic Perception Questionnaire (Frankenhaeser et al. 1969). The extroversion-introversion and active-passive aspects of task perception are measured by the Minnesota Multiphasic Personality Inventory. Somatic distress can be measured by the Brief Psychiatric Rating Scale (Overall and Gorman 1962) and the Eysenck Personality Inventory (Eysenck 1962). Anxiety can be evaluated by the Speilberger State-Trait Inventory (Goldberg 1982), depression by the Beck Depression Inventory (Giannini 1987), and obsession by the Yale-Brown Scale (Goodman et al. 1989).

An attempt at a unified measurement of these elements was provided by the Subjective Workload Assessment Technique (SWAT). SWAT measures three dimensions of cognitive workload: (1) psychological loads, (2) mental loads, and (3) temporal loads (Reid and Nygren 1988). Each aspect of the cognitive workload is ranked. Statistical analyses of the time-effort-stress relationship determine the appropriateness of the initial ranking. Contradictions are eliminated and rank data modified to determine the best fitting scale (Reid and Nygren 1988). The second phase of this test is event scoring. After a task has been evaluated, the evaluator provides a subjective score for the perceived load experienced in each dimension. These event scores are then transmitted to the previous component scores of time, effort, and stress that are combined to provide an overall workload score.

The NASA Test Load Index is another multifactor scale. It is used to measure changes in operator levels of workload. This score is based on weighted averages of mental, physical, temporal, performance, effort, and frustration demands. Similar to the SWAT, the evaluation is based on a two-part procedure. After workers have completed a group of tasks, estimates of importance of the six dimensions are obtained. The six factors are presented to the worker with 15 paired comparisons. The worker then circles the member of each pair that he or she believes contributes more to the workload. The number of times each dimension is chosen in the pairs is then added and weighted. These weights are subsequently used to produce a ranking of the importance of each task. A continuous time scale is presented on six 20-point rating scales and then multiplied by a factor of 5 to produce a range from 0 to 100. These values are added to produce an overall workload estimate (Hart and Staveland 1988).

Cognitive Workload

Cognitive information must be received and integrated for the worker to perform useful work. For successful reception to occur, a sustained focus must be placed on the information to be processed (Pashler 1994). Distraction can be produced by material that is irrelevant or perceived to be irrelevant to the task. Received information is stored as memory traces (Carrier and Pashler 1996). Once stored, links can be integrated between the different traces (Massaro 1989).

Cognitive overload can be viewed as a worker's inability to receive and integrate excessive information (Giannini et al. 1995). Overload occurs when the total amount of work per time period exceeds the worker's self-perceived abilities. Researchers have reported that perceived job exertion correlates with overload (Frankenhaeser and Gardell 1976).

In an overload situation, useful work capacity declines. Frequently, the error rate increases as workers screen out excess or perceived excess information. Workers in this situation may suffer physical complaints such as migraine headaches, cluster headaches, hypercholesterolemia, gastric and peptic ulcers, and tachycardia (Giannini 1987). Psychopathologic symptoms such as anxiety, depression, and irritability can also be produced.

Cognitive overload can be heuristically diminished by increasing receptive and integrative capacity. This can be accomplished by splitting information into abstract and concrete modalities (Pisoni 1993). Reception can also be increased by dividing information into auditory and visual components (Crowder 1993). Task repetition provides a feedback system that can modify and enhance these capacities (Gabrieli et al. 1993).

Type A and Type B Personality Moderators

A positive-feedback loop can create a dysfunctional type A behavioral pattern (Giannini 1996). The type A worker displays a behavioral pattern that demonstrates a sense of urgency and striving (Friedman and Rosenman

1974). Workers with a high activity level have a weak negative relationship between perceived job demands and satisfaction. Type A workers can over-load their capacity by assuming progressively greater workloads (Hollander et al. 1997). Thus, type A workers with a high activity level are less likely than type B workers with a low activity level to report cognitive overload in demanding work situations. The relationship between workload and stress is greater, however, for workers with type A personalities than for those with type B behavior (Wickens 1984). A high cognitive workload may cause a type B worker to think that expectations will be impossible to meet, whereas the same workload would not discourage a type A worker, who would, nevertheless, experience greater stress than his or her type B counterpart (Giannini et al. 1978; Miller et al. 1977).

Organization of Mental Space

Job tasks place demands on cognitive workload. The worker's mental space is constantly altered by changes in incoming data. Consequently, the inter-nal space is subject to continuous alteration. As decisions are made, both the external environment and mental space are altered. The major inter-faces through which this continuous adjustment occurs are perception, integration, and action (Armstrong et al. 1984; Giannini et al. 1984).

Reception is the process by which information is collected through any combination of sensory inputs. In work environments, information is often transmitted through displays such as dials, gauges, light displays, monitors, and sirens. In conducting job analysis, the occupational therapist must assist the worker in using and coordinating senses to prevent sensory overload (Scalaithe et al. 1997) (Table 5.1).

In integrating information, workers interpret and organize perceived information and initiate plans. Processing is subject to a feedback loop of multiple variables, including emotional and cognitive states, personality type, intelligence level, abstracting ability, imagination, experience, educa-tion, training, sense of responsibility, and status.

TABLE 5.1
Major Senses

Auditory	Positioning
Depth perceptive	Pressure perceptive
Figure-ground perceptive	Proprioceptive
Gustatory	Stereognostic
Kinesthetic	Tactile
Left-right discriminating	Visual
Olfactory	Visual-spatial organizing

After information is received and integrated, action is initiated. Work is often done with tools. Efficient usage depends on coordination, laterality, endurance, fine- and gross-motor coordination, strength, and visual-motor integration. Information must be processed and then coordinated with the appropriate tools and elements of the worker's mental space (Winscott 1965; Giannini 1993).

The mental space of the worker is not a fixed medium, but its limits are determined by the interaction of intellectual and genetic endowment, learning, social status, and physical development. The occupational therapist can be called on to integrate the worker's limits to job tasks, whether the professional role is job analysis for a client undergoing work hardening or ergonomic analysis for a corporate group. This can be accomplished by modifying the work parameters to suit the worker or, more challengingly, by modifying and possibly expanding the limits of the worker (Sabelli and Carlson-Sabelli 1989).

In the latter, the occupational therapist acts on the mental space. The worker's experiences are more efficiently organized and then focused on the task. The worker is taught to eliminate, reduce, or ignore extraneous data. Task perception is shifted from a negative, overwhelmed state to one of recognition and familiarity. Information is then processed according to previously learned modalities. Action proceeds as mastery of an organized cognitive and motor behavioral pattern (Savell et al. 1986).

Conclusion

Cognitive workload should be considered in the design of ergonomically sound tasks. Careful observation and measurement are necessary to access actual and perceived workloads. Occupational therapists must create situations that reduce the actual workload or, if this is not possible, assist the worker in developing mental constructs that assist in the reception or integration of incoming information. Because occupational therapists use occupation as a tool for treatment, knowledge of cognitive workload can be applied to many therapeutic situations. Cognitive workload enhances the practice of occupational therapists, as therapy often deals with issues of cognition.

References

Armstrong T, Pannett B, Ketner P (1984). Subjective worker assessment of hand tools used in automobile assembly. Am Indust Hygiene Assoc J 50:639–645.

Crowder R (1993). Auditory Memory; Thinking in Sound. Oxford, UK: Oxford University Press.

Eysenck HJ (1962). Manual for the Eysenck Personality Inventory. San Diego: Education and Industrial Testing Service.

Fiori N, Richardson J, Boain M (1991). Operator workload and system performance under different conditions of force feedback in a telemanipulation task. Ergonomics 34:193–210.

Frankenhaeser M, Gardell B (1976). Underload and overload in working life: outline of multidisciplinary approach. J Hum Stress 2:35–46.

Frankenhaeser M, Norhedon B, Sjobert H (1969). Physiological and subjective reactions to different work loads. Percept Motor Skills 28:343–349.

Friedman M, Rosenman R (1974). Type A Behavior and Your Heart. New York: Knopf.

Gabrieli J, Milberg W, Keane M, Corkin S (1990). Intact primary patterns. Neuropsychologia 27:644–664.

Gallagher S (1991). Acceptable weights and physiological costs of performing combined manual handling task in restricted postures. Ergonomics 34:939–952.

Gamberale F (1988). Maximum acceptable workloads for repetitive lifting tasks: an experimental evaluation of psychophysical criteria. Presented at the Fourth Finnish–U.S. Joint Symposium on Occupational Safety and Health. Turka, Finland. July 7–14, 1988.

Giannini AJ, Daoud J, Giannini MC, et al. (1978). Intellect versus intuition—A dichotomy in the reception of nonverbal communication. J Gen Psychol 99:19–23.

Giannini AJ, Barringer ME, Giannini MC, Loiselle RH (1984). Lack of relationship between handedness and intuitive and intellectual (rationalistic) modes of information processing. J Gen Psychol 111:31–39.

Giannini AJ (1987). Biological Foundations of Clinical Psychiatry. New York: Elsevier.

Giannini AJ (1993). Tangential symbols. J Clin Pharmacol 33:1139–1146.

Giannini AJ, Giannini JN, Melemis SM (1997). Visual symbolization as a learning tool. J Clin Pharmacol, 37:559–565.

Giannini AJ (1996). Alexithymia, affective disorders, and substance abuse: possible cross-relationships Psychol Rep 78:1389–1392.

Gillet M, Morgan W (1977). Influence of acute work activity on state anxiety. J Psychosom 15:179–181.

Goldberg R (1982). Anxiety: Biobehavioral Diagnosis and Therapy. New Hyde Park, NY: Medical Examination Publishing.

Goodman WC, Price LK, Rasmussen SA (1989). The Yale-Brown Obsessive Compulsive Scale: use and reliability. Arch Gen Psychiatry 46:1006–1011.

Hart S, Staveland L (1988). Development of the NASA Task Load Index (TLX): Results of Empirical and Theoretical Research. In PA Hancock, N Meshkati (eds), Human Mental Workload. New York: Elsevier North Holland.

Hasher L, Zacks R (1988). Working Memory, Comprehension and Aging. In G Bower (ed), The Psychology of Learning and Motivation. New York: Academic Press, 112–113.

Hermansen L, Saltin B (1956). Oxygen uptake during maximal work activity. J Appl Physiol 26:31–37.

Hollander E, Kwon JM, Rowland C (1997). Psychosocial function and economic costs of obsessive-compulsive disorder. Int J Neuropsych Med 2(10):16–25.

Kuronski W (1991). Psychophysical acceptability and perception of load heaviness in females. Ergonomics 34:487–496.

Luczah H (1991). Work under extreme conditions. Ergonomics 34:687–720.

Massaro D (1989). Experimental Psychology: An Information Processing Approach. Orlando, FL: Harcourt-Brace-Jovanovich.

Miller RE, Giannini AJ, Levine JM (1977). Nonverbal communication in man with a cooperative conditioning task. J Soc Psychol 103:101–109.

Overall JE, Gorham DR (1962). The brief psychiatric rating scale. Psychological Rep 10:799–812.

Pashler H (1994). Overlapping mental operations in serial performance with preview. Q J Exp Psychol 47:161–191.

Pisoni DB (1993). Longterm memory in speech perception. Speech Commun 113: 109–125.

Reid G, Nygren T (1988). The Subjective Workload Assessment Technique: A Scaling Procedure for Measuring Mental Workload. In PA Hancock, N Meshkati (eds), Human Mental Workload. New York: Elsevier North Holland.

Sabelli HC, Carlson-Sabelli L (1989). Biological priority and psychological supremacy: a new integrative paradigm. Am J Psychiatry 146:1541–1551.

Sanders M, McCormick E (1987). Human Factors in Engineering and Design. New York: McGraw-Hill, 341–346.

Savell JM, Twohig RT, Ruchford DL (1986). Empirical status of instruction enrichment techniques. Rev Education Res 56:381–409.

Scalaithe PO, Wilson FAW, Rakic PS (1997). Areal segregation of face-processing neurons in prefrontal cortex. Science 278:1135–1137.

Tsang P, Johnson W (1989). Cognitive demands in automation. Aviat Space Environ Med 60:130–135.

Wickens C (1984). Engineering Psychology and Human Performance. Columbus, OH: Charles Merrill.

Winscott DW (1965). Maturational Processes and the Facilitating Environment. New York: International University Press.

Wright T (1986). A History of Domestic Manners and Sentiments in England during the Middle Ages. London: Oxford University Press.

Review Questions

(Answers are found in Appendix D.)

1. The two major elements of processing cognitive information are
   (a) reception
   (b) elaboration
   (c) integration
   (d) conceptualization

2. All of the following are rating instruments used in measuring cognitive
   workload except the
   (a) Brief Psychiatric Rating Scale
   (b) Minnesota Multiphasic Personality Inventory
   (c) Bender-Gestalt test
   (d) Beck Depression Inventory

3. Three of the elements of cognitive workload are
   (a) perception
   (b) encoding
   (c) action
   (d) processing

4. All of the following are physical symptoms of cognitive overload except
   (a) cluster headache
   (b) migraine
   (c) peptic ulcer
   (d) heart attack

5. An important early investigator in cognitive workload was
   (a) Marsilio Ficino
   (b) Leonardo da Vinci
   (c) Paolo Ucello
   (d) Francesco Guicciardini

CHAPTER 6
Psychosocial Factors in Work-Related Musculoskeletal Disorders

Asnat Bar-Haim Erez and Karen N. Lindgren

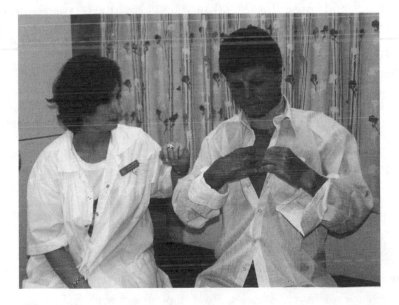

ABSTRACT

The relationship between psychosocial risk factors and work-related musculoskeletal disorders (WRMDs) is gaining attention from researchers and clinicians. This chapter defines psychosocial risk factors, including those proposed by the National Institute of Occupational Safety and Health (NIOSH) and the International Labor Office (ILO). This chaper reviews the research regarding the relationship of specific risk factors and WRMDs, along with methodologic problems. The chapter also discusses four pathways explaining this relationship, interventions for clinicians, and future directions of intervention.

Understanding the role of psychosocial risk factors is important in the intervention and prevention of disability. In 1986, NIOSH called for researchers to address the variety of risk factors thought to contribute to job stress and work-related disability in the work environment. Consequently, researchers began to study the relationship of psychosocial factors in disability. Evidence has verified the importance of the relationships between psychosocial stressors and psychological dysfunction and between psychosocial and musculoskeletal problems. In the Netherlands, these health problems (i.e., psychological dysfunction and musculoskeletal problems) are the main causes of disability in two-thirds of occupation-related disability cases (Houtman et al. 1994).

Evaluating psychosocial factors with physical and ergonomic factors is gaining support from researchers, which indicates that the use of a framework to treat WRMDs is becoming more prevalent (Sauter and Swanson 1996). Although WRMD is generally considered multifactorial, past research has focused on physical load. More recent research, however, has included an examination of the relationship between psychosocial factors and WRMD. Despite this research, no consensus has been reached regarding the definition of psychosocial factors and how such factors relate to WRMD (NIOSH 1997; Sauter and Swanson 1996).

Psychosocial Factors Defined

Several definitions of psychosocial factors have been proposed. Most definitions suggest that psychosocial factors depend on workers' perceptions, a point emphasized by Hagberg and colleagues (1995, p. 11): "Psychosocial factors at work describe how the work organization is perceived by workers and managers; work organization is the objective nature of the work process and it deals with the way in which work is structured and processed."

NIOSH (1997) defines *psychosocial factors* as a general term that identifies many variables, which can be roughly divided into three categories: (1) factors associated with the work environment, (2) factors associated with the extra-work environment, and (3) individual characteristics of the worker. Stress results from the interaction of factors from the three categories.

Risk factors associated with the work environment (or work organization) include (1) characteristics of the job (e.g., workload, job control, repetitiveness, mental demand), (2) organizational structure (e.g., communication issues), (3) interpersonal relationships at work (e.g., relationships with employer, supervisor, coworkers), (4) temporal aspects of work (e.g., shift work, cycle time), (5) financial and economic aspects (e.g., salary, benefits), and (6) community aspects of occupation (e.g., prestige, status). The second category of risk factors identified by NIOSH, extra-work environment, identifies factors that come from outside work. The third category describes individual worker characteristics, such as genetic factors (e.g., gender, intelligence), acquired aspects (e.g., social class, culture, educational factors), and disposition (e.g., personality, characteristic traits, attitudes toward life and work). Disposition often affects the way workers perceive or react to the same work situation (Hurrell and Murphy 1992).

In contrast to NIOSH, ILO (1986) and the World Health Organization, in a joint report, organized work-related psychosocial factors into five categories: (1) physical environment, (2) factors intrinsic to the job (e.g., work load, work design), (3) arrangement of work time (e.g., hours of work, shifts), (4) management or operating practices (e.g., roles of the worker, relationships at work), and (5) technological changes. This definition is similar to the NIOSH description but does not identify individual worker differences or extra-work environments.

Psychosocial Factors and Work-Related Musculoskeletal Disorders

NIOSH (1997) describes five psychosocial factors potentially related to WRMDs (back and upper extremity disorders): (1) job satisfaction, (2) intensified workload, (3) monotonous work, (4) job control, and (5) social support. NIOSH (1997) reports stronger support for the relationship between these psychosocial factors and WRMD in the back, neck, and shoulder area than in the hand and wrist area. This may be due to the fact that a larger number of studies concentrated on the back, neck, and shoulder area rather than on the hand and wrist area or that most studies done on the hand and wrist area did not consider psychosocial variables. Studies examining these relationships are reviewed in Table 6.1.

Low levels of *job satisfaction* may be associated with high levels of upper extremity musculoskeletal symptoms (Hopkins 1990; Tola et al.

TABLE 6.1
Psychosocial Factors Associated with Upper Extremity and Back Musculoskeletal Disabilities

Study (year)	Occupational Population	Control Used	Area Studied	Psychosocial Factors				
				Job Satisfaction	Workload	Monotonous Work	Job Control	Social Support
Ahlberg-Hulten (1995)	Health care workers (female)	Longitudinal (study of same group)	Back				+(with high demands)	
Bernard et al. (1992, 1994)	Newspaper workers	—	Upper extremity		+		+(for data-entry workers)	+
Bigos et al. (1991)	Aircraft plant workers	History of back injury	Back	+			+	+
Bongers et al. (1994)	—	Longitudinal	Back	+	+			
Hales et al. (1994)	Telecommunications workers	Extra-job factors	Upper extremity		+		+	+
Himmelstein et al. (1995)	General population	—	Upper extremity	+				+
Hopkins (1990)	Keyboard clerks	—	Upper extremity	+		+	+	+
Houtman et al. (1994)	General population	Physical stressors	Back Upper extremity		+[a]	+[a,b]	+[a,b]	
Hughes et al. (1997)	Aluminum smelter workers	—	Back	+				+

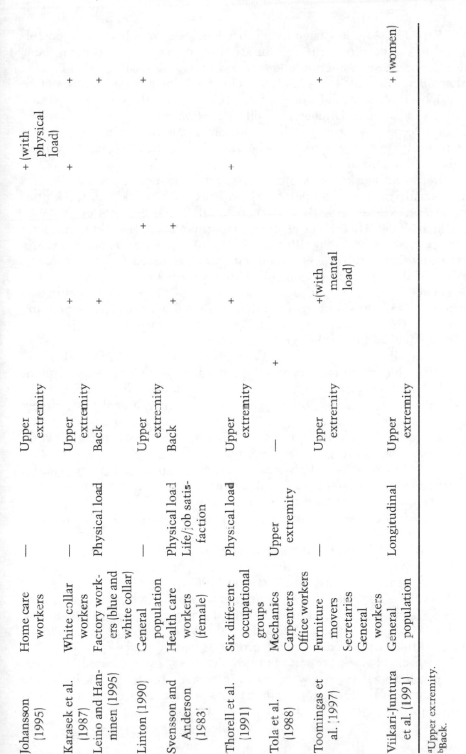

Johansson (1995) — Home care workers — Upper extremity — | — + (with physical load)

Karasek et al. (1987) — White collar workers — Upper extremity — | — +

Leino and Hanninen (1995) — Factory workers (blue and white collar) — Physical load — Back — +

Linton (1990) — General population — Upper extremity — | — +

Svensson and Anderson (1983) — Health care workers (female) — Physical load Life/job satisfaction — Back — +

Thorell et al. (1991) — Six different occupational groups — Physical load — Upper extremity — +

Tola et al. (1988) — Mechanics Carpenters Office workers — Upper extremity — | — +

Toomingas et al. (1997) — Furniture movers Secretaries General workers — | — Upper extremity — +(with mental load)

Viikari-Juntura et al. (1991) — General population — Longitudinal — Upper extremity — + (women)

aUpper extremity.
bBack.

1988). Several researchers have found that low levels of job satisfaction correspond to the development and duration of musculoskeletal symptoms, although these results did not hold true in a longitudinal study with Finnish workers (Bongers et al. 1993; Himmelstein et al. 1995; Viikari-Juntura et al. 1991): Job satisfaction did not predict neck and shoulder symptoms in a follow-up 1 year later. Hughes and colleagues (1997) found low job satisfaction (and decision latitude) to be important predictors of increased back pain in heavy-industry workers. The variation in results may be due to population differences.

Intensified workload is most consistently associated with WRMDs and is usually measured by perceived time pressure, workload, work pressure, and workload variability (Bernard et al. 1993; Bongers et al. 1993; Hales et al. 1994; Theorell et al. 1991). Houtman et al. (1994) found that a high pace of work had a significant relationship to WRMDs and primarily caused back symptoms, even when data were adjusted for the degree of physical load. A study that controlled for physical load found an association between workload and upper back and limb symptoms (Leino and Hanninen 1995). Others have found that increased workload (time pressure and greater time at a computer) was related to symptoms in the neck, shoulder, hand, and wrist (Bernard et al. 1992, 1994).

To help distinguish between various elements of workload, Lindstrom (1994) identified two types: (1) quantitative workload (large amount of work, long hours, or haste at work) and (2) qualitative workload (tasks too simple or too difficult). Both types affected workers' health negatively but through different mechanisms. Quantitative workload affects biomechanical factors and stress, whereas qualitative workload affects mental overload and thus physical well-being. Similarly, Toomingas and colleagues (1997) differentiated physical workload from mental workload. He discovered that high mental demand was related to general musculoskeletal sensitivity, especially in the neck and low back.

Monotonous work is associated with neck symptoms and low back pain (Hopkins 1990; Houtman et al. 1994; Linton 1990; Svensson and Andersson 1983). Some theorize that the rate of detection of symptoms is higher in less interesting jobs because boring work fails to distract attention from symptoms (Sauter and Swanson 1996).

Job control, one of the most consistently researched psychosocial factors, is frequently linked to musculoskeletal symptoms (Hales 1994; Svensson and Andersson 1983; Theorell et al. 1991). Bernard et al. (1994) speculated that the introduction of computers caused a lack of control over specific aspects of work, reduction of task diversity, and increased isolation. These psychosocial factors were more important predictors of hand and wrist symptoms in newspaper departments with a high concentration of data-entry workers (thought to have low-control jobs) compared to editorial workers (thought to have jobs involving more decision making and varied tasks). Ahlberg-Hulten and colleagues (1995) found that lower-back symptoms are associated with lack of job control and the presence of extremely demanding work, whereas upper-back symptoms appear to be associated with emotional and interpersonal factors. A longitudinal study of the role of psychosocial factors on neck and shoulder and low back pain among Finnish men and women found that a poor sense of job control was associated with neck and shoulder pain and fewer years of education corresponded with low back pain (Viikari-Juntura 1991). In an investigation of home care workers, decreased job control combined with high physical workload increased the prevalence of musculoskeletal symptoms in the neck and shoulders (Johansson 1995).

Although job control has been linked to musculoskeletal symptoms, the location of injuries have varied from study to study. In addition, major methodologic differences exist between studies (e.g., differences of the populations studied and definitions of job control). Individual factors, such as gender or education, may affect psychosocial factors and physical symptoms, making definitive conclusions difficult.

Social support from coworkers or supervisors has been studied in a variety of populations with fairly consistent results. Perception of poor social support is associated with increased report of symptoms, although the direction of this relationship is unclear. Himmelstein and colleagues (1995) differentiated individuals who worked with WRMDs from those who did not by noting that the individuals who did not work due to WRMD expressed more anger toward their employers (although both groups had a similar perception of the work environment). In a rare longitudinal study, Bongers and colleagues (1994) found evidence that high physical demands combined with poor social support increase symptoms. Feurstein (1985) found that decreases in coworker cohesion correlated to higher pain ratings (but not with distress). Other research supports the theory that decreased social support from coworkers and supervisors correlates with increased musculoskeletal symptoms in the upper extremities (neck and shoulder area, wrist and hand area) in a variety of occupations (e.g., furniture movers, secretaries) (Bernard et al. 1992, 1994; Hales 1994; Hopkins 1990; Toomingas et al. 1997).

Despite these fairly consistent results, several studies have not found an association between social support and symptoms such as the neck and shoulder pain or general musculoskeletal aches (Karasek et al. 1987; Theorell et al. 1991). In addition, the relationship between social support and symptoms is unclear: Perhaps symptoms lead to decreased social support. Bigos and colleagues (1991) and Leino and Hanninen (1995) have attempted to clarify this relationship. Both groups reported that dissatisfaction with social relationships at work predicted the report of musculoskeletal symptoms.

Theories Explaining the Relationship between Psychosocial Factors and Work-Related Musculoskeletal Disorders

Several theories attempt to explain the influence of psychosocial factors on the development of musculoskeletal symptoms. Most of these theories assume that psychosocial factors help cause symptoms, although some suggest other relationships. Four main theories are reviewed in this section.

One of the most popular explanations suggests that psychosocial factors increase muscle tension and exacerbate existing biomechanical strain on the musculoskeletal system through increased mental stress (Bernard et al. 1994; NIOSH 1997; Waersted et al. 1991). In one study, increased electromyographic activity was recorded from the muscles of the neck (trapezius) and the erector spine muscles during mentally stressful activities (Toomingas et al. 1997). Electromyographic activity increased with ergonomic loads and increased further when psychological loads were added, which supports the theory of increased muscular tension due to mental stress. Absence of relaxation mediates the effects of poor psychosocial work conditions (Lundberg et al. 1994). Bongers and colleagues (1993) suggest that psychosocial factors directly influence mechanical loads through changes in posture due to stress. For example, people tend to change posture when pressured by deadlines (e.g., hunched trunk, elevated shoulders). In addition, stress originating from the combination of few variables, such as poor job control or poor social support joined with a poor capacity to cope, may increase muscle tone and, in the long run, lead to musculoskeletal disorders. Theorell and colleagues (1991) demonstrated that increased mental demands are associated with increased worry, fatigue, and difficulty sleeping. These symptoms correspond with behavior that increases muscle tension, which is associated with back, shoulder, and neck discomfort.

Sauter and Swanson (1996) suggest an ecologic model describing a pathway leading from work organization to musculoskeletal outcome in office workers. The pathways included in this model are based on research with a specific population (computer workers). The model identifies a direct path between work technology (tools and work system) with both physical demands (including ergonomics) and work organization. A direct path also exists between physical demands and work organization, suggesting that physical demands are exacerbated by organizational demands (i.e., increased job specification increases repetition). Another path identified in the model exists between work organization and psychosocial strain (i.e., stress). This path is suggested to affect musculoskeletal outcomes in two ways. First, stress increases muscle tension and autonomic processes and adds to the biomechanical strain that already exists. Second, cognitive processes mediate the relationship between biomechanical strain and musculoskeletal symptoms (i.e., the process of detecting and interpreting symptoms can further influence stress at work). Stress-related arousal may increase sensitivity to normal musculoskeletal sensation: The worker becomes aware of any small sensation that in other situations would be suppressed. Workers involved in stressful work conditions may also attribute normal musculoskeletal sensation to work conditions and believe such sensations to be a sign of injury and illness. Musculoskeletal disorder is influenced by environmental forces that include medical, societal, and cultural factors; legal and compensation systems; and workplace relationships. The cognitive-perceptual process may lead to interpretation of discomfort as an underlying injury and may develop into sickness and lead to disability.

The demand-control-support model (Karasek 1979; Karasek and Theorell 1990) provides another technique for identifying the relationship between psychosocial factors and WRMDs. According to this model, psychological demands have adverse affects on a worker if they occur jointly with low decision latitude. Low decision latitude is identified by the absence of authority to decide what to do and how to do it and by the lack of intellectual discretion (i.e., the opportunity to use and develop skills at work). The social support component in this model refers to the support available in the workplace that is thought to mediate the demands and the symptoms. Research of this model supports the assumption that these components are relevant to the development of musculoskeletal disorders (Theorell 1996).

A major problem reported due to musculoskeletal symptoms, *pain* is a complex phenomenon that may trigger dysfunction of both the physiologic and psychological systems. Himmelstein et al. (1995) suggested that individuals who report high levels of pain and symptoms appear to have more difficulty coping with pain and associated loss of function, thus contributing to their prolonged disability. The perception of pain and the cognitive processes used to explain and deal with pain and disability may contribute to pain perception in several ways. Fear of increased pain may lead to avoidance of activities. Fear of reinjury can lead to gross inactivity, muscular reconditioning, stress, and maladaptive beliefs (Flor et al. 1985; Keefe and Egert 1996). An example is turning the pain into a catastrophe ("it's the end of the world"). This may increase anxiety about pain and lead to the reporting of higher pain levels.

NIOSH (1997) notes that changes in physical and biomechanical demands frequently occur simultaneously with changes in psychosocial demands, making it difficult to delineate the causal relationships between them. This often causes methodologic problems.

Methodologic Problems

Interpretation of the research is complicated by the different designs used, populations studied, and type of psychosocial factors and WRMDs examined.

Several methodologic problems are included here to clarify research techniques. Most of the research examining the relationships between psychosocial risk factors and WRMDs use cross-sectional designs, making causality impossible to determine (Bongers et al. 1993; Himmelstein et al. 1995).

Few studies have considered the confounding effect of physical stressors (static load and repetitive work) when assessing the relationships between psychosocial risk factors and WRMDs (Bongers et al. 1993; Houtman et al. 1993; Sauter and Swanson 1996). An exception is the study done by Theorell et al. (1991), who did control for physical stressors when assessing factors such as social support.

Another problem arises from tools used to measure psychosocial factors. Psychosocial factors are difficult to measure with objective measurements and are usually subjective, assessed through surveys or self-report techniques. Cognitive theorists suggest that the individual is a filter through which the environment is observed. For instance, Lazarus (1974) emphasizes the cognitive and affective functions of the individual identifying work demands. Thus, determining whether risk factors are colored by one's perception or are reflective of the "true" situation is difficult. The lack of standardized and reliable methods of measuring psychosocial factors also contributes to research difficulties (Houtman et al. 1993; Lindstrom 1994; NIOSH 1997; Sauter and Swanson 1996).

Although many studies found the relationships to be significant, the strength of these relationships is modest (NIOSH 1997; Sauter and Swanson 1996). This prevents definitive conclusions or solutions when creating and using programs for workers suffering from WRMDs.

Sauter and Swanson (1996) suggest ways to improve research by (1) developing longitudinal studies, (2) improving the tools used to assess health and psychosocial factors, (3) improving analytical methods to separate the effects of the psychosocial factors, and (4) examining the suggested pathways explaining the relationships.

Assessment: The Occupational Stress Inventory

The occupational stress inventory (OSI) (Osipow and Spokane 1987) was designed (1) to measure occupational stressors that apply across different occupational levels and environments and (2) to provide measures for the theoretical model linking work-related stress with the psychological strains experienced by the worker as a result of stressors and for the coping resources available to the worker to deal with the stressors and the psychological strain. The OSI is only in research stages and not intended for clinical use. However, it shows promise as an instrument for assessing occupational stress.

The OSI measures three dimensions in occupational adjustment: occupational stress, measured by six scales of the occupational roles questionnaire; psychological strain, measured by four scales of the personal strain questionnaire; and coping resources, measured by four scales of the personal resources questionnaire.

Occupational roles questionnaire scales include (1) role overload (how much job demands exceed resources and whether the worker can accomplish the expected workloads), (2) role insufficiency (appropriateness of the worker's training, education, skills, and experience to job requirements), (3) role ambiguity (the level of the worker's understanding of the expectations and evaluation criteria), (4) role boundary (the extent the worker experiences conflicts in role demands or loyalties), (5) responsibility (the amount of responsibility perceived by or given to the worker to ensure the performance and welfare of others on the job), and (6) physical environment (the frequency at which the worker is exposed to extreme conditions [e.g., high levels of environmental toxins]).

Personal strain questionnaire scales include (1) vocational strain (the amount of difficulty the worker is having in work quality or output), (2) psychological strain (the effect of any emotional problems), (3) interpersonal strain (the amount of disruption in interpersonal relationships), and (4) physical strain (complaints about physical illness or poor self-care habits).

Personal resources questionnaire scales include (1) recreation (pleasure and relaxation derived from regular recreational activities); (2) self-care (the frequency with which the worker engages in personal activities that reduce or alleviate chronic stress); (3) social support (the extent the individual feels support and help from those around him or her); and (4) rational and cognitive coping (how frequently the individual uses cognitive skills to deal with work-related stress).

These three sets of scales indicate the dynamics between work-related stressors, strain experiences, and coping resources. Such an assessment tool can help clinicians understand different aspects of work that affect well-being. Clinicians can plan a specific treatment and configure it to the individual worker based on the worker's coping resources.

Interventions

Psychosocial factors alone cannot account for disability. Excluding them in the evaluation and prevention processes, however, may inhibit successful intervention. The nature of the psychosocial risk factors and their distribution among workers may suggest the direction and level of intervention (i.e., individual or organizational). Himmelstein and colleagues (1995) suggested that early intervention to prevent work disability might benefit from focusing on reducing employer-employee conflicts, improving medical management of pain, and enhancing the ability to cope with residual pain and distress and avoiding unnecessary surgery.

Lindstrom (1994) describes a research-based model for creating a good work organization based on psychosocial intervention. The need to optimize quantitative workload and qualitative workload is emphasized, and the level of autonomy and freedom at work is maximized because they are thought to decrease stress and hence musculoskeletal symptoms. Improving interpersonal relationships among workers and improving communication between employees and supervisors is encouraged. Coping skills are improved either through mental exercises or increased mastery of work. The organization of the entire workplace is evaluated and altered by occupational health professionals. Workers at risk are provided with support and skills to deal with the work demands through group workshops, new skills–development workshops, and individual support from occupational psychologists.

The Rochester model of work disability also emphasizes the complexity of issues created by work disability. This model identifies four categories of variables that may affect work disability and work re-entry: (1) medical status, (2) physical capabilities (including work tolerance), (3) work demands (biomechanical, metabolic, psychological), and (4) psychological or behavioral resources (worker traits, pain management, readiness to work). This model recommends evaluation and intervention to prevent disability and assist in work re-entry (Fitzgerald 1992; Moon 1996).

Most of the intervention programs use cognitive-behavioral methods, such as relaxation and cognitive restructuring, to provide the worker with coping skills (Feurstein 1996; Spence 1991). Cognitive strategies include focusing on the source of the stress and paying close attention to its interpretation, examining the attribution style after symptoms and stress occur, and adopting alternative methods for addressing problems. Cognitive-behavioral strategies also help improve pain management by altering cognitive, behavioral, and affective responses. The techniques used include relaxation (including using biofeedback), activity pacing, cognitive restructuring, and imagery and distraction to deal with pain (Keefe and Egert 1996). These techniques require a clinical psychologist who is able to assess and treat within the framework of cognitive-behavioral therapy.

Future Directions

The role of psychosocial factors in WRMDs has received increased attention from researchers and clinicians. However, the field needs standardized instruments to measure psychosocial factors to further cross-study comparisons. In addition, clinical tools should be developed to assess work-related psychosocial factors and treatment outcomes.

References

Ahlberg-Hulten GK, Theorell T, Sigala F (1995). Social support, job strain and musculoskeletal pain among female health care personnel. Scand J Work Environ Health 21:435–439.

Bernard B, Sauter S, Fine L (1993). Hazard evaluation and technical assistance report. NIOSH Report No. HHE 90-013-2277. Cincinnati: U.S. Department of Health and Human Services, Public Health Service, Centers for Disease Control and Prevention, National Institute for Occupational Safety and Health.

Bernard B, Sauter S, Fine L, et al. (1992). Job task and psychosocial risk factors for work-related musculoskeletal disorders among newspaper employees. Scand J Work Environ Health 18(suppl 2):119–120.

Bernard B, Sauter S, Fine L, et al. (1994). Job task and psychosocial risk factors for work-related musculoskeletal disorders among newspaper employees. Scand J Work Environ Health 20:417–426.

Bigos SJ, Battie MC, Spengler DM, et al. (1991). A prospective study of work perceptions and psychosocial factors affecting the report of back injury. Spine 16:1–6.

Bongers PM, Winter CR, Kompier MAJ, Hilderbrandt VH (1993). Psychosocial factors at work and musculoskeletal disease. Scand J Work Environ Health 19:297–312.

Feuerstein M (1996). Workstyle: Definition, Empirical Support, and Implications for Prevention, Evaluation, and Rehabilitation of Occupational Upper-Extremity Disorders. In SD Moon, SL Sauter (eds), Beyond Biomechanics: Psychosocial Aspects of Musculoskeletal Disorders in Office Work. Bristol, PA: Taylor & Francis, 177–206.

Feuerstein M, Sult SC, Houle M (1985). Environmental stressors and low back pain: life events, family, and work environment. Pain 22:295–307.

Flor H, Turk DC, Birbaumer N (1985). Assessment of stress-related psychophysiology reactions in chronic back pain patients. J Consult Clin Psychol 53:354–364.

Hagberg M, Silverstein B, Wells R, et al. (eds) (1995). Work Related Musculoskeletal Disorders (WMSDs): A Reference Book for Prevention. London: Taylor & Francis.

Hales TR, Sauter SL, Peterson MR, et al. (1994). Musculoskeletal disorders among video display terminal users in a telecommunications company. Ergonomics 37:1603–1621.

Himmelstein JS, Feurstein M, Stanek FJ, et al. (1995). Work-related upper-extremity disorders and work disability: clinical and psychosocial presentation. J Occup Environ Med 37:1278–1286.

Hopkins A (1990). Stress, the quality of work, and repetitive strain injury in Australia. Work Stress 4:129–138.

Houtman ILD, Bongers PM, Smulders PGW, Kompier MAJ (1994). Psychosocial stressors at work and musculoskeletal problems. Scand J Work Environ Health 20:139–145.

Hughes RE, Silverstein BA, Evanoff BA (1997). Risk factors for work-related musculoskeletal disorders in an aluminum smelter. Am J Ind Med 32:66–75.

Hurrell JJ, Murphy LR (1992). Psychological Job Stress. In WN Rom (ed), Environmental and Occupational Medicine (2nd ed). New York: Little, Brown, 675–684.

ILO (1986). Psychosocial Factors at Work: Recognition and Control. Geneva: ILO.

Johansson JA (1995). Psychosocial work factors, physical workload and associated musculoskeletal symptoms among home care workers. Scand J Psychol 36:113–129.

Karasek RA (1979). Job demands, job decision latitude, and mental strain: implications for job redesign. Admin Sci Q 24:285–307.

Karasek RA, Gardell B, Lindell J (1987). Work and non-work correlates of illness and behavior in male and female Swedish white collar workers. J Occup Behav 8:187–207.

Karasek RA, Theorell T (1990). Healthy Work. New York: Basic Books.

Keefe FJ, Egert JR (1996). A Cognitive-Behavioral Perspective on Pain in Cumulative Trauma Disorders. In SD Moon, SL Sauter (eds), Beyond Biomechanics: Psychosocial Aspects of Musculoskeletal Disorders in Office Work. Bristol, PA: Taylor & Francis, 159–175.

Lazarus RS (1974). Psychological stress and adaptation and illness. Int J Psych Med 8:225–241.

Leino PI, Hanninen V (1995). Psychosocial factors at work in relation to back and limb disorder. Scan J Work Environ Health 21:134–142.

Lindstrom K (1994). Psychosocial criteria for good work organization. Scan J Work Environ Health 20:123–133.

Linton SJ (1990). Risk factors for neck and back pain in a working population in Sweden. Work Stress 4:41–49.

Lundberg U, Kadefors R, Melin B, et al. (1994). Stress, muscular tension and musculoskeletal disorders. Int J Behav Med 1:354–370.

NIOSH (1986). Proposed National Strategy for the Prevention of Musculoskeletal Injuries. Washington, DC: U.S. Department of Health and Human Services.

NIOSH (1997). Musculoskeletal Disorders and Workplace Factors. Washington, DC: U.S. Department of Health and Human Services, Public Health Service, Centers for Disease Control and Prevention, National Institute for Occupational Safety and Health.

Osipow SH, Spokane AR (1987). Manual for the Occupational Stress Inventory. Odessa, FL: Psychological Assessment Resources.

Sauter SL, Swanson NG (1996). An Ecological Model of Musculoskeletal Disorders in Office Work. In SD Moon, SL Sauter (eds), Beyond Biomechanics: Psychosocial Aspects of Musculoskeletal Disorders in Office Work. Bristol, PA: Taylor & Francis, 3–21.

Spence SH (1991). Cognitive behavior therapy in the treatment of chronic, occupational pain of the upper limbs: a two-year follow-up. Behav Res Ther 29:503–509.

Svensson H, Anderson GBJ (1983). Low-back pain in 40- to 47-year-old men: work history and work environment factors. Spine 8:272–276.

Theorell T (1996). Possible Mechanisms Behind the Relationship Between the Demand-Control-Support Model and Disorders of the Locomotor System. In SD Moon, SL Sauter (eds), Beyond Biomechanics: Psychosocial Aspects of Musculoskeletal Disorders in Office Work. Bristol, PA: Taylor & Francis, 65–73.

Theorell T, Harms-Ringdahl K, Ahlberg-Hulten G, Westin B (1991). Psychosocial job factors and symptoms from the locomotor system: a multicausal analysis. Scand J Rehabil Med 23:165–173.

Tola S, Riihimaki H, Videman T, et al. (1988). Neck and shoulder symptoms among men in machine operating, dynamic physical work and sedentary work. Scand J Work Environ Health 14:299–305.

Toomingas A, Theorell T, Michelsen H, Nordemar R (1997). Association between self-rated psychosocial work conditions and musculoskeletal symptoms and signs. Scand J Work Environ 23:130–139.

Viikari-Juntura E, Vuori J, Silverstein BA, et al. (1991). Life-long prospective study on the role of psychosocial factors in neck shoulder and low-back pain. Spine 16:1056–1061

Waersted M, Bjorklund RA, Westgaard RH (1991). Shoulder muscle tension induced by two VDU-based tasks of different complexity. Ergonomics 34:137–150.

Review Questions

(Answers are found in Appendix D.)

1. The difference between the NIOSH and the ILO definitions of work-related factors is that
   (a) ILO includes the physical and ergonomics environment
   (b) NIOSH includes extra-work factors and ILO does not
   (c) NIOSH includes organizational factors and ILO does not
   (d) no difference exists
   (e) both a and b

2. The psychosocial factor(s) most consistent with WRMDs is (are)
   (a) social support
   (b) job satisfaction and job control
   (c) social support, workload, and job control
   (d) monotony at work

3. What is the most common explanation for the relationship between psychosocial factors and WRMDs?
   (a) Physical demands increase the biomechanical stress on muscles, leading to WRMDs
   (b) Cognitive processes cause musculoskeletal symptoms to be magnified
   (c) Psychosocial factors increase mental stress, which in turn increases muscle tension that exacerbates existing biomechanical strain on the musculoskeletal system
   (d) Work organization affects social support

4. Why is it difficult to find a causal relationship between psychosocial factors and WRMDs?
   (a) Most studies use a cross-sectional design, making it difficult to determine causality
   (b) Changes in physical and biomechanical demands frequently occur together with changes in psychosocial demands, making it difficult to determine causality
   (c) Both a and b
   (d) Not enough research exists to determine causality

CHAPTER 7
Environmental Design

Peter Picone

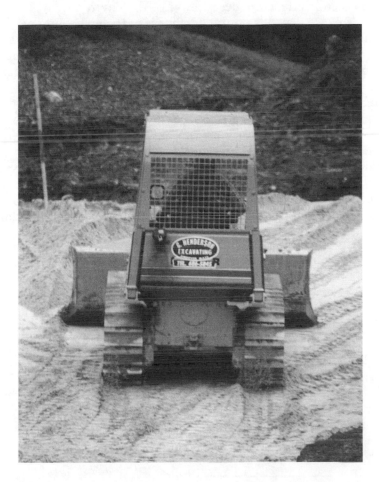

ABSTRACT

Practitioners must consider people, environment, and equipment in the design of a workplace. The design should be user-centered and optimized for task performance. Environmental variables and equipment limitations function as design constraints. The ergonomist or designer must compensate for variables such as vibration, noise, illumination, and temperature to ensure a successful design.

In ergonomics, all forms of system design, analysis, or review require the understanding that task performance is a function of three factors: (1) the person performing the task, (2) the equipment used, and (3) the environment in which the operator and the equipment interact (Figure 7.1). The factors shown in Figure 7.1 are inseparable for the purposes of analysis and design.

Many factors affect the description of the environment. How factors affect performance depends on the harshness of the environment, the skills and abilities of the operator, and the importance or complexity of the tasks. For example, in the design of a commercial airplane, the operational environment of the pilot differs significantly from that of the passenger. Based on the importance of tasks and the physical and cognitive requirements of each user, the design of the area around each varies widely. The pilot requires a steering wheel and access to the throttles, but passengers, who are not required to perform critical tasks such as flying the plane, have neither. Conversely, the passenger, whose task is to enjoy himself or herself during the flight, has a tray table to hold food and a seat-back pocket to hold a book. The pilot should not have many of these same design requirements.

Several environmental variables inherent in many industrial workplaces must be considered by the designer. This chapter describes and quantifies vibration, noise, illumination, and temperature and discusses the impact of each variable on design.

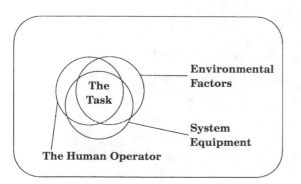

FIGURE 7.1.   Task performance environment.

Vibration

Vibration affects almost everyone regardless of job or activity. In the work-place, vibration is felt most commonly with tasks that involve machinery and vehicles. It can take the form of whole-body vibration, usually trans-mitted to the person through a vehicle seat or through the shop floor, or can be transmitted segmentally and isolated locally, as with arm and hand vibration that occurs when using a powered hand tool, such as a drill, a grinder, or a saw. Vibration can be of low or high frequency and of a wide variety of intensities and can occur in combinations of single frequencies and resonant harmonic frequencies.

Terminology and Measurement

Mechanical vibration can be measured and described in units of frequency and time. These measurements include Fourier analysis, modal analysis, transfer function analysis, and mechanical impedance analysis. The details of these methods can be found in a good mechanical engineering text, such as Cannon's *Dynamics of Physical Systems* (1967). Concepts important in the discussion and understanding of the effects of vibration are frequency, amplitude, form factor, resonance, and harmonics.

Frequency

The frequency of a sound or vibration is the number of complete cycles per second (hertz [Hz]). In Figure 7.2, vibration A completes one full cycle per second. Its frequency is therefore 1 Hz. Vibration B completes only half of its complete cycle in 1 second; therefore, its frequency is 0.5 Hz.

Amplitude

The amplitude of a vibration is represented by the amount of movement from a mean position to either the positive or negative extreme. It is a measurement of the power or force of the vibration. In Figure 7.2, if the

FIGURE 7.2. Characteris-
tics of a sound or vibration.

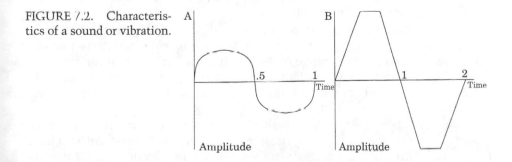

units of the amplitude scale are the same for vibration A and vibration B, vibration B has a greater amplitude than vibration A.

Form Factor

Form factor is the differentiation in shape of a vibration. In Figure 7.2, vibration A has a smooth form and vibration B a jagged form. If these vibrations were musical tones, the clean sinusoidal shape of vibration A would sound like a note from a flute or a guitar string, whereas vibration B would have a rougher sound, like a harmonica.

Resonance

Resonance is the vibrating frequency (hertz) at which maximum mechanical energy is transferred from the vibrating source to a person. At resonance frequency, the person is maximally "tuned" to the vibrating source, and the movement of human tissue (when properly synchronized) amplifies the power produced by the vibrating source.

Harmonics

A harmonic vibration is a vibration whose frequency is an integral multiple of the fundamental or base frequency. For example, if the fundamental frequency is 50 Hz, the first harmonic is 100 Hz, the second harmonic is 150 Hz, the third harmonic is 200 Hz, and so on.

Differentiation between Noise and Whole-Body Accelerations

Vibration can affect the human body in many ways. Airborne vibration striking the ear causes the eardrum to vibrate in resonance with the incoming changes in air pressure, and the vibration is perceived as sound. Mechanical vibrations also interact with the human body, and parts of the body respond by vibrating in resonance with the external vibration. This resonance effect often amplifies the incoming vibration and can cause damage to the part of the body in resonance. Exposure limits and recommended tolerances can be found in the *Guide for Evaluation of Human Exposure to Whole-Body Vibration*, compiled by the International Organization for Standardization (1974).

Based on their composition and mass, different parts of the body resonate at different frequencies. In the vertical direction, the body (mostly the torso) resonates in the range of 4–8 Hz (usually at 5 Hz). In the horizontal and lateral directions, resonance is in the range of 1–2 Hz (Coermann 1962). The head and shoulders tend to resonate at 10–20 Hz, and the eyeballs resonate at 60–80 Hz (Grether 1971).

The effects of vibration on task performance are difficult to quantify. Different frequencies impact various parts of the body differently. These effects fall into three general categories: (1) general discomfort, (2) disruption of visual acuity, and (3) tickling sensation in the hands and feet (at frequencies greater than 100 Hz). General discomfort has negative motivational and physiologic effects on operator performance. Disruptions in visual performance can result in degradation of any task that requires eye-hand coordination, especially tasks in which reading and writing are important. Loss of visual acuity can become extremely hazardous in some occupations. For example, a helicopter pilot with a vibration-induced loss of visual acuity may not see high-tension electrical wires in his or her path.

The severity of the tickling sensation in the hands and feet is related to the duration and intensity of the vibration. When intensity is high and duration is long, as in the case of chainsaw and other power tool operators, physiologic damage can occur. The threshold for this type of damage is approximately 1g (amplitude) at 100 Hz, and the rise thereafter is 6 dB per octave (May 1978). At lower intensities and shorter durations, fine manipulative skills can be disrupted; the extreme case is the development of "dead hands" (Raynaud phenomenon of occupational origin, vibrational white fingers). In its early stages, this syndrome causes occasional tingling, numbness, and blanching of the fingers. With repeated exposure, the disease acquires a peripheral vascular component (intermittent blanching and cyanosis of all fingertips except the thumb), episodes of which last 15–30 minutes. In its extreme form, the disease progresses to gangrene of the affected fingers. Cold temperatures tend to trigger the attacks, and both fevers and smoking exacerbate the problem (Salvendy 1987).

Noise

Although sound is simply exposure to oscillating mechanical vibrations in the form of pressure changes at the ear, the impact of sound on a human operator and general performance can be quite different from that of other direct, coupled mechanical vibrations. Evaluating sound and vibration in a work environment involves examination of the system from two perspectives: (1) the direct physical attributes of the sound and vibration and (2) the subjective responses of the person to those physical attributes. Each of these perspectives should directly influence design strategies.

Terminology and Measurement

Sound Pressure Level

The sound pressure level (SPL) of the energy that impinges the ear is measured in decibels (dB). Mathematically, it is defined as follows:

$$SPL = 20 \log_{10} P_n \parallel P_{ref}$$

where P_n is the root mean square sound pressure produced by the source being measured and P_{ref} is a standard reference value that corresponds roughly to the minimum pressure detectable by the human ear, usually considered to be 20 µPa (2×10^{-5} Pa = [2×10^{-5} N]/m^2 = 2×10^4 µbar). Thus, the SPL is an absolute ratio of two pressure magnitudes with respect to the minimum audible SPL (International Labor Office 1980). This is an excellent physical measurement, but because the human ear does not perceive sound equally across the entire range of audible frequencies, the definition is often modified to accommodate frequency biases of the ear. Modifying the weighting in some of the frequency bands results in a sound level that to some extent correlates with the loudness of a sound as heard by the listener. The weighted scales dB(A) and dB(C) are used to measure the "loudness" of a sound as opposed to its SPL or direct pressure ratio. This modification allows evaluation of sound or environmental noise based on the way it is perceived by the ear and the operator's response to the sound.

Loudness, Noisiness, and Annoyance

Loudness is the subjective magnitude of a sound. This refers only to how intensely the sound is perceived, not how the listener evaluates its content. The "unwantedness" of the sound should not be considered loudness. The degree to which a sound is considered noisy is the level of unwantedness of the sound and is considered separately from loudness. Different reactions to music fall into this category. For example, a parent may consider classical music played at the same loudness as their children's rock music to be much less noisy than the rock music. The noisiness of a sound results in an associated degree of annoyance. *Annoyance* is the overall unwantedness of a sound heard in a natural situation. A person's judgment of the annoyance of a sound includes the noisiness inherent in the sound and variables related to the situation in which the sound is heard (Peterson and Gross 1978). A sound heard during the night can be much more annoying than the same sound heard during the day. Anyone who has ever tried to sleep listening to a dripping faucet or running toilet is well aware of this phenomenon. Similarly, a repeated sound may be more annoying when a worker is concentrating on a task than when the worker is more relaxed. That same sound can also become more annoying when the listener is unable to remove the sound. When they have the option of turning off an alarm or other auditory warning, machine operators consider the sound less objectionable than when they are forced to listen to it until a supervisor turns off the alarm.

Speech Interference and Intelligibility

Speech interference is a function of the loudness of a sound, not simply its SPL. Measurements of interference and intelligibility are generally based on a calculation of the percentage of words, phrases, or sentences correctly understood over a specific speech communication system in a particular noise environment. This can pertain to both human-to-human communication and to human-to-machine speech recognition systems (Picone

1983). Interference and intelligibility are typically measured with either the Phonetically Balanced Monosyllabic Word Intelligibility Test or the Modified Rhyme Test. In the former test, a list of 1,000 words is dictated by a source (usually a tape recording), and the listener responds by crossing off or marking a word on a preformatted list. In the Modified Rhyme Test, a source reads a list of 300 words, and a listener selects one of six words from a prepared multiple-word list as the word heard for each word spoken. For example, the speaker says, "Would you please circle the word *gold* now." The listener then selects the word from a group that consists of the words *mold, bold, sold, gold, hold,* and *cold.*

Speech intelligibility also may be predicted by the articulation index. The peak speech-to-root mean square noise ratio is calculated in selected frequency bands. The bands range from 200 to 7,000 Hz (the range of frequencies that contain the most information with regard to speech content). The articulation index is a measurement of the peak amplitude of speech in relation to the "average" amplitude of the background noise. What is being measured is the degree to which a sound containing information necessary for the interpretation of that sound as speech is being masked by background noise. In the case of the two phonetic lists, degradation that has occurred in a communication system is measured directly (even if the system is in an open-air, face-to-face environment). In the case of the articulation index, a predictive measurement is made of the anticipated decrement in speech performance based on the amount of meaningful sound energy available over the background clutter.

Auditory Effects of Noise

Audible Frequencies

The human auditory system has an extremely wide range of sensitivity to the spectrum of sound amplitude. The need to cover the full range of human sensitivity requires sound intensity to be measured by a logarithmic scale (the decibel). Human sensitivity to the range of sound frequencies is much lower than the sensitivity to amplitude. The full range of frequencies perceivable by a human covers the bands from approximately 20 Hz on the low end to 20,000 Hz on the high end. This range varies widely with factors such as age or hearing loss due to physical damage to the auditory system (Woodson 1981).

Hazardous Noise Limitations

Two types of sound must be considered in the assessment of noise hazards: (1) continuous noise and (2) impact noise. Continuous noises are what people most commonly encounter in their daily activities. These are repetitive sounds of a slowly fluctuating intensity that have relatively slow rise and fall times. Examples include a noisy street or background noise in an office. Impact noise, however, is a sound with an almost instantaneous rise and fall time; it usually reaches a very high intensity for a very short time. Examples include gunshots, cars backfiring, hands clapping, or noises made by some factory machines, such as automated looms or presses.

Hazardous Properties of Noise

Hazardous noise should be evaluated by the following characteristics:

- Damage to a particular frequency band is caused by a sound an octave below that region. For example, exposure to intense sound at a frequency of 8,000 Hz causes damage to the listener's sensitivity at 16,000 Hz.
- Very-low-frequency noise energy tends to be less damaging to hearing than middle-frequency noise.
- Susceptibility to noise-induced hearing loss varies from person to person.
- High sound intensity and long exposure times often produce extensive hearing loss. In occupations for which such exposures are common, a large percentage of an exposed group have extensive hearing losses in similar frequency bands.
- Hearing loss due to noise is most pronounced and most susceptible at about 4,000 Hz but spreads over the frequency range as exposure time and level increase.

Over the years, studies have isolated properties of extended sound exposure that contribute most heavily to the destruction of neurologic elements of the ear and to subsequent hearing loss. Of these properties, the most critical are the overall sound pressure level, the spectral distribution of the sound, the total duration of exposure, and the temporal distribution of the exposure.

Sound Pressure Level

A sound pressure level less than 80 dB(A), although potentially annoying, usually does not cause any temporary or permanent hearing damage. With a sound pressure level greater than 80 dB(A), other criteria must be assessed before the sound is defined as hazardous.

Sound Spectrum

The sound spectrum is the range of component frequencies of the sound. As mentioned, the frequency at which damage occurs in the presence of excessive SPLs depends on the frequencies of the stimulus causing the damage. A single sound may have many different component frequencies, and each of those frequencies may be present at a different level of intensity. If one of the components is of a damaging magnitude, then damage will most likely occur relative to that frequency rather than to any of the others.

Duration of Exposure

Brief exposure to relatively high SPLs, regardless of the frequency of the sound, may often be tolerated without long-term damage. The most hazardous exposure is one in which exposure occurs throughout a full period of work (e.g., an 8-hour day). The Department of Labor has adopted a recommended allowable exposure level (Table 7.1). The long-term allowance begins at 90 dB(A) for an 8-hour day and decreases in allowable exposure time as the intensity of the sound rises. However, even short exposure to extremely high SPLs can be damaging.

Temporal Distribution

Temporal distribution is exposure to a sound over time during which the exposure is not uniform. For example, airport ground crews are exposed to very loud jet engine noises (115–125 dB[A]) for very short periods (2–3 minutes) every time a plane pulls in or takes off from the gate. Although this noise falls well within the exposure guidelines, a strong possibility exists that such exposure may prove damaging in the long term. Because of this risk, airport ground crews or anyone else exposed to a similar noise environment should always wear hearing protection.

Exposure and Frequency Relationships

Keeping hazardous and unwanted noise and vibration levels in the workplace below the recommended maximum levels is always prudent. Efforts to remove or isolate unwanted noise and vibration always have a positive impact on design. When redesigning the environment is impossible, steps should be taken to restructure the task or protect the operator. Techniques for obtaining a better design include reducing exposure time, using personal protective hearing devices whenever possible, and combining both measures.

When the opportunity to redesign the work environment does exist, methods of control include reduction of a sound or other vibration at its

TABLE 7.1
Allowable Sound Exposure Levels

Duration (hrs/day)	Sound Level (db[A])	Example
8	90	Subway car at 20 ft
6	92	
4	95	A passing motorcycle
3	97	
2	100	Blow-dryer or chainsaw motor
1.5	102	
1	105	Car horn
0.25 or less	115	Jet engine

source and prevention of propagation, amplification, or reverberation. Methods for preventing propagation typically involve the use of acoustic or mechanical dampening materials or devices. Even minor changes can often have a large effect on controlling auditory environments. For example, the sound characteristics of a room can be altered by changing the density of a carpet, adding acoustic tile to a ceiling, using screens or sound-proof partitions, or hanging sound-dampening materials on walls. Vibration can often be controlled by mounting vibrating equipment on dampening platforms to isolate the equipment from the floor or by providing noise-isolating enclosures for the equipment.

When altering the environment is impossible, workers should wear hearing protection. The type of protection used should be considered carefully. Although some devices offer better protection than others, the protective device should not interfere with the tasks to be performed and should be compatible with any other equipment the operator uses. For example, safety glasses may interfere with the effectiveness of earmuff-type protective devices, because the temple piece of the glasses may break the seal at the ear when the two devices are worn together. Providing workers with hearing-protection devices does not ensure they will use them. General hygiene factors should also be considered. Each worker should have his or her own hearing-protection device, especially if earplugs are used. When possible, disposable ear protection is preferred over reusable devices. Additional care should be given to training the worker on the proper use of the device. For example, foam inserts lose a large percentage of their effectiveness when the incorrect size is used or when they are improperly inserted into the ear canal. Employers and supervisors should monitor and encourage use and ensure that the workers are using devices properly.

Use of Auditory Displays

Audio displays are typically used when the information to be provided is short, simple, and transitory and requires an immediate response. Typically these responses are used to warn, alert, or cue an operator that a response is required (Military Standard 1989). Audio displays fall into two categories: verbal and nonverbal. A verbal auditory display usually is preceded by a nonverbal tone to attract the operator's attention. A well-known example of this type is used in automobiles to warn that the car door is open: A tone sounds and a synthesized voice immediately states, "Your door is ajar." Nonverbal displays are either pure periodic tones, such as a beep from a computer, or more complex sounds, such as doorbell chimes. Design considerations for both verbal and nonverbal displays include the following:

1. Frequency range used (e.g., an ambulance or police car siren)
2. How frequently the signal occurs

3. Intensity of the signal
4. Compatibility of the signal with the ambient acoustic environment
5. Compatibility of the signal with operator constraints or limitations (e.g., whether the operator wears hearing protection or a protective mask or headgear)
6. Ease of discernment between the signal and other auditory displays
7. Onset and SPL of the signal and the distance over which the signal must be heard
8. Ear to which the signal is presented (if headsets are used)

Illumination

In its most technical form, detailed lighting and illumination design is best left to lighting specialists. This portion of the chapter therefore focuses on the concepts required to make a basic assessment of the lighting in a work situation. A brief discussion of the relationship between lighting factors and operation of computers is also provided.

Terminology and Measurement

The *Illuminating Engineering Society Lighting Handbook* (Kaufman and Haynes 1984) begins with a 40-page dictionary of lighting terminology essential for practicing lighting engineers. Because of its size, summarizing it here in a few paragraphs is impossible. However, studying this source before attempting any lighting design or redesign project is encouraged.

Light can be defined as any radiant energy capable of exciting the human retina and producing a visual sensation. In physics, visible light is regarded as that portion of the electromagnetic spectrum that lies between wavelengths of 380 and 770 nm. As with the auditory system, these upper and lower limits of perceived wavelength vary from person to person, as well as with the colorblind, who misinterpret different portions of that spectrum. Radiant energy in this band of the electromagnetic spectrum makes visible anything from which it is emitted or reflected in sufficient quantity to activate the receptors of the eye (Kaufman and Haynes 1984). Responses from the receptors of the eyes are then interpreted by the brain as visual perception. Associated with this perception are all of the perceptual and psychological factors to which the brain is often subject. Radiant energy is measured in a number of ways. Two of the most common are radiant flux and luminous flux.

Radiant Flux

Radiant flux is the rate of flow of radiant energy. It is usually expressed in watts or joules per second. Light bulb strength is measured in watts, or the amount of radiant energy given off in a certain period.

Luminous Flux

Luminous flux is the rate of flow of light. In the Système International (SI), it is measured in lumens. A light bulb is often rated in terms of the average number of lumens as well as the wattage. The radiometric evaluation of luminous flux is based on the amount of radiant power. The photometric evaluation is based on the luminous flux emitted within a unit solid angle (1 steradian) by a point source that has a uniform luminous intensity of 1 candela. A candela is the SI measurement of luminous intensity. One candela is equal to 1 lumen per steradian. A much more specific definition examines the wavelength of the light and the power density of the light. The following terms refer to what happens to light energy after it has been generated.

Reflectance
Reflectance is the amount of incident light not transmitted or absorbed by a surface. It is usually described as the ratio of reflected light to incident light.

Transmittance
Transmittance is the amount of light that passes through a surface or a body. When struck by light, a pane of glass reflects some light and allows some light to pass through. The amount of light that passes through is described by the transmittance level.

Absorption
Absorption is the amount of light not transmitted or reflected by a surface. It is the general term for the process by which incident light is converted into another form of energy, usually heat. An example of this phenomenon can be seen merely by putting one's hand next to a light bulb and feeling the incident light turning to heat as it is absorbed by the hand.

Glare
Glare is the sensation produced by light in a visual field that is considerably brighter than the light level to which the eyes are accustomed. Glare usually results in annoyance, discomfort, and loss of visual performance or visibility.

Luminous Environment and Visual Task–Oriented Design

Two general approaches are prevalent in lighting design: designing in relation to the luminous environment and designing in relation to visual tasks. They are fully compatible, and both should be considered in any evaluation.

General Guidelines

Spatial Function
Lighting must conform to activity. In a warehouse, activities may be driving a forklift and reading large package labels. In a law office, they may

include reading fine print in a contract. Both require different lighting levels, types, and coloration.

Quality and Quantity of Illumination
The designer should consider not only where a task is performed but also how the periphery is perceived. For example, the designer must determine how many lights are needed, how they should be shielded, and whether they will produce glare on any surface in the area.

Lighting Systems, Lighting Sources, and Luminaries
A practitioner involved in the redesign of an environment should consider not only the engineering specifications of the amount of lighting required and where it should be placed, but also whether the lighting should be local, general, supplemental, or task-ambient and whether the quality of the fixture should be direct, indirect, diffuse, or a combination of these qualities. The designer also must recognize other physical and environmental constraints, such as the amount of dust or dirt in the area and how color balancing will influence the task or the perception of space.

Control Systems
The designer must determine whether the lighting should be controlled in groups of lights or individually, where controls should be located in relation to traffic flow, and whether the controls should be discrete (on-off switch) or continuously dimmable.

Economics
The designer should consider the client's budget. For example, a solid brass fixture on a gold chain may complement marble floors, but less expensive recessed-can lighting may perform just as well. Although lighting plays a very important part in the overall perception of the environment and interaction within that environment, economic reality ultimately becomes a factor.

Integration with Mechanical and Acoustical Systems
The design of one system cannot be separated from that of the entire environment. Often, the ideal place for a lighting fixture is already occupied by an air-conditioning duct or sound barriers. Likewise, the location of a built-in fixture could force the relocation of a workstation and the disruption of an entire floor plan. All systems and the operational environment should be coordinated in the planning phase or closely examined, as would be the case in a retrofit design effort.

Integration with Furniture
In many work environments, ceiling lighting can also serve as supplemental lighting, and lighting fixtures can be built into the workstation furniture for tasks requiring more light. The built-in fixtures can serve as direct

task lighting, or they can throw diffuse lighting toward the ceiling to obviate the need for other freestanding fixtures.

Luminous Environment Design

Luminous environment design primarily focuses on aesthetics and is less oriented to tasks performed in the work space. The approach is typically implemented in three major steps.

Step 1: Determine the Visual Composition
Visual composition of space concerns focal centers, the overhead zone, the perimeter zone, the occupied zone, transitional zones, and levels of sensory stimulation.

Step 2: Determine the Desired Appearance of Objects
The appearance of objects in the design space is affected by light diffusion, sparkle, and apparent color rendition.

Step 3: Select Lighting to Accomplish Steps 1 and 2
The selection process is performed by reviewing an engineering study, an architectural study, and the architectural context of the lighting features.
    The engineering study examines

- Distribution characteristics and coloration of light
- Dimensional characteristics and form
- Lighted and unlighted appearance of other materials
- Initial and operating costs
- Maintenance
- Energy consumption

The architectural study examines

- Brightness, color, scale, and form
- Compatibility with the period of the design
- Space requirements and architectural detailing
- Coordination with other environmental systems

The architectural context of the lighting examines

- Visually subordinate lighting systems
- Visually prominent lighting systems

Reviewing the above steps and studies should help in the initial production of the intended design. Subsequent processes include mock-up, review, and design revision.

Visual Task–Oriented Design

The general approach of the visual task–oriented design is the same as that of the luminous environment design, but the focus is on enhancing the performance of tasks rather than making the environment aesthetically pleasing. The steps are typically as follows:

Step 1: Analyze Tasks for Their Visual Components

1. Identify common visual tasks performed in the environment.
2. Consider illumination methods required for these tasks:
   Diffuse or directional lighting
   Importance of shadows to provide a three-dimensional effect
   Susceptibility of the task to veiling reflections
   Importance of coloration of the lighting (e.g., does the lighting need to be daylight balanced)

Step 2: Analyze the Area Where Tasks Are Performed

1. Measure the dimensions of the area and determine the reflective qualities of the surfaces.
2. Determine the surface luminance required to minimize transition adaptation effects without providing a bland environment.
3. Determine whether the surfaces produce unwanted glare.
4. Determine whether uniformity in illumination is desirable, or whether spot effects could be used to focus attention more effectively.

Step 3: Select Light Fixtures

1. Determine the type of light distribution, control mechanism, and spectral quality needed to perform the task and provide a visually comfortable environment.
2. Determine the type of fixture needed to illuminate the work surfaces.
3. Decide how the lighting fixture should look and how it should be mounted.
4. Determine the atmosphere of the area and therefore the maintenance requirements; dusty, dirty, and greasy environments put specific demands on the type of fixture used and determine how often the fixtures need to be cleaned or replaced.
5. Determine the cost of the lighting system in relation to the budget.

Step 4: Calculate, Lay Out, and Evaluate

1. Arrange the lighting fixtures to best portray the task. Consider illuminance, direction of illumination, veiling reflections, and disabling glare.

2.   Arrange fixtures to provide the most comfortable situation for the worker. Consider visual and thermal effects and direct and reflected glare. Mobility and traffic patterns may also be factors here.
3.   Provide an aesthetically pleasing arrangement without impairing any of the prior design considerations.
4.   Determine energy management requirements.

Both the luminous environment design and visual task–oriented design approaches have merits. Regardless of the background of the analyst—architect or ergonomist—each approach should produce similar results when applied to most industrial or commercial environments. In most cases, both perspectives should be examined.

Light and the Use of Computers

With the introduction of computers and terminals to the work environment, some workers have assumed tasks and functions that have such a high degree of specialization that general guidelines not only do not suffice but also may do more harm than good. One such environment that has received much attention is the computer workstation. More than 50 million Americans use computers on a regular basis. Many of them often experience difficulty focusing on distant objects, a general blurring of vision beyond close range, eyestrain, irritated eyes, headaches, and intermittent blurring of images on the screen.

The two most common of these problems are the result of breakdowns of eye focus and abnormalities in eye coordination. In addition to physical symptoms, problems related to the visual stress of the task include posture-related changes such as neck, shoulder, and back pain; frequent loss of place while trying to concentrate; and excessive fatigue and irritability (Godnig and Hacunda 1991).

The problems associated with the use of a computer can be segmented into two categories: hardware related and software related. In some situations, the areas overlap. For example, the colors on the screen are generated by the hardware, but the specifications for the color are generated in the software. Beyond the physical problems of neck and back strain, psychological, perceptual, and other performance-related problems can be traced to either of these sources. For example, a common perceptual problem in the use of computers is color shift. After an operator views a source of light, such as a computer, for some time, an afterimage of the display remains in the user's vision. This is similar to but not as severe as the spot that remains in front of your eyes after your photograph is taken with a flash camera. In the case of a computer, the afterimage takes on the complementary color of the viewed image. For example, if you use a green screen background, a pinkish glow may persist for some time after looking away from the screen. Although this afterimage is harmless and dissipates in time, effects such as these may become important if supplemental tasks require the recognition of color-coded warnings.

Another perceptual problem that affects human performance during use of a computer is polarity. Polarity relates to the use of black letters on a bright screen or bright letters on a black screen. The most common configuration on many older computers was bright letters on a black screen. However, more recently, for tasks such as word processing, the foreground-to-background contrast provided by reverse polarity (black letters on a bright screen) and the similarity of this presentation style to that of print on paper makes text more readable than when the older, more conventional polarity is used. Unfortunately, that is where the similarity to paper ends. Looking at text on a computer screen is essentially equivalent to looking directly into a floodlight (rather than the ambient light reflected off this printed page). To eliminate the potential impact of eye fatigue, the user should be given the option of reversing the polarity or controlling the screen colors to fit various tasks.

A hardware-related problem that affects user performance is the luminance and contrast ratios of the screen and the interaction with the operating environment. Most monitors allow the user to adjust the brightness and contrast levels of the display. The user should be able to adjust the monitor to best perform in the ambient light. A standard for evaluating these limits is the 10-3-1 rule: the contrast ratio between the text on the screen and its background should be 10 to 1 (text 10 times brighter than the background). The overall brightness of the ambient environment should be three times brighter than the screen background (Godnig and Hacunda 1991).

Many other guidelines are associated with hardware in the design and use of computers as well as with general workstation design. Graphic interfaces and new software designs increase the use of pointing devices such as mice, trackballs, pen interfaces, and thumb balls. An entire field of design is developing for both hardware and software (American National Standards Institute 1987; International Organization for Standardization 1998).

Temperature

To remain alive, humans must be able to regulate their internal body temperature by keeping it within a very small range of temperatures. This balance is maintained by either taking in, retaining, or putting out heat from the body under the control of the body itself or the effects of the environment. The heat-balance equation that governs this process states that the body's metabolic heat production added to the retained heat from the external environment must equal the body's heat dissipation. Dissipation can take the form of evaporation, radiation, conduction, or convection. All these methods of dissipation depend on the internal and external environments of the body, and none can be fully defined without some reference to the environment.

Terminology and Measurement

Evaporation

The rate of evaporation of liquid from a surface is expressed as the volume of liquid dissipated from an area of that surface in a unit of time. A sample evaporation rate is 2 ml of water per minute per square inch of skin. Critical environmental factors involved in evaporation include surface air velocity, the relative and absolute temperatures of both the air and the evaporative surface, the composition of the surface, the amount of liquid at the surface available for evaporation, and the relative humidity of the air. The process of cooling by evaporation can be broken into two stages. The first is the conduction of fluid to the evaporative surface and the transformation of the fluid to a vapor. The second is the removal of the newly formed vapor by surface air currents. The first stage is commonly called *perspiration*; the second is known as *convection* and is related to the ambient air velocity.

Temperature

Temperature is a measurement of heat energy. It is also a measurement of the ability of one body to transfer heat to or receive heat from another body. In a two-body system, the body with the higher temperature loses heat to the other body. In environmental design, one body is typically the human operator in a system and the other body is either the mass of air that surrounds the operator or a piece of equipment the operator must use. In this context, a continuous exchange of heat occurs between the two bodies. Temperature is measured with a thermometer in degrees Celsius, Fahrenheit, or Kelvin. Two types of liquid-in-glass thermometers are commonly used for measuring temperature: dry-bulb and wet-bulb. Dry-bulb thermometers are conventional thermometers, with which most people are familiar. A wet-bulb thermometer is a dry-bulb thermometer whose bulb is surrounded by a water-soaked muslin wick. The wet-bulb measurement accounts for the evaporative quality of the air. As water evaporates from the wick, it takes the latent heat from the bulb with it. This cools the bulb and lowers the measured temperature by an amount that depends on the humidity of the surrounding air. The difference between the wet-bulb and dry-bulb temperatures is used to determine the relative humidity of the air.

Wet-Bulb Globe Temperature
One of the methods of heat exchange and dissipation is radiation. A body begins to radiate its own energy as it receives heat energy from another

body (such as the sun or a hot industrial furnace). According to the Stephan Boltzman law, radiant heat energy is a function of the gradient between the two temperatures raised to the fourth power. This law also applies to "black bodies"—those that radiate the maximum amount for a given temperature. For evaluating the radiative heat environment, a third type of thermometer, the black globe thermometer, is used to measure the globe temperature. This thermometer is a standard dry-bulb thermometer placed inside a black copper globe, adjacent to the wet- and dry-bulb thermometers.

When regulatory agencies examine environmental conditions, the wet-bulb globe temperature (WBGT) index is used as the most relevant parameter. It is calculated using the following equations:

- Indoor exposure or outdoor exposure with no solar load:

$$WBGT = 0.7\ WB + 0.3\ GT$$

- Outdoor sunlit exposure with solar load:

$$WBGT = 0.7\ WB + 0.2\ GT + 0.1\ DB$$

WB is the wet-bulb temperature obtained with a wetted sensor exposed to the natural air movement (unaspirated); *GT* is the globe temperature measured at the interior of a 6-in. black globe; and *DB* is the dry-bulb temperature (U.S. Department of Health, Education, and Welfare 1972.)

Effective Temperature
Effective temperature is an arbitrary index that combines the effects of temperature, humidity, and air movement to reflect the sensation of warmth or cold felt by the human body. The numerical value is the equivalent of the temperature of still, saturated air, which would induce an identical sensation.

Thermal Comfort

Thermal comfort is a function of both the effective temperature and a person's degree of acclimation to the particular environment.

Acclimation

Acclimation is an adaptive process of the body that results in reduced severity of the body's reactions to the stresses of exceptionally high or low temperatures. When first exposed to a hot environment, a person may have an impaired ability to work and may show evidence of physiologic strain. If the exposure is repeated for longer durations (e.g., over several days), the ability to work returns, and the evidence of physiologic strain decreases. Within the first 4–7 days after initial exposure, a dramatic improvement occurs in the ability to work, and physiologic responses such as body temperature and average heart rate decrease, blood pressure becomes stable, the subjective reaction of discomfort is reduced, and sweat is profuse and diluted. In general, a person who is in good physical condition will acclimate quickly, and an obese or overweight person will find adapting more difficult.

Design for Hot Environments

Designing for a hot environment requires consideration of the level of acclimation of the operators and the psychological effects of exposure to heat. Even a fully acclimated person who shows no decreased ability to perform physical work in a hot environment may still be affected by the heat and may show decreased psychological capability, including loss of mental initiative; decrease in accuracy of work performed (especially in an operator who was poorly motivated already); the need for greater concentration to perform a task; and the possibility of general personality changes (including irritability and a shortened temper). In addition to the design constraints imposed by the hot environment, many of the common items found in the work environment also serve to heighten the effects of the heat and pose a barrier to what might normally be a simple design problem. Care should be taken to investigate all of the barriers imposed by the work/task environment. These include protective gloves (which reduce an operator's ability to perform fine manipulative tasks and necessitate that equipment controls be farther apart than usual to allow for operation by a gloved hand) and possibly protective masks (which may reduce visibility and hearing and increase effects of heat).

Design for Cold Environments

When surroundings are exceptionally cold, the body must increase its metabolic output to maintain the heat-balance equation and may alter its internal blood distribution to protect the vital organs. The body begins to shiver and experiences pain and numbness and reduces blood flow to the extremities. All of this may result in a severe reduction in the ability to perform fine manipulative tasks. As in a hot environment, care should be taken to ensure that a system operator in a cold environment is fully acclimated before he or she assumes responsibility for any task. Additional clothing may restrict the operator in much the same way protective clothing does in a hot environment. In addition, operators in a cold environment may experience decreased mobility if additional clothing is required to stay warm.

Conclusion

Ergonomics requires the incorporation of knowledge of diverse topics. Additional research is almost always necessary to properly apply principles to new problems. The designer must remember that the environment is only one of the three factors that should be considered before a design is complete. Ignoring the role of human limitations, task performance requirements, or characteristics of equipment can be just as hazardous as ignoring the role of the environment.

References

American National Standards Institute (1987). Human Factor Standards for VDT Workstations. ANSI-STD-8001. Washington, DC: American National Standards Institute.

Cannon RH Jr (1967). Dynamics of Physical Systems. New York: McGraw-Hill.

Coermann RR (1962). The mechanical impedance of the human body in sitting and standing positions at low frequencies. Hum Factors 4:225–253.

Godnig EC, Hacunda JS (1991). Computers and Visual Stress: Staying Healthy. Grand Rapids, MI: Abacus.

Grether WF (1971). Vibration and human performance. Hum Factors 13:203–205.

International Labor Office (1980). Protection of Workers against Noise and Vibration in the Working Environment. ILO Codes of Practice. Geneva: International Labor Office.

International Organization for Standardization (1974). Guide for the Evaluation of Human Exposure to Wholebody Vibration. Report No. ISO 2631. International Organization for Standardization. New York. American National Standards Institute.

International Organization for Standardization (1998). Ergonomics Requirements for Office Work with Visual Display Terminals (VDTs). Report No. ISO 9241. International Organization for Standardization. New York: American National Standards Institute.

Kaufman JE, Haynes H (eds) (1982). Illuminating Engineering Society Lighting Handbook: Application. Baltimore: Waverly.

Kaufman JE, Haynes H (eds) (1984). Illuminating Engineering Society Lighting Handbook: Reference. Baltimore: Waverly.

May DN (1978). Handbook of Noise Assessment. Van Nostrand Reinhold Environmental Engineering Series. New York: Van Nostrand Reinhold.

Military Standard. Human Engineering Design Criteria for Military Systems, Equipment and Facilities (1989). MILSTD1472D. Washington, DC: U.S. Government Printing Office.

Peterson APG, Gross F.F. (1978). Handbook of Noise Measurement. Concord, MA: GENRAD.

Picone P (1983). Learning Systems and Pattern Recognition in Industrial Control. In EJ Kompass, TJ Williams (eds), Proceedings of the 9th Annual Advanced Controls Conference. Purdue University. Sept. 21–23, 1983. Barrington, IL: Dunn & Bradstreet.

Salvendy G (1987). Handbook of Human Factors. New York: Wiley, 650–669.

U.S. Department of Health, Education, and Welfare (1972). Criteria for a Recommended Standard: Occupational Exposure to Hot Environments. Washington, DC: U.S. Government Printing Office.

Woodson WE (1981). Human Factors Design Handbook: Information and Guidelines for the Design of Systems, Facilities, Equipment, and Products for Human Use. New York: McGraw-Hill.

Review Questions

(Answers are found in Appendix D.)

1. The three most important elements in ergonomic task design are
   (a) user, system equipment, and task
   (b) user, system equipment, and environment
   (c) task, system equipment, and environment
   (d) task, cost, and environment
   (e) cost, user, and environment

2. What frequency represents the third harmonic of a 500-Hz tone?
   (a) 125 Hz
   (b) 1,000 Hz
   (c) 1,500 Hz
   (d) 2,000 Hz
   (e) 5,000 Hz

3. Which of the following measures does not involve perception of (response to) a sound?
   (a) Noisiness
   (b) Loudness
   (c) Annoyance
   (d) Sound pressure level
   (e) All of the above

4. Luminous flux is the same as radiant flux.
   (a) True
   (b) False

5. Which measurement(s) should be used when evaluating a work site for thermal compliance with Occupational Safety and Health Administration standards?
   (a) Dry-bulb
   (b) Wet-bulb
   (c) Effective temperature
   (d) WBGT
   (e) All of the above

CHAPTER 8

Human Factors in Medical Rehabilitation Equipment: Product Development and Usability Testing

Valerie J. Berg Rice

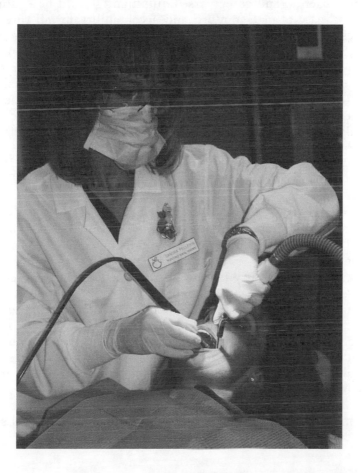

ABSTRACT

This chapter examines the development of an assistive walker to illustrate usability (user-acceptance) testing and to describe the process of usability testing. Product development has three phases: (1) initial development, (2) efficacy testing, and (3) comparison testing. These phases are equivalent to pilot, laboratory, and field testing and help ensure that the final product does what it was designed to do, is acceptable to the people who use it, and can be used easily. Each of these phases of product development involves a nine-step testing process. The objective of usability testing is to match the product with human capabilities, limitations, and acceptance to produce an environment or product that is user friendly.

Three groups that use medical and rehabilitation equipment are medical personnel, patients, and caregivers. Equipment should be evaluated for effectiveness, ease of use, comfort, and acceptability for all three groups. This process is called *usability testing* (also known as *evaluative testing* or *development research*). Usability is most effective when implemented throughout the development process. If necessary, however, it can be implemented during any of the stages of product development (Meister 1989). Usability testing provides valuable information for equipment design, recommendation, and purchase. Usability testing that helps provide an appropriate equipment design or work process can help prevent injuries, reduce human error during product use, and increase product sales.

Overview

Usability testing is the systematic evaluation of the "interaction between people and the products, equipment, environments, and services they use" and "is the fundamental principle that underpins all ergonomics" (McClelland 1990, p. 218). Usability testing also has been called *user-acceptance testing*, *user trials*, and *usability engineering* and is usually conducted by human factors engineers. Many products are developed by designers or engineers who assume their products are functional, easy to use, and acceptable. This assumption is often based on the designer's own knowledge or on the fact that the designer can easily use the product. Usability testing makes no such assumptions; it makes the user the most important influence on product design.

Usability testing typically focuses on evaluating the interface between user and machine. Examples include evaluating controls and displays on

automobile consoles or in aircraft cockpits, designing user-friendly software, and designing human-computer interfaces. Usability testing also can
be applied to products that are not considered machines, such as workstations (Davies and Phillips 1986; Stubler and Bernard 1986). Both complex
(e.g., anesthesia monitors and mammography machines) and simple (e.g.,
walkers and splints) equipment can benefit from experimental evaluation
that concentrates on users. User testing may or may not be conducted by
the equipment manufacturer. If such testing is not done, evaluation by a
team that includes medical, rehabilitation, and human factors/ergonomics
personnel can be beneficial.

Considerations

Users of health care equipment have different skills, abilities, knowledge,
and requirements (Bogner 1998); they range from physicians, technicians,
and rehabilitation specialists to patients and nonprofessional providers, such
as friends and family members. Caregivers caring for an older patient may
have impairments themselves. The physical and cognitive characteristics of
each user group, along with any symptoms of disease processes, must be
considered in the design of equipment. For example, diabetic retinopathy
may impair a diabetic person's ability to read the small pen and credit card
design displays on blood glucose meters (Bogner 1998). If the product is to be
used internationally, usability evaluations must be conducted in a variety of
settings. In many cases, adequate information about the target population is
not available, especially for special populations such as those with life-long
disabilities (Kumar and Rice 1998). Usability evaluations involving the
intended users are crucial in the design of medical and rehabilitation equipment to ensure safety and efficacy.

Usability testing applies equally to the design of procedures, processes,
and systems. A macroergonomic systems perspective addresses the entire
problem, rather than a small part. For example, standard operating procedures (SOPs) for patient treatment written for worst-case scenarios must
target ease of use, easy comprehension, availability, training, and so forth. If
a rehabilitation facility is located in a region with a significant Hispanic
population, emergency SOPs should also be printed in Spanish and employees should be able to communicate and understand emergency messages in
Spanish. Procedures guiding medical decision making can do much to prevent human error. Considering errors as evidence of the failure of a system
rather than the failure of an individual has been a more effective alternative
in reducing medically related human errors (Leape 1994; Reason 1990).

The context of device use is important (Moray 1994), and ecologic
validity (how closely the testing environment resembles the actual environment) is a significant consideration during usability testing. If users are

expected to operate equipment in adverse conditions, such as providing emergency medical care while on board an aircraft, the design should take factors such as lighting, print size, and equipment layout into account. Inadequate staffing, shift work, double shifts, or using contractors who are unfamiliar with particular devices or SOPs are relatively common and can result in failure to follow proper instructions, inadvertent operation of controls, failure to recognize critical circumstances, poor decision making, or lack of attention (Hyman 1994). Fail-safe designs may have multiple safety features to help avoid improper use of equipment or prevent the improper attachment of two pieces of equipment, which could occur in emergency (i.e., hurried) situations. Human factors/ergonomics considerations in the design of equipment and processes should be preventive. Demands of equipment set-up and adjustment, durability, maintainability, and interaction with other devices should be considered.

Iatrogenic injuries or illnesses are adverse effects resulting from medical procedures or medication that are not a direct or indirect complication of a patient's injury or illness (Perper 1994). Sometimes, iatrogenic injuries are the result of errors facilitated by inadequate labeling of a device or medication, inherent defects in the design of the device, or improper use of the equipment. Medical equipment associated with user problems and errors ranges from the relatively simple (syringes) to the complex (computer-controlled diagnostic equipment) (Nickerson 1992). Although the U.S. Food and Drug Administration has worked with both the industrial and the medical communities on human factors issues, most of these efforts focus on improvement of user performance instead of improving the design of the equipment itself (Hyman 1994). Well-designed usability testing is important, as the design of the equipment and the instructions for using the equipment may influence the occurrence of errors. Appropriate design may assist in preventing human error, even as proper design of rehabilitation equipment can encourage independence, boost self-esteem, and broaden abilities in activities of daily living, such as in the design of a lift-seat wheelchair (Bloswick et al. 1998).

Process

The first step in the usability testing process is to identify subject-matter experts (SMEs) and the user population (Figure 8.1, step 1). An SME is any person who can be a valid judge of a design by virtue of his or her experience, education, or research of system operations, job performance, or task dimensions. The investigators, SMEs, and representatives from the user group meet to define the project and ask questions about the product (see Figure 8.1, step 2). During this meeting, the groundwork is laid for development of design objectives and task and function analysis. Techniques used during meetings with user groups can include focus groups and user workshops (Jor-

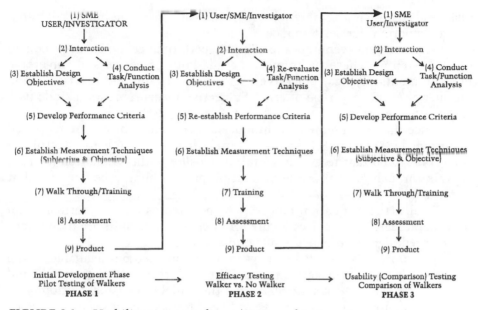

FIGURE 8.1.   Usability test procedures. (SME = subject-matter expert.)

dan 1994), informal discussions, interviews (structured or open-ended), questionnaires, brainstorming, checklists, and observations (Vianen et al. 1996).

The next two steps, which can occur simultaneously, are to identify design objectives and to conduct a task and function analysis (see Figure 8.1, steps 3 and 4). Design objectives focus on product features that affect performance, safety, expense, acceptance, comfort, ease of use, and aesthetics. Inclusion of these objectives in initial product development helps confirm that the product is effective, safe, and accepted by user groups before expensive investments are made in product creation. Changes are not easy to implement when the product is being manufactured. Design should be closely related to task and function analysis provided by investigators, users, and SMEs as a team. These are the critical success factors. Establishing critical success factors for the users and the producers of the equipment identifies usability as essential to ensuring a successful product. This lets the user and producer know that their problems and concerns are the focus of the design. During a task and function analysis, the task to be performed is evaluated according to the aspects that are most demanding, frequent, and essential for task completion. The analysis also identifies the pattern and sequence of tasks and subtasks.

The design objectives and the information from the task and function analysis are used for the fifth step, the development of performance criteria. Performance criteria should closely resemble the requirements of the task and should be performance oriented (action oriented). For example, a task analysis of an assembly job might indicate that fine-motor coordination is important for performance.

Measurement techniques to quantify performance are chosen (see Figure 8.1, step 6). These techniques include both objective and subjective measurements. Typical objective measurements include reaction time, number of errors, and type of error. Subjective measurements include user ratings of comfort, convenience, ease of use, and aesthetics.

Once the measurement techniques are chosen, subjects are recruited and trained (see Figure 8.1, step 7). Completing steps 1–6 before recruiting subjects is important to guarantee full disclosure of the evaluation process. A walk-through or trial of the evaluation process should be conducted at this time.

Finally, the evaluation process is conducted as either a formal or an informal research project (see Figure 8.1, step 8). The results are used to critique or redesign the product (see Figure 8.1, step 9).

The process is repeated as new information becomes available or the design is changed. A design is proposed, tested, rejected (or accepted), and revised repeatedly (Meister 1985). During the initial design and development, a number of prototypes may be developed and tested. Designs can be assessed using product description, mock-ups, prototypes (partial or full), or complete functional products. One or two design options are then chosen for rigorous evaluation. The evaluations can be categorized as experimental or nonexperimental, formal or informal, two-dimensional or three-dimensional, and nonperformance or performance oriented (Meister 1985).

An experimental evaluation requires measurement of subject performance under contrasting conditions in a controlled environment and use of experimental and statistical controls. A nonexperimental evaluation does not require contrasting conditions or strict controls. For example, evaluating a subject's reaction time and subjective reaction to several versions of a product in a laboratory is experimental. Having subjects complete a subjective rating scale while using a single product on the job is nonexperimental. Formal assessments have definite procedures and are well defined; informal assessments have less defined objectives and procedures. For example, a questionnaire is formal, but an open-ended group discussion is informal. Two-dimensional evaluations examine a product's attributes through checklists, whereas three-dimensional evaluations may use mock-ups or prototypes and can incorporate either nonperformance or performance measurements (Meister 1985).

An experimental evaluation of two or more prototypes determines which design is better or best according to user performance and preference. If only one product is evaluated, the assessment addresses the same design questions of effectiveness, ease of use, accomplishment of the mission, and deficits or areas that need improvement, but only for that one product.

As mentioned, an important aspect of usability testing is that it is performed during each stage of development. Even after the product is on the market, usability assessment can be conducted to ensure the product remains useful and effective. If product development occurred without usability testing, evaluation may be the first step in determining whether change is needed. The user population, especially patients, may not voice their concerns about the effectiveness of a product. This leaves the responsibility with the developers and SMEs. The information gained from a usability evaluation after the product is on the market can determine the need for product redesign and assist medical personnel in making recommendations. Information regarding the effectiveness, efficiency, and ease of use of a product is important in the recommendation of a product for purchase by a patient, a patient's family, or a medical facility.

Product Development, Efficacy Testing, and Comparison Testing of an Assistive Walker

Many patients use walkers to increase mobility. Many types of walkers are available. Some have features such as baskets, pouches for carrying small items, and drink holders. Some are balanced at the center handle; these walkers are designed for patients with hemiplegia and thus with limited use of one hand. Wheeled walkers may be especially beneficial during the early rehabilitation process, but it is difficult to know whether one with front wheels only or one with three wheels will best serve a patient. Other important features are the weight, portability, and stability of the walker and the height, shape, and size of the grip handles.

A therapist (investigator), for example, has an idea for a new walker design. Three iterations of the usability process are conducted. During the first iteration (product development), several variations of the new walker design are constructed and evaluated. This is prototype or pilot testing. Both the walker design and the testing process are evaluated. The information gained from the pilot test is used in the second iteration of the usability process, in which the best walker design (as determined during the pilot test) is evaluated (efficacy testing). This phase involves a more formal process of performance testing in a controlled setting to determine the effectiveness of the new walker. The final phase (comparison or field testing) involves a field study to determine user acceptance and performance. This testing is conducted in a setting similar to the environment in which the walker will be used (see Figure 8.1).

Each phase is considered usability testing. *Usability testing* means that the product is evaluated by obtaining information from representative users, often while they use the product. The goals of usability testing are to develop a product that (1) accomplishes the purpose for which it was designed, (2) is easy to use, and (3) will be used. The third goal involves factors, such as aesthetics, that influence whether a person chooses to use the product. In addition, the best design is one that does not require the user to study an instruction manual; instead, the design should guide the user's actions, so its use is intuitive.

First Iteration: Product Development

The goal of product development is to produce several design alternatives and to select one for additional evaluation. The first step is to identify the SMEs, users, and investigators (see Figure 8.1). This group could include product developers, medical personnel who have prescribed walkers for patients, therapists and nurses who work closely with patients who use walkers, family members of patients who use walkers, and the patients themselves. A target group of patients should be identified, because the needs of various groups, such as patients with hemiplegia and those with cerebral palsy, differ. For example, a patient who has problems with balance and coordination may not want wheels on his or her walker, and a patient who quickly becomes fatigued may need an attachable seat that folds while the patient is walking. Identification of a target group should be based on demographics; knowledge, skills, and experience; attitude; lifestyle; cognitive and physical abilities; and cultural background.

The second step is the interactive process between the investigators and the SMEs and users (see Figure 8.1). During this interaction, deficiencies in existing walker designs are identified and consequent research questions are developed. Positive aspects of existing walker designs may be identified and incorporated into the design objectives (see Figure 8.1, step 3). If the producers of the equipment have different aims, these also need to be identified. Such aims could include high sales, marketability, production location or costs, and user education or manual development.

Design objectives are developed as a result of the observations, replies to questionnaires, and discussions among SMEs, users, and investigators (Table 8.1). Design objectives should include any items considered important to enable full, practical use of the walker. The development of design objectives should answer the question, "What design features are important for a walker to be used by this target population?" The purpose of a walker is to assist people in walking by allowing them to stabilize themselves by putting some of their weight on the walker handles. Thus, the first objective should be stability. Secondary characteristics of the design are those that are important to a user but that may not influence the primary purpose of the product. An example is making the walker easily collapsible for placing in a car. Tertiary items include attractiveness and convenience. Convenience characteristics of a walker might include baskets or pouches for personal items and attachable trays to hold food or drinks.

Labeling design objectives as primary, secondary, and tertiary does not mean one level is more important than another. Secondary and tertiary items are important because they influence whether the product will be accepted and used. A product may help patients accomplish a task but be

TABLE 8.1
Design Objectives for Product Development

Primary
  Walker
    Lightweight
    Adjustable height
    Adjustable width
    Stability
  User
    Appropriate weight distribution
    Ability to maintain erect posture during use
Secondary
  Comfort
  Ease of use
  Ease of adjustment
  Ease of storage
  Portability
  Optimum grip height
    Shape
    Size
Tertiary
  Attractiveness
  Convenience

---

so difficult, inconvenient, or unattractive to use that people choose to do without it. The importance of individual design objectives should be determined by the combined interaction of the SMEs, users, and investigators.

While design objectives are being defined, a task and function analysis should be accomplished (see Figure 8.1, step 4). Information gained from establishing the design objectives should be used in conducting the task and function analysis and vice versa. The task and function analysis is based on input from users and SMEs. The investigator who conducts the assessment should observe the user performing a typical task and break the task into its component parts. These components should be described using action phrases. The design objectives and the information gained from the task and function analysis are used to develop performance criteria (see Figure 8.1, step 5).

Representative tasks are identified on the basis of criticality, frequency, and difficulty. The selected tasks can be used as independent variables (the different walkers are also independent variables). For this situation, the tasks chosen could include walking and maneuvering around items that block the user's path; entering, using, and exiting a rest room; and using a small set of stairs. The first task is used to test the walker prototypes. Performance criteria are developed from the selected task.

TABLE 8.2
Dependent Measurements for Product Development

Objective
  Walker weight
  Height adjustment
  Percentage of the target population who can use the walker
  Distance between walker legs
  Biomechanical analysis of weight distribution
  Material strength
Subjective
  Perceived stability
  Perceived comfort
  Perceived pain or strain
  Perceived exertion
  Perceived ease of use
  Perceived ease of adjustment
  Perceived portability
  Forced-choice rankings

The sixth step is to establish subjective and objective measurements. Because the first iteration is the development phase, only one task may be used to select the new design for the walker. Similarly, only the design objectives deemed most important may be used. The breadth and depth of the evaluation during the product-development stage are determined by the investigator. Consideration of costs and benefits assists the investigator in making the determination. For example, if construction of the walkers for additional testing is expected to be expensive, the testing should be thorough. If construction and possible alterations are relatively inexpensive, the prototype study may be smaller in terms of breadth and depth (or complexity).

Design objectives (dependent measurements) require both objective and subjective measurements. Dependent measurements for the sample situation are listed in Table 8.2. In addition to the measurements listed, the base and depth of the walker should be measured to determine walker stability. Many manufacturers list the weight capacity of walkers. If more information is required, however, material strength can be determined through consultation with an engineer familiar with the materials and construction of walkers. Subjective measurement techniques may include interviews, questionnaires, rankings, Likert scale ratings, or ratings by means of techniques such as magnitude estimation (Cordes 1984). Group interviews, rather than open-ended individual interviews, are often used to promote discussion (McClelland 1990). Forced-choice rankings, especially useful in the comparison of several designs, require the user to rank the designs in order of preference. Observations and ratings by the investigator can be helpful, but the investigator must take care not to bias the results.

Subject training and a walk-through of the testing process constitute the seventh step (see Figure 8.1). Enough training should be done to eliminate a learning (or practice) effect. Subjects should not continue to improve with time, regardless of experimental condition.

The eighth step is the actual assessment; in this case it involves a comparison study of several prototype walkers. Subjects perform one or more of the reference tasks, and the investigator collects and analyzes objective and subjective information. On the basis of the analysis, one design is usually selected for the next phase, efficacy testing. In the example, the walking task is evaluated in a nonexperimental, formal-informal, three-dimensional, and performance-oriented context. *Nonexperimental* means no statistical controls, even though contrasting conditions are used (one walker design compared with another). The comparison study contains both formal and informal elements: A formal procedure and questionnaire are used in addition to an informal interview session. The process is three-dimensional because prototypes of the walkers are used in a realistic task.

The goal of the evaluation (to identify one walker for additional testing) can be met with a relatively small number of participants. Subjects receive a detailed briefing, undergo a medical screening, and sign an informed-consent form. Each hospital or nursing facility usually has a human-use committee that determines the requirements for briefing, screening, and the format and contents of the consent form.

The experimental design is a repeated-measurements design, counterbalanced for order. The term *repeated-measurements design* means that each subject served as his or her own control and completed the task under each of the experimental conditions (various walker designs). Counterbalancing for the order in which each walker is used can be accomplished by using a balanced Latin-square design. This means each treatment condition (each walker design) is immediately preceded and followed once by each of the other conditions (Winer et al. 1991). This is often the preferred method to counterbalance a design without having to conduct tests of all possible ordering combinations. Another method of controlling for order effects is to randomize the order of administration.

Analysis of the subjective data can be accomplished by the use of nonparametric statistical analysis (Siegel 1956; Winer et al. 1991). Nonparametric statistical analysis is a useful tool for usability studies that collect subjective data and use small sample sizes. Parametric statistical analysis can be used for objective data when proper experimental design and sufficient population sampling are used. Considerable debate exists about using parametric statistics with subjective data (Anderson 1961; Gaito 1987; Westermann 1983).

TABLE 8.3
Hypothetical Results from Product Development

	Design 1	Design 2	Design 3
Load	6 lb	7 lb	16 lb
Height	17–37 in.	32–37 in.	30–38 in.
Weight distribution	Good	Good	Good
Material construction	350-lb capacity	375-lb capacity	500-lb capacity
Posture	Good	Good	Good
Stability	17.5*	12.2	14
Comfort	14.5	15.8	16
Pain or strain	12.1*	14.2	14.6
Ease of use	10.3	12.2	16.8*
Ease of adjustment	18.7*	16	14.8
Portability	16.5*	13.9	9.8
Ranking	1.25*	2.25	2.5

*Significantly different from other two walkers (p <.05).
Note: All ratings (except ranking) used a Borg-type scale with anchored subjective ratings 0–20 (Borg 1962). The lower number indicates less and the higher number indicates more of the given quality. Rankings were 1–3.

The results should clearly indicate the preferred design on the basis of user preference and performance data. The investigator may give a weighting factor to items considered to be of primary importance. For example, object load, adjustability, use by the greatest percentage of the target population, and biomechanical advantage may be weighted more than convenience and aesthetics.

As a result of the first iteration, design 1 is selected for additional testing (Table 8.3). The design is selected because it has the largest height range and is considered the most stable, adjustable, and portable. Its use caused the least pain and strain, and it was ranked the preferred walker. Note that design 1 was selected despite being the most difficult to use.

Second Iteration: Efficacy Testing (Controlled Setting)

The goal of efficacy testing is to determine whether the walker improves the user's ability to walk and maneuver through the activities of daily living. Therefore, testing consists of having subjects use the walker, as opposed to not using a walker, while performing several representative tasks. If the investigator believes that walkers have been shown to be effective ambulation tools and that such an evaluation would be superfluous, this phase can be eliminated. If this phase is eliminated, usability testing begins with a comparison between the new design and existing designs (usability [comparison] testing; see Figure 8.1, phase 3).

Identification of the SMEs and users was accomplished in the beginning of phase 1 (pilot testing); the experimental subjects now are added to the group as SMEs (see Figure 8.1, step 1). The interaction among SMEs, users, and the investigator should focus on the results of the pilot test (see Figure 8.1, step 2).

The design objectives for the walker most likely will remain the same as those identified in the development phase (see Table 8.1; see Figure 8.1, step 3). However, additional objectives can be identified in the pilot testing and in the interactions among the subjects, SMEs, and users.

The task and function analysis should be re-evaluated (see Figure 8.1, phase 2, step 4). The representative tasks can be altered on the basis of information gained during the development phase. For the second iteration of the process (efficacy testing), all three representative tasks are used to ascertain whether the new walker meets the functional goals. The tasks identified during the task or functional analysis are walking and maneuvering around items that block the user's path; entering, using, and exiting a rest room; and using a small set of stairs. Each task is completed in a controlled laboratory setting. In each task, performance criteria should provide information essential to successful performance and include objective and subjective data (see Figure 8.1, step 5). When the same criteria are used for product development, efficacy testing, and comparison testing, performance standards can be developed and product improvement can be monitored. Additional dependent measurements in the example include time to complete each element of the task, time to complete the entire procedure, heart rate, and perceived exertion (Borg 1962, 1970, 1978) (Table 8.4).

In the example, the same objective and subjective measurement techniques used during the development phase are used during efficacy testing (see Table 8.2; see Figure 8.1, step 6). The first task is walking and maneuvering around items that block the user's path and involves the following procedures: rising from an easy chair, turning right, walking 5 feet and maneuvering to the left of a chair that blocks the path, walking 4 feet and maneuvering right to avoid a child's toy, walking another 5 feet, and sitting in a kitchen chair.

In addition to the primary task of walking, important secondary tasks should be included in the testing procedure. For example, if the walker is used to enable someone to move between a desk and a filing cabinet, such a task pattern should be incorporated into the testing procedure.

Again, subjects should be trained in each task used in the test procedure (see Figure 8.1, step 7). Because more than one task is being studied (walking, maneuvering in a rest room, and using stairs), the order of the tasks should be balanced to control for order effects, such as transfer of learning or a conditioning effect. Training of test subjects in testing procedures also decreases the likelihood that learning effects will influence the study results.

TABLE 8.4
Hypothetical Results from Efficacy Testing: Walking and Maneuvering Task

	Walker	*No Walker*
Total time	9.2 mins	15.6 mins
Get up	1 min	2 mins
Turn right	0.45 min	1.2 mins
Walk 5 ft	1.5 mins	2.6 mins
Walk around chair	0.6 min	1.5 mins
Walk 4 ft	1.3 mins	2 mins
Avoid toy	1 min	1.9 mins
Walk 5 ft	1.77 mins	2.9 mins
Sit in chair	1.4 mins	1.5 mins
Heart rate	145 beats/min	155 beats/min
Perceived exertion	15.8*	18.3
Stability	19.7*	5.1
Comfort	18.5*	6.7
Pain or strain	5.5*	14.2

*Significantly different from no walker ($p < .05$).
Note: All ratings (except ranking) used a Borg-type scale with anchored subjective ratings 0–20 (Borg 1962). The lower number indicates less and the higher number indicates more of the given quality.

After training, the actual assessment (experimental evaluation) takes place. Task performance should be evaluated by timing and accuracy data. In the example, efficacy testing is experimental, formal, three-dimensional performance testing. As with any research method, consistency in experimental testing must be ensured in subject training, measurement techniques, and data compilation. Two excellent resources on these topics are Winer et al. (1991) for laboratory studies and Cook and Campbell (1979) for field studies.

During efficacy testing, the number of subjects will probably be greater than the number who participated in the pilot test. Adequate results can be obtained with a relatively small number of subjects, especially because this is a repeated-measurements study. Statistical analysis can include a repeated-measurements analysis of variance and post hoc testing.

The results should give the investigator clear information about the efficacy of use of the walker (as opposed to no walker) in terms of both the subjects' performances and their preferences. Efficacy testing provides information on the benefits and limitations of using the walker in three different situations for men and women. Initial results suggest that the walker is beneficial (see Table 8.4). The subjects performed the task more quickly; experienced less subjective exertion, less pain and strain, more stability, and more comfort; and had a lower heart rate when they used the walker than when they did not use the walker. The final output is the product (see Figure 8.1, step 9), which is re-evaluated by the research team.

Third Iteration: Comparison Field Testing

The second iteration of the usability cycle (efficacy testing) revealed that the walker was helpful in improving ambulation and maneuvering in using a rest room. However, the following concerns were identified during testing:

1. The gripping edge of the walker was uncomfortable and caused pain on the thenar eminence during ambulation.
2. Subjects requested a handle material that does not feel cold to the touch and comes in different colors.
3. Subjects requested detachable accessories, such as a tray for holding objects, a recessed cup holder, and a basket with adjustable sections.
4. The fold-up seat was weak and unstable and did not have appropriate contour or padding.

The concerns must be discussed by SMEs, subjects, users, and investigators (see Figure 8.1, steps 1 and 2). The cost of product development and the purchase price must be considered along with the preferences expressed. The changes that can be made are incorporated, and a new walker is constructed (see Figure 8.1, step 3). The new design must then be re-evaluated in the type of environment in which it is to be used. In addition, the investigator should compare this design with that of other walkers available on the commercial market (usability [comparison] testing; see Figure 8.1, phase 3).

A review of the task and function analysis reveals that the assistance provided by the walker is most pronounced during the walking task. Because both the old and the new design objectives can be tested by walking, this task is chosen as representative (see Figure 8.1, step 4). The purpose of the comparison field testing is to compare one or more designs with each other in a realistic environment. The investigator can compare the findings obtained when a subject uses the new walker design with the findings obtained when no walker is used to verify the results of the efficacy test in a realistic environment.

The task in comparison testing should be similar to the task used during efficacy testing in the laboratory. The tests can be conducted in nursing homes where throw rugs, narrow halls, and wheel chairs are obstructions. It can also be conducted in a work setting where storage cabinets are located in the halls, ramps are located between split-level floors, and low-level ambient light is used. The most appropriate setting for the target group is determined by the users, SMEs, and the investigator. If users are required to perform additional tasks or carry objects, these tasks are included in the evaluation (see Figure 8.1, step 5). The objective and

172   *Ergonomics for Therapists*

TABLE 8.5
Hypothetical Results of Walker Subjective Ratings

	New Design	Walker A	Walker B
Stability	18.8	17.7	19
Comfort	15.3*	12.3	14
Pain or strain	8.9*	17.3	16.2
Ease of use	15	15.9	16.5
Perceived exertion	16.4	15	15.2
Ranking	1.25*	2.5	2.25

*Significantly different from other two walkers (p <.05).
Note: All ratings (except ranking) used a Borg-type scale with anchored subjective ratings 0–20 (Borg 1962). A lower number indicates less and a higher number indicates more of the indicated quality. Rankings are 1–3.

subjective measurement techniques are the same as those used during efficacy testing to verify results (see Figure 8.1, step 6).

Training and walk-through of the test situation are conducted because the conditions have changed from a laboratory-based evaluation to a field test. Training helps prevent mistakes during testing and eliminates a learning effect (see Figure 8.1, step 7). The assessment is the eighth step, and applying the data obtained to the product design is the ninth step.

The results of the comparison test in the example were as follows: The new design was ranked as the preferred walker compared with the other two walkers. The subjects' heart rates were lower with the new design. Subjects completed the task faster when they used the new design; however, time to stand and sit was slower. Subjects found the new design easier to use. Use of the new design increased comfort and decreased pain and strain. No differences were found for ratings of stability, perceived exertion, or performance of ancillary tasks. These results showed the new design to be superior for ambulatory assistance as measured by user preference and performance (Table 8.5).

Conclusion

Usability testing of medical or rehabilitation equipment is an essential component of product development but is often neglected. This neglect becomes obvious when practitioners or patients attempt to use the product. Without user testing, products are often difficult to use, cannot be used intuitively, are not comfortable, and demonstrate that they are not made for all categories of users, such as technicians, medical practitioners, and patients. The importance of usability testing of medical equipment has become widely recognized, as evidenced by its consideration as one criterion for approving products and setting international and national standards (McClelland 1990). Fortunately, testing and designing evaluative and treatment equipment (Jeng and Radwin 1998), devices for special populations (Bull et al. 1989; Das 1998; Everly et al. 1998), and technology for groups that consider themselves technically challenged (Czaja 1998) have gained the attention of a number of human factors/ergonomics practitioners.

Medical professionals often design equipment based on their experience with patients or according to individual patient needs but fail to complete the design sequence by conducting systematic user tests. Rather than have complete knowledge of the success of the product, they have two sets of opinions: their own and those of the patients with whom they work. Little attempt is made to make the product effective for a broad patient population.

Usability testing provides a mechanism to evaluate a product from a user's perspective. The procedure should be used to assess all rehabilitation and medical equipment. Usability testing should include factors such as ease of operational learning, effectiveness, efficiency, flexibility, maintainability, durability, safety, and task matching with user characteristics. Manufacturers, practitioners, and instructors in professional programs should begin introducing the concepts and procedures of usability testing to improve patient care.

References

Anderson NH (1961). Scales and statistics: parametric and nonparametric. Psychol Bull 58:305–316.

Bloswick DS, Shirley B, King E (1998). Medical and Rehabilitation Equipment Case Study: Design, Development, and Usability Testing of a Lift-Seat Wheelchair. In VJB Rice (ed), Ergonomics in Health Care and Rehabilitation. Boston: Butterworth–Heinemann, 249–262.

Bogner MS (1998). An Introduction to Design, Evaluation, and Usability Testing. In VJB Rice (ed), Ergonomics in Health Care and Rehabilitation. Boston: Butterworth–Heinemann, 231–247.

Borg GA (1962). Physical Performance and Perceived Exertion. Lund, Sweden: Gleerup.

Borg GA (1970). Perceived exertion as an indicator of somatic stress. Scand J Rehabil Med 2:92–98.

Borg GA (1978). Subjective aspects of physical and mental load. Ergonomics 21: 215–220.

Cook TT, Campbell DT (1979). Quasi-Experimentation: Design and Analysis Issues for Field Settings. Boston: Houghton Mifflin.

Cordes RE (1984). Use of Magnitude Estimation for Evaluating Product Ease-of-Use. In E Grandjean (ed), Ergonomics and Health in Modern Offices. New York: Taylor & Francis.

Czaja SJ (1998). Gerontology Case Study: Designing a Computer-Based Communication System for Older Adults. In VJB Rice (ed), Ergonomics in Health Care and Rehabilitation. Boston: Butterworth–Heinemann, 143–154.

Das B (1998). Physical Disability Case Study: An Ergonomics Approach to Workstation Design for Paraplegics. In VJB Rice (ed), Ergonomics in Health Care and Rehabilitation. Boston: Butterworth–Heinemann, 123–142.

Davies DK, Phillips MD (1986). Assessing User Acceptance of Next Generation Air Traffic Controller Workstations. In Proceedings of the Human Factors Society. 30th Annual Meeting. Santa Monica, CA: Human Factors Society.

Everly JS, Bull MJ, Stroup KB (1998). Consumer Product Case Study: Development of Child Safety Seats for Children with Hip Dysplasia. In VJB Rice (ed), Ergonomics in Health Care and Rehabilitation. Boston: Butterworth–Heinemann, 279–286.

Gaito J (1987). Measurement scales and statistics: resurgence of an old misconception. Psychol Bull 101:159–165.

Hyman WA (1994). Errors in the Use of Medical Equipment. In MS Bogner (ed), Human Error in Medicine. Hillsdale, NJ: Erlbaum, 327–347.

Jeng O, Radwin RG (1998). Development of a Functional Test Battery for Carpal Tunnel Syndrome. In VJB Rice (ed), Ergonomics in Health Care and Rehabilitation. Boston: Butterworth–Heinemann, 263–278.

Jordan PW (1994). Focus Groups in Usability Evaluation and Requirements Capture: A Case Study. In SA Robson (ed), Contemporary Ergonomics 1994. Bristol, NJ: Taylor & Francis, 449–453.

Kumar S, Rice VJB (1998). Ergonomics for Special Populations: An Introduction. In VJB Rice (ed), Ergonomics in Health Care and Rehabilitation. Boston: Butterworth–Heinemann, 113–122.

Leape LL (1994). The Preventability of Medical Injury. In MS Bogner (ed), Human Error in Medicine. Hillsdale, NJ: Erlbaum, 13–26.

McClelland I (1990). Product Assessment and User Trials. In JR Wilson, EN Corlett (eds), Evaluation of Human Work: A Practical Ergonomics Methodology. New York: Taylor & Francis.

Meister D (1985). Behavioral Analysis and Measurement Methods. New York: Wiley.

Meister D (1989). Conceptual Aspects of Human Factors. Baltimore: Johns Hopkins University Press.

Moray N (1994). Error Reduction as a Systems Problem. In MS Bogner (ed), Human Error in Medicine. Hillsdale, NJ: Erlbaum, 67–91.

Nickerson RS (1992). Looking Ahead: Human Factors Challenges in a Changing World. Hillsdale, NJ: Erlbaum.

Perper JA (1994). Life-Threatening and Fatal Therapeutic Misadventures. In MS Bogner (ed), Human Error in Medicine. Hillsdale, NJ: Erlbaum, 27–52.

Reason J (1990). The Contribution of Latent Human Failures to the Breakdown of Complex Systems. Philo Trans Royal Soc London 327:475–484.

Siegel S (1956). Nonparametric Statistics for the Behavioral Sciences. New York: McGraw-Hill.

Stubler WF, Bernard TE (1986). Office Ergonomics: Design Methodology and Evaluation. In Proceedings of the Human Factors Society. 30th Annual Meeting. Santa Monica, CA: Human Factors Society.

Westermann R (1983). Interval-scale measurement of attitudes: some theoretical conditions and empirical testing methods. Br J Math Statistic Psychol 36:228–239.

Winer BJ, Brown DR, Michels KM (1991). Statistical Principles in Experimental Design. New York: McGraw-Hill.

Suggested Reading

Bailey RW (1982). Human Performance Engineering. Englewood Cliffs, NJ: Prentice Hall.

Benel DCR, Pain RF (1985). The Human Factors Usability Laboratory in Product Evaluation. In Proceedings of the Human Factors Society. 29th Annual Meeting. Santa Monica, CA: Human Factors Society.

Bogner MS (1994). Human Error in Medicine. Hillsdale, NJ: Erlbaum.

Brown CR, Schaum DL (1980). User-Adjusted VDU Parameters. In E Grandjean, E Vigliani (eds), Ergonomic Aspects of Visual Display Terminals. New York: Taylor & Francis.

Kantowitz BH, Sorkin RD (1983). Human Factors: Understanding People-System Relationships. New York: Wiley.

Jordan PW, Thomas B, Weerdmeester BA, McClelland IL (1996). Usability Evaluation in Industry. Bristol, PA: Taylor & Francis.

Rice VJB (1998). Ergonomics in Health Care and Rehabilitation. Boston: Butterworth–Heinemann.

Salvendy G (ed) (1987). Handbook of Human Factors. New York: Wiley.

Schneiderman B (1987). Designing the User Interface: Strategies for Effective Human-Computer Interaction. Reading, MA: Addison-Wesley.

Whiteside J, Bennett J, Holtzblatt K (1988). Usability Engineering: Our Experience and Evolution. In M Helander (ed), Handbook of Human-Computer Interaction. Amsterdam: North Holland.

Review Questions

(Answers are found in Appendix D.)

1. A friend has asked you to define usability testing to her son and daughter who are in high school. Do so in five sentences or less.

2. In usability testing on medical and rehabilitation equipment, what user groups should be considered?

3. If a patient inadvertently injures him- or herself when using a product at home, why would the health care worker not just retrain the patient or warn him or her that such a mistake could cause an injury?

4. What are *context* and *ecologic validity*? Why are they important in usability testing?

5. Why is usability testing considered an "iterative" process?

6. What are the steps recommended for usability testing?

PART **III**

Special
Considerations

CHAPTER 9
Lifting Analysis

Diane Aja and Krystal Laflin

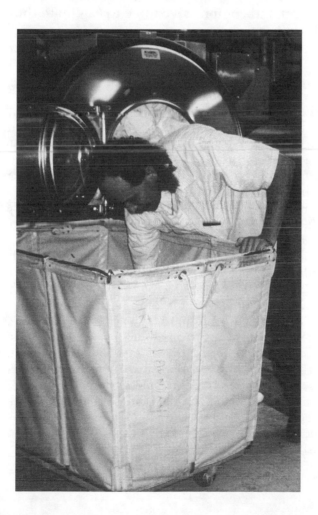

ABSTRACT

Lifting is one of the most common physical tasks in work environments. Therapists involved with injury prevention and injury management programs should be familiar with the causes of lifting injuries, personal risk factors as they relate to lifting, types of lifting techniques, and the variety of lifting assessments. This chapter reviews two methods for assessing safe lifting. The 1981 lift formula published by the National Institute of Occupational Safety and Health (NIOSH) has been revised on the basis of research and recommendations from health care providers and ergonomics specialists; the new formula (NIOSH 1991) changes some of the original criteria and includes methods to account for asymmetric lifting and coupling. A second formula, developed by Bloswick, uses the concepts of moment and compressive force to calculate the impact of lifting and lowering tasks, including moving clients.

The treatment and prevention of low back pain (LBP) has received increased attention. Much research has gone into the biomechanical analysis of structure and function of the back in lifting. As a result, a number of models have been presented for assessing individual lifting capacity and predicting lifting stresses through task analysis. Despite these efforts, back injuries have continued to occur at an alarming rate. In 1989 in the United States, an estimated 45 million days (approximately 40% of all work days missed) were missed because of back pain, costing an estimated $14 billion (Peterson 1990). In addition, a total of $20 billion is spent on the management of LBP annually (Webster and Snook 1990).

Injuries occur when physical demands of a job exceed the worker's strength (Anderson 1985). Lifting injuries account for 15–65% of work-related LBP. Eighty percent to 90% of those with idiopathic back pain recover within 6 weeks. The remaining 5–10% account for 70–80% of societal costs caused by lifting injuries (Nachemson 1992). Regular heavy lifting has been shown to result in injury rates eight times those of the normal population (Mayer et al. 1988). Post–job offer screening tests have been one method used to correctly identify persons who possess the capabilities of meeting or exceeding the job requirements, reducing the risk of injury by as much as two and one-half times (Keyserling et al. 1980; Laflin et al. 1997; Perry et al. 1994). The significant role psychosocial factors play in incidence and recovery from injury should also be kept in mind (Nachemson 1992).

Causes of Lifting Injuries

Lifting injuries can be caused by traumatic events, overexertion, and cumulative stress. In addition to prolonged sitting and psychosocial stresses, activities that involve pushing, pulling, using extreme postures such as forward flexion, and cyclic loading (whole body vibration) are associated with the development of LBP and impairment. Bending combined with lifting has been shown to be the most common cause of LBP. Lifting done above the chest may cause excessive stress to the shoulder and wrist joints as well as increase arching of the back, resulting in increased loading on the facet joints. The most efficient height for lifting is 40–60 in. Combinations of lifting and twisting increase the risk of herniated discs by loading the posterior annulus. Pushing and pulling can also result in high disc loads. The friction between shoes and the floor has a significant effect on static and dynamic strength relative to push-pull tasks. The ideal height for push-pull tasks is 35.5–44.5 in. Prolonged sitting or standing increases muscle fatigue and stress to the disc. Repeated stress from compressive loads is thought to cause microtrauma to the vertebral end plate and cartilage and lead to weakening of the annulus fibrosus, which may eventually protrude into the spinal canal. Some claim that 70–80% of all chronic LBP is due to discogenic problems either resulting in nerve root encroachment or facet dysfunction caused by altered biomechanics. Shear forces resulting from flexion, extension, lateral flexion, and rotation during lifting tasks are resisted by the annulus and the facet joints. Any disc changes, such as narrowing, result in increased facet joint stress. Compressive strength of the vertebral body depends on the weight lifted relative to the projected compressive strength and the duration and rate of the applied stress. With repetitive loading below 30% of compressive strength, the spine can tolerate up to 5,000 cycles compared to only a few cycles at loads above 70% of compressive strength.

Acute traumatic events may be caused by slips, trips, falls, unexpected weight shifts, equipment failure resulting in loss of grip, or unexpected motions to catch an object or regain balance. Although regular safety training can enhance awareness and responsibility for environmental conditions, total elimination of these incidents is unlikely. Traumatic injuries can be severe and often lead to chronic disability (NIOSH 1981).

Overexertion occurs when the task exceeds worker strength or the physiologic limit of a structure. Many authors have documented the effects of lifting stresses on various anatomic structures, including ligaments, muscles, vertebral bodies, intervertebral discs, facet joints, and the vertebral end plates. The use of the NIOSH lift formula in conjunction with normative tables for lifting as developed by Snook and Ciriello (1991) can predict safe lifting limits and aid in job redesign. Lifting injuries related to overexertion can also be minimized through post–job offer screening.

The term *cumulative trauma disorder*, often associated with upper extremity injuries, has also been used to describe low back disorders. Cumulative stress from repeated forces over a prolonged period to the same muscle group, joint, or tendon can result in soft-tissue microtears and trauma. An inflammatory response is initiated as a result of these injuries. Prolonged inflammation may lead to tendon and synovial disorders, muscle tears, ligamentous disorders, excessive scar tissue development, degenerative joint disease, bursitis, or nerve entrapment. Genaidy et al. (1993) developed a formula to calculate spinal compression tolerance limits, defining *spinal compression tolerance* (also known as *compressive strength*) as the maximum compressive load imposed on the spine before the compression leads to the failure of one or more of its parts (e.g., vertebral body, intervertebral disc, and vertebral endplate). The lumbar spine has the highest spinal compression values, followed by the thoracic spine and the cervical spine. Many researchers have supported the theory that the compressive strength of the vertebral bodies is much lower than that of the intervertebral discs. Complex loading such as bending and twisting result in much lower spinal compression tolerance limit values. Because it is used to calculate the load at which microtrauma occurs, the formula developed by Genaidy et al. may be more protective than the NIOSH lift formula, which is used to calculate the load at which failure may occur (Laflin and Aja 1995). The Genaidy et al. formula was designed to be used as an adjunct to biomechanical approaches, such as those proposed by Chaffin and Anderson (1984) and Bloswick (1993), in calculating compressive forces of a given task.

Variables that contribute to increased stress and cumulative trauma must be considered in designing lifting tasks. In addition to the variables outlined by NIOSH (horizontal reach, vertical height, travel distance, asymmetry of motion, coupling, and frequency), physiologic factors must also be considered. Muscle effort greater than 40% of maximal voluntary contraction affects blood flow and the rate of local muscle fatigue. Inadequate recovery time also can impair circulation and muscle recovery, contributing to fatigue and strain. Tasks should be designed to keep maximum voluntary effort low and avoid sustained awkward positions. Personal risk factors complicate the stresses on the low back. These include, age, gender, anthropometry, physical fitness level, medical history, smoking, psychosocial factors, and lifting technique.

Personal Risk Factors

Age

Muscle strength peaks between the ages of 20 and 30 and decreases progressively thereafter. Lower body strength declines more than upper body strength does. In a study cited by Hogan (1980), the maximal strength of a

65-year-old person is 80% of his or her original strength at age 20. With age, bone density decreases, a generalized decline in range of motion occurs, gel is lost from the nucleus, and disc degeneration increases. The majority of studies have shown that the incidence of LBP is highest in the 30s and 40s, increases up to age 49, then drops substantially. Recurrences, duration of symptoms, and length of disability increase with age (Garg et al. 1990).

Gender

On the average, women's lifting strengths (primarily arm and torso) are about 60% of men's. Women's lower extremity strength and cardiovascular endurance is 70% of men's. Generally, the larger the cross-sectional area of a muscle, the greater the maximal strength. Men's muscles generally tend to be larger than women's. Specific analysis of upper extremity and lower extremity differences reveal a much greater range that may have implications in job design. Strength differences have been analyzed based on static and dynamic measures. In static analysis, women demonstrate a higher percentage of strength in pulling versus pushing. Static upper extremity strength of women varied between 35% and 79% of men, with a mean of 55.8%. In dynamic assessment of the upper extremity, women's strength ranged from 59% to 84% of men's, with a mean of 68.6%. Static trunk strength for women was between 37% and 70% of men's, with an average of 63.8%. Lower extremity static strength for women was between 57% and 86% of men's, with a mean of 72%. These differences should be considered when assessing job risk and performance for men and women relative to a specific task. Overall, greater fatigue and physical stress can be expected when women are required to perform equally to men in medium-heavy to heavy job categories (Garg et al. 1990).

Anthropometry

Little evidence exists to support the notion that body weight or size has a direct correlation to frequency of back incidents. Body weight does contribute to increasing joint stress and can lead to premature degenerative changes that may increase the biomechanical stress on the low back and result in LBP. Large stature, especially a protruding abdomen, can prevent proper positioning on the job, increasing horizontal lifting stresses that increase compressive forces on the back. Heavier individuals exert more energy to lift and carry loads, thereby increasing fatigue and leading to strain. Mass generally confers an advantage in pushing-pulling and counterbalancing loads (Garg et al. 1990).

Job-site demands can be greater for the short or tall worker, increasing biomechanical stress. Most work environments are designed for an average-sized man (5 ft 9 in. tall) and an average-sized woman (5 ft 5 in. tall) (Grandjean 1988). Horizontal loads, vertical stress, and awkward positioning are more likely for individuals outside of the "normal" range.

Medical History

Recurrence of back symptoms has been reported to be between 50% and 60% in the first 5 years and to taper off after that. Individuals with a history of back pain have an increased risk for injury and should not engage in heavy lifting (Nachemson 1992).

Smoking has been thought to be related to a higher incidence of back pain and a slower recovery time from injury. Speculation about the physiologic reason has varied. Frymoyer et al. (1983) suggest that smoking may reduce the vertebral-body blood flow, impairing vertebral body and disc nutrition, increasing these structures' susceptibility to injury, and slowing healing.

Psychosocial factors have been shown to play a major role in incidence of injury as well as the extent of disability from an injury. Job satisfaction, relationship with employees, and home stress have also been shown to predict back-injury claims and length of disability (Frymoyer and Cats-Baril 1987).

Lifting Technique

The combination of lifting, bending, and twisting is the most frequent cause of back injury. In 25–70% of back injuries, lifting, lowering, pushing, pulling, and carrying have been implicated as causes (NIOSH 1991). The weight of the load, force required, frequency, shape, size of the load, stability of the load, asymmetry of the lift, and sudden unexpected maximal efforts are some of the factors that have been reported to increase the likelihood of injury. Marras and Mirka (1989) showed that as trunk asymmetry increases, overall strength (isometric, concentric, and eccentric) decreases at the rate of 8–9% of maximum for every 15 degrees of asymmetry increase. Trunk strength was found to be greatest at 22.5 degrees of flexion and was shown to decrease 7–10% as the trunk became more upright or more flexed.

Several lifting strategies have been described: the back or stoop lift (knees straight and back bent), deep squat lift with back straight or flexed back (knees flexed more than 90 degrees), freestyle or partial squat with back straight (knees flexed no more than 90 degrees), trunk kinetic lift (from a deep squat, the hips and pelvis move first), two-stage leg lift or leg roll (from a deep squat, the weight is transferred to one or both thighs, then lifted), and the golfer's lift for very light loads (one arm is used as support while the lifter is bending forward with a straight back pivoting around the hip joint of the straight leg) (Brooks 1995; NIOSH 1991). The most popular styles discussed in the literature are the squat lift with the back either in slight lordosis or the back more kyphotic, the freestyle posture, the bent or stooped lift, the weight lifter's lift, and the golfer's lift for light loads. NIOSH has reported that little evidence exists to identify one lifting technique as correct. Rigidity in teaching can often lead to more stress on the spine as well as other structures, such as the knees and the cardiovascular system. Because of the variability of compliance in the workplace with rote teaching of lifting techniques (Carlton 1987; St. Vincent et al. 1989), a more reasonable approach would be to teach concepts related to the ergonomics of lifting, paying particular attention to the horizontal load, which is the major contributor to spinal stress during lifting. Adaptation of technique should consider an individual's leg strength, body size, cardiovascular status, and condition of the spine and other bony structures. The stresses on the patella femoral structures, determined by moment arm calculations, can be very high and potentially damaging with a squat lift. In addition, repetitive lifting from a squat position is metabolically more demanding and can lead to earlier fatigue.

The training programs that result in increased job satisfaction and compliance are those that actively involve the employees in design and implementation of ergonomic solutions. Lecture alone can lead to increased job dissatisfaction, particularly if management does not implement ergonomic changes, and an increase in injury reporting can occur (King et al. 1997). This theory is supported in part by Carlton (1987) and St. Vincent et al. (1989), who found that instructions in body mechanics and practice in the clinic had no carryover in the work environment. The technique taught was very rigid and advocated a straight back and deep squat. McCauley (1990) found that body mechanics practice at work did result in carryover in the work environment. A weakness of McCauley's (1990) and Carlton's (1987) studies is that the time frame between teaching and testing was only 1 month.

Lifting speed can affect the degree of compression on the lumbar spine. An assessment of three different lifting strategies and their effects on control of the motion patterns and external joint loads stated that the average speed per a submaximal lift was 1.4 seconds (Hsiang and McGorry 1997). Although weight lifters may use inertia and speed to their advantage to keep the weight accelerating, decreasing the amount of exertion needed at the transitional level around waist height, high-speed lifting and jerking especially with a twist may easily tear the capsular ligaments of the facet joint. An increase in speed associated with lifting results in a decrease in maximum voluntary muscle strength. In general, the literature reports that lifts should be done as close to the body as possible in a slow, controlled manner (Garg et al. 1990).

Squat Lift

The squat lift with a straight or slightly lordotic back (back bowed in) or with the back horizontal or flexed at the hips appears to be most popular in client educational programs. The premises of this lift are as follows:

1.   The object can be held close to the body, thereby minimizing the compressive forces and spinal bending moment on the back.
2.   Erector spinae (ES) muscle activity is thought to reduce the stress on the posterior inert structures of the spine.
3.   The legs are at a mechanical advantage to assist with lifting of the load.
4.   The weight of the body is used to initiate horizontal motion during the lift (Delitto et al. 1987).

Proponents of a more kyphotic (i.e., back bowed out) position for lifting contend that the ES muscles are more quiescent during the lift, thereby reducing the compressive forces on the spine. This posture also minimizes the flexion movement of the spine by tension in the posterior ligaments, lumbodorsal fascia, and latissimus muscle, which results in decreasing ES muscle activity. NIOSH (1991) reports that a bent spine increases the shearing forces on the L5-S1 disc, the articular facets, and the annulus fibrosis.

Shear force is described in two ways: load shear and joint shear. *Load shear* defines those shearing forces parallel to the plane of the L4-L5 disc that are the result of gravity acting on the flexed upper body and hand-held load. *Joint shear* defines the estimated shear force experienced by the joint. Joint shear force is calculated as the load shear force minus the shear forces supported by the muscles. In assessing weight-lifting strategies with the lifters using a sumo or dead lift, joint shear force was estimated to be about 35% lower than load shear force. A sumo lift resulted in 8% lower load shear forces than a conventional dead lift and therefore may be advocated as the lift of choice in individuals recovering from a back injury (Cholewicki et al. 1990).

Rose et al. (1987) contend that the ES muscle activity during lifting is critical in minimizing the anterior shear forces on the lumbar spine. Their research indicated that ES activity was found to be greatest during the first half of the back-bowed-in lift and decreased through the second half of the lift. This relationship was reversed when using a rounded or slightly kyphotic lifting strategy (ES activity lower in the first half of the lift and greater in the second half of the lift). With the back arched, as the load increased, the ES activity increased more than for the kyphotic lift. Rose et al. contend that the greatest load on the intervertebral joints occurs in the initial portion of the lift, when the body must overcome the inertial forces necessary to complete the lift. Although this contraction causes compression forces on the spine, ES activity is speculated to offset the shear forces that are more damaging and less well tolerated by the spine. The decrease in ES activity with increasing loads in the kyphotic lift may place the muscles and ligaments at greater risk of injury, particularly with sudden or unexpected load shifts.

The oblique abdominal muscles were more active in the first half of the lift and increased with lifting load for both of the lifting techniques. The oblique muscles help support the spine during lifting through intraabdominal pressure and tensing of the thoracolumbar fascia.

Whether considering back-bowed-in or -out and straight or stooped positions, the key component remains the horizontal location of the load at the initiation of the lift. In the squat lift, whether the back is held straight or slightly flexed (stooped) as in a weight lifter's stance, the object must be placed between the legs to decrease the high compressive forces caused by the horizontal location of the load. The stooped position has been shown by Chaffin and Anderson (1984) to produce the lowest compressive force on the L5-S1 disc, because the object can be held more closely to the body without the interference of the legs and ES activity is decreased. This position also decreases the stress to the lumbodorsal fascia. Maintaining a strictly upright position requires a deeper squat to reach the object, increasing the stress on the knees. The deep squat results in decreased stability because the feet may not be flat, and decreased leverage results if the feet are not placed far enough apart. Knee extensor muscles often are a weak link in the lifting process, resulting in use of asymmetric positions to bring the load upright. Asymmetric lifting results in use of significantly lower maximum voluntary muscle strength and higher compressive force, disc pressure, myoelectrical activity, and antagonistic activity of trunk muscles, resulting in complex and potentially hazardous stresses to the lumbar column (Marras and Mirka 1989; NIOSH 1991).

Weight Lifter's Lift

Cholewicki et al. (1990) analyzed the reaction moments at the knee, hip, and L4-L5 joints, and the compressive and shearing forces on L4-L5, using male and female weight lifters performing dead lifts at the Canadian Power Lifting Championship in 1989. The dead lift requires the barbell to be lifted off the floor in one continuous motion until the knees and hips are locked straight and shoulders are pulled back. Sumo and conventional techniques are commonly used. In the sumo technique, a wide stance is adopted and the lifter grips the barbell with the arms passing between the knees. In the conventional lift, the stance is narrower and the arms pass on the outside of the knee. In both techniques, the back is kept straight or slightly arched. The calculated compressive forces on the spine for the dead lifters were beyond any of the documented tissue tolerance limits described in cadaveric studies. Despite these extreme forces, weight lifters often train several times a week without any apparent injury.

The sumo (wide stance) dead lift style resulted in decreased loads on the lumbar joint. The wide foot stance allows the lifter to keep the load closer to the body, shortening the moment arm. Body segment length may influence technique and load stress. Torso length influences the amount of moment necessary to support the weight. The more vertical the torso, the shorter the moment arm.

Load shear force is the result of gravity's acting on the flexed upper body and hand-held load. Load shear force depends on the trunk angle, the weight of the upper body, and the barbell load. Joint shear is calculated as the load shear minus the forces supported by the biomechanical models outlining muscle architecture. A portion of the anterior shear force was offset by the muscular action of the extensors—more so for the sumo lift than the conventional lift.

The lifting strategy used and length of body segment varies the forces acting on the knee, hip, and L4-L5. In the lifting of a 205.5-kg barbell, disc compressive forces were found to be as high as 10,405 N, exceeding the maximum compressive force tolerated, 3,432 N, per NIOSH. The discrepancy between load tolerances in living studies versus cadaveric studies is due to a number of factors. Cadaveric samples are often older men, compared to live models of young men. Also, bone mineral content and body mass have been shown to correlate with the axial compressive strength of the lumbar spine unit. Extreme loads on the spine caused by heavy weight lifting are hypothesized to result in skeletal adaptation in the form of increased bone strength (Cholewicki et al. 1990).

Golfer's Lift

The golfer's lift is often taught as a strategy for lifting light objects or for performing tasks such as emptying the washing machine. The golfer's lift is performed with one leg on the ground; as the trunk is flexed forward, rotation occurs around the hip joint of the weight-bearing leg while the contralateral leg is allowed to rotate posteriorly, maintaining the normal spine contours. One hand is used to support the body's weight while lifting is done with the other hand.

Wilson et al. (1997) used a dynamic model to compute joint reaction forces and net muscle moments of the ankle, knee, hip, and L4-L5 articulations of the weight-bearing side, comparing the golfer's lift to a double support lift and to flexing at the trunk in chronic back pain clients. In both lifts, the weight was negligible and one arm was used for support and push-off. Subjective pain ratings were compared using a 0–10 scale, 0 corresponding to no pain and 10 corresponding to worst pain ever experienced. No differences in pain rating were reported using the golfer's lift, whereas an increase in pain was reported using the back-bowed-in lift. The golfer's lift required less spinal extensor activity (reduced flexion moment) than the back-bowed-in lift.

The golfer's lift is useful for everyday light load lifting. It reduces the stresses on the vertebral column, hips, and knees and therefore may help decrease the cumulative stress on these structures caused by repetitive light load lifting.

Lifting Tests

Lifting assessment is a common part of occupational and physical therapy. Lifting incidents account for 15–65% of work-related LBP episodes (Mayer et al. 1988).

Lifting assessment is performed in the clinic for a variety of purposes. Whether this assessment is to be used in a functional capacity evaluation, a progress report, to upgrade work restrictions, or as part of a post–job offer screening, the tests should be valid and reliable indicators of function. Lifting assessment is broken down into four categories in the literature: static (isometric), isokinetic, psychophysical, and isoinertial.

Both NIOSH and the Americans with Disabilities Act have set guidelines that must be met when performing strength tests, particularly when used for post–job offer screening. These criteria include

1. Safety: The test should be safe to administer. The potential risk and exposure to the person should not outweigh the value of the data to be gained.
2. Reliability: The reliability of the tests must be documented.
3. Validity: The test should measure what it is intended to measure and should predict future performance and injury.
4. Practicality: The test should be practical from cost and procedural standpoints.
5. Focus: Only the tasks required or needed to perform the job should be tested.

Test termination has been described by a number of authors. In the lifting tests described by Mayer et al. (1988) and Matheson et al. (1985), reasons for termination include

- High-risk work style
- Inability to safely complete the task, based on changes in posture and muscle recruitment
- Exceeding the heart rate limit
- Self-perception report that the load is at maximum for the performance target
- Achievement of psychophysical rating scale
- Achievement of load guideline with no reason to continue, or indication that the worker is not likely to be safe or competent at higher loads
- Achievement of target load
- Attainment of weight above recommended limits for body weight

Static Strength Testing

Static strength, as defined by Chaffin (1975), is the capacity to produce torque or force by a maximal voluntary isometric muscular exertion. Some debate exists in the literature as to the reliability and validity of static strength testing. Keyserling et al. (1980) were able to provide evidence that isometric strength testing of the back and arms demonstrated predictive validity related to musculoskeletal injuries in industry. Marras et al. (1989)

found that static exertions in the trunk resulted in trunk torques 20–30% greater than concentric or eccentric contractions. Peak torque occurred at 40 degrees of flexion, compared to 22.5 degrees for dynamic exertions.

Keyserling et al. (1978) showed static testing to be highly reliable when specific testing criteria are met. These criteria include consistent instruction about body posture, avoidance of jerky motions, and maintenance of the force for 4–6 seconds. Ideally, the strength-measuring device should be capable of averaging the force or torque produced by the person during the steady state. The device should not influence the ability to exert maximally due to localized discomfort at the interface between the subject and the machine. Adequate rest between exertions is necessary to prevent fatigue.

Cable tensiometers, most frequently used and accessible in clinics, require greater effort to ensure consistent use of instructions, consistent body placement, and consistent setup to produce reliable data. To enhance reliability, a description of the test conditions should include

1. Parts of the body and muscles functioning
2. Position of the body during the exertion; drawings or photographs are most useful
3. Description of how the body is being supported against the reaction forces
4. Description of the operational characteristics of the strength measuring and recording device (Chaffin 1975; Garg et al. 1990; Keyserling et al. 1978)

Although isometric strength testing has been shown to reduce injury rates due to overexertion caused by a mismatch between worker's strength and the job requirements, the components of lifting related to the acceleration of the lift, placement and transfer of the object, load size and consistency, coupling, frequency, or duration cannot be tested. NIOSH reports on dynamic models of lifting indicate that the peak compressive forces in the disc and peak dynamic forces in the back muscles are two to three times greater than those predicted by a static model. As with all tests, constant clinical research is needed to validate data, using tools that are reliable, substantial, and predictive.

Isokinetic Testing

Isokinetic devices allow individuals to exert as much force and angular movement as they can generate up to a predetermined velocity. When a limb's angular rate of movement equals or exceeds the preset velocity limit, the dynamometer produces an equal counter force to ensure a constant movement rate. The results of an isokinetic evaluation involve analysis of the subject's ability to generate torque, work, and power.

Torque is the moment of force that a muscle produces, measured about the joint's axis of rotation during a contraction. Torque may be reported as either a peak or average value. The force and distance of a given muscle contraction allows the calculation of work. *Power* is determined by assessing the time required to perform work within single or several repetitions. *Endurance* is defined as the capacity of a muscle to produce force over a series of consecutive isokinetic contractions. Isokinetic endurance can be quantified by the number of repetitions required for the maximum torque value in a repetition to fall below 50% of the maximum value recorded in the first repetition or by the percent decline over a certain number of repetitions or amount of time (Perrin 1993).

Maximal muscle torque in isometric and isokinetic contractions has been shown to be related to gender and age as well as to the variables of speed and trunk angle. Back extensors are generally stronger than abdominal musculature. Individuals with strong abdominal muscles were found to have strong back muscles. In general, abdominal and back muscles were found to decline equally with age. Trunk muscles are more easily fatigued by a sustained contraction than by repeated contractions, and abdominal muscles are more easily fatigued than back muscles (Hasue et al. 1980).

Dueker et al. (1994) performed isokinetic trunk testing on male and female applicants for heavy labor jobs in a steel mill. Subjects were tested standing, with gravity compensation for trunk weight at 60, 120, and 180 degrees per second. These speeds contrast with the work of Marras and Mirka (1989), who found that eccentric strength increased with trunk velocity up to 30 degrees per second. Dynamic lifting velocities generally did not exceed 30 degrees per second. In Dueker's study, the difference in strength between women and men was with the literature: The strength of women was approximately 60% that of men. Results of the study showed no difference in injury rate between women who did not meet the isotonic lifting criteria and women who were able to lift 100 lb (required on the job). Over a 6-year follow-up, no difference existed between the isokinetic scores of workers who experienced occupational low back injury and those workers who did not. Marras found that injury risk generally increases with increased range of motion and increased velocity. Asymmetric motion reduces trunk strength and increases muscle loading.

Safety of administration is important in strength tests. In the study by Dueker et al. (1994), three of the subjects required transportation to the emergency room for test-related problems. Tests by Langrana and Lee (1984) reported good reliability with isokinetic trunk testing in sitting, with no reports of pain.

Psychophysical Tests

Psychophysical lifting models have been shown to be the best predictors of actual lifting capacity. Psychophysical lifting assessment allows the subject to determine his or her maximum acceptable weight, given the frequency of the lift, the size of the container, and the starting height and vertical range over which the load is lifted. The degree of lifting asymmetry and styles of lifting also have been studied by this method (Matheson et al. 1995).

Psychophysics, the study of the functional relationships between the body and mind, is based on the premise that intensity of sensation grows as the stimulus increases. "Equal stimulus ratios produce equal subjective ratios. In every sense modality, sensation is a power function of stimulus" (Garg et al. 1990). Psychophysics is used to determine the maximum acceptable weight that can be lifted. Subjects adjust the task variables to determine either the maximum weight that can be lifted or the maximum weight that can be repetitively lifted for an 8-hour shift. This method also applies to lowering, pushing, pulling, holding, and carrying activities. Psychophysical lifting may result in greater weights for infrequent maximal lifting than the biomechanical model. In repetitive lifting, the maximum acceptable weights for psychophysical testing are lower at low lifting frequencies and higher at high frequencies than when a physiologic model is used (Garg et al. 1990).

In psychophysical testing, subjects are asked to rate lifts. Rating scales such as the Borg scale are used to assess the lift in terms of perceived maximum and perceived capacity to repetitively lift a certain weight throughout the work day. Research has shown strong reliability and validity of perceived effort for task performance with correlation between effort and true metabolic cost of the task. No difference was found in the reliability of methods for rating effort between men and women (Hogan 1980).

Isoinertial and Progressive Isoinertial Lifting

Isoinertial testing uses psychophysics to determine the maximum weight that a person can handle. The lifter rates the perceived strain acceptable for safe performance of a task and is allowed to use any posture for the testing. Research by Kroemer (1983) showed that test-retest results obtained with a dynamic lift test are more reliable than those of static strength tests. Progressive isoinertial lifting (PILE), as defined by Mayer et al. (1988), involves a sequence of incremental weight lifting identical for individuals of the same gender. The end point of the lifting test is determined by fatigue (subjective complaint of discomfort or inability to complete the four lifts required in 20 seconds), an aerobic end point defined by exceeding a heart rate of 85% of an age-adjusted maximum (unless on beta-blocking medication or using previously set cardiac limits), or a safety end point if the weight being lifted is more than 55–60% of the lifter's body weight.

The PILE protocol was designed for cervical and lumbar testing. The cervical test is performed from waist (30 in.) to shoulder (54 in.), and the lumbar test is performed from floor to waist (30 in.). Women begin with an 8-lb load (the weight of an empty milk crate) and men begin with a 13-lb load (the weight of a custom-built wooden box similar to that described by

Blankenship [1986]). Subjects start the lift with the empty box, performing four lifts in 20 seconds. At the completion of each cycle of four lifts, the pulse is taken and, if the aerobic end point has not been met, a 5-lb weight is added for women and a 10-lb weight for men. This sequence is continued until the subject asks to end the test, cannot complete the four lifts (psychophysical end point) or reaches his or her heart rate limit (aerobic end point), or the weight exceeds 55–60% of the subject's body weight (safety end point). Results are recorded as follows:

1. Repetitive weight lifted at end of testing: Clinically, this weight describes an individual's frequent lifting capacity. According to the Department of Labor, this is defined as lifting for 67–100% of the day at a rate of up to one lift per 5 minutes.
2. Endurance time to end of the test.
3. Final and target heart rate: A final heart rate well below the maximum may be an indicator of effort, although subjective pain complaints may have been the reason for termination of testing.
4. Total work (TW) done: Work equals force times distance. The distance traveled for each 20-second portion of the lifting cycle is 10 ft for lumbar testing and 8 ft for cervical testing. TW is the sum of forces times distance. For example, a female subject completes 100 seconds of lifting for a lumbar test. The final force equals the final weight lifted in the last 20-second cycle, which is 28 lb:

$$TW = (8 + 13 + 18 + 23 + 28) \times 10 \text{ ft} = 900 \text{ ft-lb}$$

5. Power consumption: Total power consumption (TP) is the work performed divided by the unit of time represented:

$$TP = TW/t = 900 \text{ ft-lb}/100 \text{ sec} = 9 \text{ ft-lb/sec or } 12.4 \text{ W}$$

The PILE protocol is a reliable and valid tool that is easily used in any clinical setting. It allows more realistic projections of repetitive lifting for an 8-hour day than extrapolation from maximum lift data. Use of heart rate responses allows some thoughts to be formulated relative to effort and cardiovascular condition level.

Maximum Lift Assessment

Maximum lift assessment determines the maximum weight one can lift at a given time. Usually this weight is considered the weight one can safely lift at a frequency of once an hour for an 8-hour day. Frequency of lift is then extrapolated using 70% of the maximum for occasional lifting (33–66% of an 8-hour day) and 40% for frequent lifting (67–100% of an 8-hour day).

Matheson (1985) and Blankenship (1986) have been proponents of maximum lift assessment for many years. Their protocol uses a 14 in. × 14 in. × 14 in. wooden box with cut-out handles and a center bar to support the weight. Subjects are asked to lift the empty box from floor to waist height, using the squat or power (weight lifter's) lift. If that lift is easily done, the therapist adds weight in 5- or 10-lb increments until maximal effort is achieved. The test is completed when the lifter can no longer maintain correct body mechanics or stops due to pain or fatigue. This maximum lift protocol can also be applied for waist-to-shoulder, waist-to-overhead, or shoulder-to-overhead lifting or any other position that needs to be assessed for determining work capacity (Blankenship 1986).

Combining the PILE lift test and the maximum lift test can provide more valid and useful information than either of the tests used alone. Evaluation of lifting tasks should consider strength, anthropometric attributes, gender, and lifting style with biomechanical analysis of the job to determine safe lifting limits. The NIOSH formula uses the individual in task analysis and thus incorporates stature and lifting technique into the assessment. Other tools use strictly a theoretical model and may not be as representative of the stressors without evaluation of the individual.

Methods for Assessing Safe Lifting During Functional Tasks

In 1985, a scientific review panel identified the prevention of work-related injuries to the lower part of the back to be included in the *Proposed National Strategy for the Prevention of Musculoskeletal Injuries* (NIOSH 1986). This document serves as a blueprint for musculoskeletal research at NIOSH. The consensus was that, despite changes in the engineering and design of work sites, training in lifting techniques, and worker placement and evaluation, the number of injuries continued to increase. A report from the U.S. Department of Labor Bureau of Labor and Statistics (1982) provided the following data:

- Back injuries account for nearly 20% of all injuries and illnesses in the workplace.
- Back injuries account for nearly 25% of annual workers' compensation payments.

A 1988 report by the National Safety Council revealed the following:

- Overexertion is the most common cause of occupational injury and accounts for approximately 31% of all injuries.
- The back is the most frequently injured part of the body (22% of 1.7 million injuries).

Three concepts have been generally accepted:

1. Many workers who perform manual lifting are at risk for injuries to the lower part of the back.
2. If the task exceeds the worker's physical capacity, LBP is likely to occur.
3. Workers who perform the same job show great variation in physical strength and limitations (Waters et al. 1994).

Work Practices Guide 1981

In 1981, NIOSH published the *Work Practices Guide for Manual Lifting*, which proposed that overexertion injuries occur when job demands exceed worker capabilities. The theory of overexertion injury led to the following lifting model:

$$\text{Strain index (SI)} = \frac{\text{Job demands}}{\text{Worker capacity}}$$

Under ideal work conditions, SI is less than or equal to 1, which indicates that worker capacities are greater than or equal to job demands. The risk for injury increases as job demands exceed worker abilities (SI >1). A simple example of the strain index is a job that requires a 70-lb (32-kg) lifting standard to be done by a worker who can lift only 35 lb (16 kg) comfortably:

$$(SI) = \frac{70}{35}$$

$$SI = 2$$

This indicates a high risk for overexertion injury.

The *Work Practices Guide for Manual Lifting* reviewed lifting-related research through 1981, presented recommendations to control risks associated with lifting, and introduced an equation for calculating the recommended weight in the performance of symmetric, two-handed lifting. For the equation, the lifting task needed to be smooth with good coupling, provide unrestricted lifting posture, and take place in a favorable environment. Further, the width of the object lifted could not exceed 30 in. (76.2 cm). Two parameters were calculated with the formula: the action limit (AL) and the maximum permissible limit (MPL). AL was defined as the estimated average weight of lift for a given job that could be safely handled by 99% of the male working population and 75% of the female working population and was determined by the lifting equation. The MPL was the AL multiplied by three (NIOSH 1981).

After the equation was applied to the task, the actual weight of the object being lifted was compared to the AL and the MPL. In situations in which the lifting task was greater than the MPL, the lifting task was deemed unacceptable and required re-engineering. If the AL were less than the lifting task and the lifting task were less than the MPL, the lift would be deemed unacceptable if it had no administrative or engineering con-

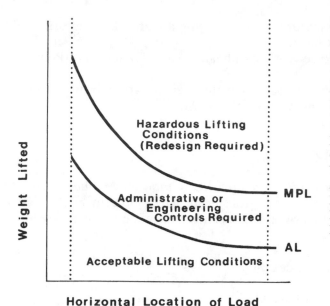

FIGURE 9.1.   Weight in relation to horizontal location of the load during a lift. (MPL = maximum permissible limit; AL = action limit.) (Reprinted from National Institute for Occupational Safety and Health. Work Practices Guide for Manual Lifting. U.S. Department of Health and Human Services. NIOSH Technical Report No. 81122. Cincinnati: NIOSH, 1981.)

trols. Administrative controls included worker selection and training to decrease the risks associated with hazardous lifting, and engineering controls included ergonomic modifications of the workplace to enhance worker safety. Lifting tasks calculated to be less than the AL represented nominal risk to most industrial work forces. Figure 9.1 compares the MPL and AL in relation to weight lifted and horizontal location of the load.

The specific lifting equation outlined in the *Work Practices Guide for Manual Lifting* was as follows:

$$AL = 90 \times (6/H) \times [1 - (0.01 \ |V - 30|)] \times [0.7 + (3/D)] \times [1 - (F/F_{max})]$$
(U.S. Customary)

$$AL = 40 \times (15/H) \times [1 - (0.004 \ |V - 75|)] \times [0.7 + (7.5/D)] \times [1 - (F/F_{max})]$$
(Metric)

H is the horizontal distance of the load from the worker, V the vertical distance of the load at the beginning of the lift, D the distance traveled during the lift, F the frequency of lifting, and F_{max} the frequency coefficient based on a 1- or 8-hour day. (The frequency coefficient is from Table 9.2.)

Revised Lifting Equation

Impetus for Revising the Lifting Equation

The first 4 years after the introduction of the 1981 NIOSH lift formula brought both positive and negative criticism. Health care providers and safety specialists, who were pleased to finally have an objective way to evaluate lifting jobs, praised the formula. In a field study designed to test the validity and applicability of the NIOSH formula, data on 101 different lifting jobs were collected over several years. The authors used the AL method to identify jobs that were causing problems in terms of injury rate and higher cost of medical and wage compensation when an injury did occur. The authors concluded that "the NIOSH method has a high potential for reducing the incidence and severity of manual materials handling injury" (Liles and Mahajan 1985, p. 60).

What frustrated investigators who tried to use the 1981 formula, however, was the definition of *lifting tasks*. Few industrial settings incorporate symmetric, two-handed lifting in the sagittal plane with good hand-to-object coupling. On the contrary, most industrial lifting tasks are asymmetric and require the load to be lifted at the side of the body. Mitral and Fard (1986) investigated the effects of symmetric and asymmetric lifting on the maximum lifting ability and physiologic effort. Results with 18 young male subjects indicated that acceptable lifting weight was reduced by approximately 8.5% when asymmetric lifting was performed. In addition, lower maximum acceptable weights were lifted when the loads were lifted asymmetrically. The subjects stated that asymmetric lifting was more physically stressful than symmetric lifting and, thus, was not their preference for performing lifting tasks. From a physiologic perspective, negligible differences in oxygen uptake or heart rate could be detected when subjects lifted asymmetrically as opposed to symmetrically.

Variations in hand-to-object coupling could not be incorporated into the 1981 formula. The reality of most industrial settings is that good hand-to-object coupling is rare. Since 1980, Drury et al. have investigated the role of hand placement and characteristics in box handling tasks. The results of their study revealed that having no handles was the worst scenario in symmetric lifting and lowering. Handles near the top center of the box were most helpful in floor-to-waist lifting. In loading and unloading pallets, in which all heights are involved, the ideal handle location varied according to the weight of the object being moved (Drury et al. 1989).

Procedures Used for Revision

In 1985, a panel of experts and experienced users were asked to review the *Work Practices Guide for Manual Lifting* and identify background data for the equation's revision. Five public meetings were held between 1987 and 1990 to discuss the following questions:

- Do the existing methods and the equation provided in the *Work Practices Guide* yield a realistic assessment of the potential for overexertion injury in two-handed repetitive lifts in the sagittal plane?
- Can asymmetric lifting tasks be explained by expanding the 1981 formula?

- Can new data on manual lifting hazards be reflected in a revision of the 1981 formula (Putz-Anderson and Waters 1991)?

A three-step process was undertaken to revise the 1981 method and equation to answer these questions. The first step involved an extensive review of the lifting literature since 1981. The following four reports were compiled to summarize the research on the physiologic, biomechanical, psychophysical, and epidemiologic aspects of lifting:

- *Physiological Basis for Manual Lifting Guidelines* (Rodgers and Yates 1991)
- *Biomechanical Basis for Manual Lifting Guidelines* (Garg 1991a)
- *Psychophysical Basis for Manual Lifting Guidelines* (Ayoub 1991)
- *Epidemiological Basis for Manual Lifting Guidelines* (Garg 1991b)

The second step of the revision involved identifying research articles that contained key data on lifting limitations when the load varied in horizontal and vertical placement. Some of the more well-defined studies had subjects perform lifting activities while varying frequency and duration. From these data, summary tables of acceptable load weights for specified population percentiles were tabulated (Batti'e et al. 1989; Garg 1989; Garg and Badger 1986; Ruhmann and Schmidtke 1989; Snook and Ciriello 1991).

The third step involved developing the three critical technical components of the lifting equation: the standard lifting location (SLL), the load constant (LC), and the multipliers or coefficients that represent the task factors. The SLL characterizes a worker's lifting posture; the SLL for the 1981 formula was determined to be a vertical height of 30 in. (76 cm) and a horizontal distance of 6 in. (15 cm) (measured from the midpoint between the ankles). Studies such as that performed by Ruhmann and Schmidtke (1989) supported an ideal vertical lifting height of 30 in. (76 cm), but the 6-in. (15-cm) horizontal distance was disputed. Garg (1989) used a laboratory study to compare the actual lifting ability of male college students with those calculated with the NIOSH lifting formula. He also compared the MPLs based on measured horizontal distances with those based on recommendations:

$$H = \left[6 + \left(\frac{w}{2}\right)\right] \text{ in.}$$

H is the horizontal distance, and *w* is the distance of the load away from the body measured in the horizontal axis (Figure 9.2).

The results showed that the measured horizontal distance was much greater than the horizontal distance generated by the formula in the 1981 NIOSH lifting guidelines. This research and that of others supported increasing the horizontal factor from 6 in. (15 cm) to 10 in. (25 cm). Workers tend to hold objects farther away from the body than originally believed; the revised formula protects them with an increased horizontal factor.

FIGURE 9.2. Vertical, lateral, and horizontal axes. (L = left; R= right.) (National Institute for Occupational Safety and Health. Scientific Support Documentation for the Revised 1991 NIOSH Lifting Equation: Technical Contract Reports. Springfield, VA· U.S. Department of Commerce, Technical Information Service, 1991.)

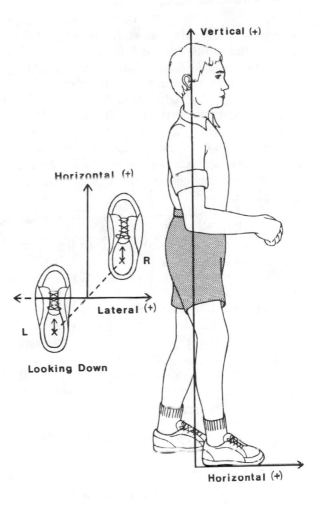

The second critical component of the equation evaluated by the panel was the LC. The LC is the maximum weight value for the SLL, based on selected conditions and constraints associated with manual lifting (Putz-Anderson and Waters 1991). The LC established for the 1981 equation was 90 lb (41 kg). When the lifting formula was revised, the LC was reduced to 51 lb (23 kg). Part of the need to lower the LC was related to the increase in the horizontal factor from 6 in. (15 cm) to 10 in. (25 cm). In addition, research by Snook and Ciriello (1991) revealed that the maximum acceptable lifting capacity of female workers was less than estimated when the 1981 formula was developed. The revised LC of 51 lb (23 kg), combined with optimal SLL conditions such as no twisting and good coupling, would be acceptable to 75% of female workers and 99% of male workers. By lowering the LC from 90 lb (41 kg) to 51 lb (23 kg), the revised formula was thought to provide a greater degree of protection for the industrial work force.

The revised lifting equation contains multipliers or coefficients similar to the task variables presented in the 1981 formula. Six multipliers involved in the actual task of lifting are used in the 1991 lifting formula: (1) horizontal, (2) vertical, (3) distance, (4) asymmetric, (5) frequency, and (6) coupling. The role of the multipliers is to reduce the maximum weight value of the LC to compensate for lifting conditions that are not ideal. Each multiplier can vary from 1.0 for optimal lifting conditions to 0 for high-strain lifting conditions. The 1991 lifting formula can be described in the following way:

$$RWL = LC \times HM \times VM \times DM \times AM \times FM \times CM$$

RWL is the recommended weight limit, *LC* the load constant, *HM* the horizontal multiplier, *VM* the vertical multiplier, *DM* the distance multiplier, *AM* the asymmetric multiplier, *FM* the frequency multiplier, and *CM* the coupling multiplier.

The research that led to the development of each multiplier can be found in the publications in parentheses: horizontal (Garg et al. 1983; Snook and Ciriello 1991), vertical (Punnett et al. 1987; Snook and Ciriello 1991), distance (Gary et al. 1978; Snook and Ciriello 1991), asymmetry (Garg and Badger 1986; Garg and Banaag 1988), frequency (Garg et al. 1978), and coupling (Garg and Saxena 1980; Smith and Jiang 1984).

Comparison of 1981 and 1991 Formulas

Similarities

The 1981 and 1991 formulas used research data in the areas of biomechanics, work physiology, psychophysics, and epidemiology available at the time. Both equations allow the lift to be broken into variables that can be altered to determine a safe lift. In addition, a safe lift can be calculated from both versions using a multiplicative lifting equation, which allows for regulated interaction between a number of factors (e.g., horizontal distance, lifting frequency). Both equations also provide a zone of acceptable lifting strain to which engineering or other interventions should be applied. Figure 9.3 is a graph of the cut-off zone for the 1991 equation, which can be compared with the 1981 cut-off zone in Figure 9.1 (Putz-Anderson and Waters 1991).

Differences

The differences between the two equations are presented in Table 9.1. Two differences are most notable. The first is that the 1991 formula contains two additional task factors: asymmetry and hand-container coupling. The second difference is that the 1991 formula provides one RWL, whereas the 1981 formula provided two (AL and MPL).

FIGURE 9.3. Weight lifted in relation to horizontal location of load during lifting. (RWL = recommended weight limit.) (Reprinted from V Putz-Anderson, TR Waters. Revisions in the NIOSH Guide to Manual Lifting. Presented at the National Conference for a National Strategy for Occupational Musculoskeletal Injury Prevention: Implementation Issues and Research Needs. April 1991. Ann Arbor, MI.)

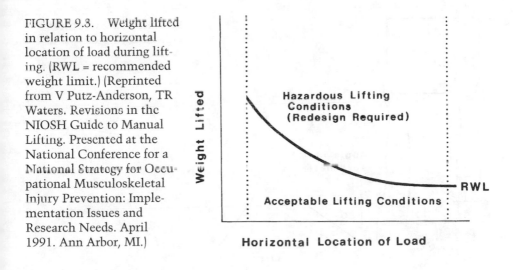

Horizontal Location of Load

Implementation of the 1991 Equation

$$RWL = 51 \text{ lb} \times (10/H) \times [1 - (0.0075 \ |V - 30|)] \times [0.82 + (1.8/D)] \times (1 - 0.0032 \ A) \times$$
$$(FM \text{ from table}) \times (CM \text{ from table}) \quad (U.S. \text{ Customary})$$
$$RWL = 23 \text{ kg} \times (25/H) \times [1 - (0.003 \ |V - 75|)] \times [0.82 + (4.5/D)] \times (1 - 0.0032 \ A) \times$$
$$(FM \text{ from table}) \times (CM \text{ from table}) \quad (Metric)$$

H is the horizontal distance of the hands from the midpoint between the ankles. It is measured from the midpoint of the line that joins the ankles to the midpoint at which the hands grasp the object while in the lifting position at the origin and destination of the lift (see Figure 9.2).

TABLE 9.1
Comparison of National Institute for Occupational Safety and Health Lifting Equations

	Multiplier	
Factor	*1981 Equation*	*1991 Equation*
Load constant	90 lb	51 lb
Horizontal	6/H	10/H
Vertical	$1 - (0.01 \ |V - 30|)$	$1 - (0.0075 \ |V - 30|)$
Distance	0.7 + 3/D	0.82 + 1.8/D
Frequency	$1 - F/F_{max}$	From Table 9.2
Asymmetry	—	$1 - 0.0032 \ A$
Coupling	—	From Table 9.3

H = horizontal distance; V = vertical height; D = distance; F = frequency; F_{max} = frequency coefficient; A = angle of asymmetry.

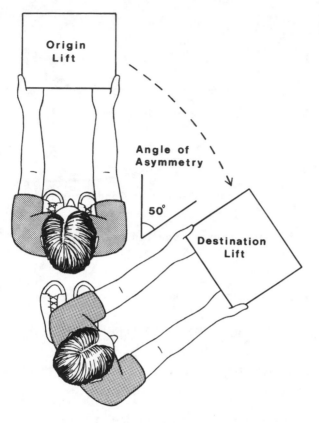

FIGURE 9.4.   Overhead view of asymmetric lift.

V is the vertical distance of the hands from the floor. The distance is measured from the floor to the point at which the hands grasp the object at the origin and the destination of the lift (see Figure 9.2).

D is the vertical travel distance between the origin and the destination of the lift. *V* origin is subtracted from *V* destination to obtain *D* (absolute value of the difference).

A is the angle of asymmetry, the angular displacement of the load from the sagittal plane. A plumb line is dropped to the floor at the beginning of the lift. The examiner uses the plumb line to draw on the floor (in chalk) the direction of the lift at the origin and the destination of the lift. Cardboard Xs also can be used to mark the plumb line measurements. A goniometer is used to measure the angle of asymmetry in degrees (Figure 9.4). Asymmetric lifting is more likely to cause injury and should be replaced by symmetric lifting whenever possible.

FM, the frequency multiplier, is the average frequency of lifting measured in lifts per minute and is determined by the frequency and duration of the lift. The duration of the lift is defined as short, moderate, or long. For a lift to be classified as *short*, lifting may be continuous for as long as 1

TABLE 9.2
Frequency Multipliers

Frequency (lifts/min)	≤8 Hours		≤2 Hours		≤1 Hour	
	V <30	V ≥30	V <30	V ≥30	V <30	V ≥30
0.2	0.85	0.85	0.95	0.95	1.00	1.00
0.5	0.81	0.81	0.92	0.92	0.97	0.97
1	0.75	0.75	0.88	0.88	0.94	0.94
2	0.65	0.65	0.84	0.84	0.91	0.91
3	0.55	0.55	0.79	0.79	0.88	0.88
4	0.45	0.45	0.72	0.72	0.84	0.84
5	0.35	0.35	0.60	0.60	0.80	0.80
6	0.27	0.27	0.50	0.50	0.75	0.75
7	0.22	0.22	0.42	0.42	0.70	0.70
8	0.18	0.18	0.35	0.35	0.60	0.60
9	0	0.15	0.30	0.30	0.52	0.52
10	0	0.13	0.26	0.26	0.45	0.45
11	0	0	0	0.23	0.41	0.41
12	0	0	0	0.21	0.37	0.37
13	0	0	0	0	0	0.34
14	0	0	0	0	0	0.31
15	0	0	0	0	0	0.28
>15	0	0	0	0	0	0

Values of vertical height (V) are in inches. Inches are converted to centimeters by multiplying by 254 and dividing by 100.
Source: Reprinted from TR Waters, V Putz-Anderson, A Garg. Application Manual for the Revised National Institute for Occupational Safety and Health Lifting Equation. Cincinnati: U.S. Department of Health and Human Services, 1994;26.

hour and followed by a recovery period of at least 120% of work time. For example, if an employee lifts for 30 minutes, a minimum of 36 minutes should be spent in nonlifting work. *Moderate lifting* is defined as continuous lifting for up to 2 hours followed by a recovery period of at least 30% of work time. For example, if an employee lifts for 2 hours, nonlifting work activities should be performed for at least 36 minutes. Lifting of *long* duration is continuous lifting up to 8 hours with no fatigue allowances other than normal breaks. For Table 9.2 to be used accurately, all criteria used to determine the frequency and duration of the lift must be met.

CM, the coupling multiplier, can be determined using Table 9.3. The maximum force a worker can exert on an object is greatly affected by the nature of hand-to-object coupling. Good coupling can reduce the maximum grasp forces required and increase acceptable lifting weight. Poor

TABLE 9.3
Coupling Multipliers

Coupling	V <30 in. (75 cm)	V ≥30 in. (75 cm)
Good	1.00	1.00
Fair	0.95	1.00
Poor	0.90	0.90

V = vertical height.

coupling requires higher grasp forces and decreases the acceptable lifting weight. Because lifting is dynamic, the quality of hand-to-object coupling may vary throughout the lift. An average has to be taken to establish the overall effectiveness of coupling during the entire lift. If any doubt exists about how to classify a particular coupling design, the most stressful classification should be selected.

Good Coupling

- Handles are 0.75–1.50 in. (2–4 cm) in diameter, are more than 4.5 in. (11 cm) long, have 2 in. (5 cm) of clearance, are cylindrical, and have a smooth, nonslip surface.
- Handhold cut-outs should be 3 in. (8 cm) high, 4.5 in. (11 cm) long, and semi-oval and have 2 in. (5 cm) of clearance and a smooth, nonslip surface. The container must be at least 0.43 in. (1 cm) thick.
- Container should be at least 16 in. (40 cm) long in front and no taller than 12 in. (30 cm) and have a smooth, nonslip surface.
- If the load is not boxed, the worker should be able to comfortably wrap a hand around the object with no wrist deviation, no awkward postures, and no excessive force in the grip.

Fair Coupling

- Handles or handhold cut-outs are of less than optimal design.
- Worker is able to clamp the fingers at nearly 90 degrees under the container if no handles or cutouts are available.

Poor Coupling

- Container is 16 in. (40 cm) or longer in front and 12 in. (30 cm) or more high; has a rough or slippery surface, sharp edges, or an asymmetric center of mass; holds unstable material; or requires use of gloves.
- Container has no handles or cut-outs.

Figure 9.5 can be used to classify coupling multipliers.

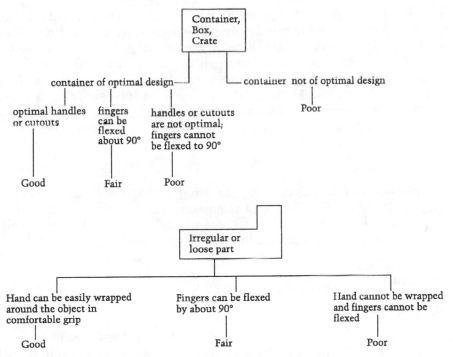

FIGURE 9.5. Classification of coupling multipliers.

Limitations of the 1991 Lifting Equation

The 1991 lifting formula applies only to lifting tasks that fit the following conditions:

1. Work environment has a favorable temperature, such as 65°–80°F (18°–27°C) with no more than 50% humidity.
2. Other work tasks do not require a high expenditure of energy.
3. Lifting task is two-handed and is not performed in a high-speed, jerky manner. The formula does not assess tasks involving one-handed lifting, lifting while seated or kneeling, lifting in a contained work space, lifting persons or wheelbarrows, or shoveling.
4. Worker-floor coupling has friction similar to that between a smooth, dry floor and the sole of a clean, dry leather work shoe.

Lifting Index

The lifting index (LI) provides a simple estimate of the hazard of overexertion injury for a manual lifting job. The use of a single number for report writing may be useful for therapists when they share information with workers. Long mathematical formulas and calculations may be confusing and intimidating, as well as time-consuming. The LI can be used as a relative measure of job severity and can help companies with numerous ergonomic problems decide which issues to address first. In addition, companies can focus on a long-term lifting problem by using the LI to break the problem into short-term issues. For example, if the LI for a specific lifting task is 4, the short-term goal could be to reduce that number to 3, with a long-term goal to reach 1 or less.

$$LI = L/RWL$$

L is the weight of the object being lifted and *RWL* is the number calculated in the 1991 lifting formula. If LI is greater than 1, overexertion injury is likely, because job demands exceed recommended weight. If LI is less than 1, the job presents minimal risk for overexertion injury.

Case Study 1

Job Description

Harold works as a cook and order-taker at a fast-food restaurant. He is 6 ft 4 in. (193 cm) tall, of slender build, and the primary provider for his family. After suffering sporadic LBP for several years, Harold received the diagnosis of acquired spinal stenosis with shooting pain in the right leg. Harold experiences the most pain when he repetitively hands trays of food to customers during a busy lunch hour. The counter is 36 in. (91 cm) wide, 48 in. (122 cm) high at the customer service end and 36 in. (91 cm) high where the worker fills the trays with food. The filled trays of food weigh as much as 5 lb (2.3 kg), and the worker is not allowed to slide the tray of food across the counter.

Job Analysis

The calculations using the 1981 formula are as follows:

$$AL = 90 \times (6/H) \times [1 - (0.01 \ |V- 30|)] \times [0.7 + (3/D)] \times [1 - (F/F_{max})]$$

H origin = 18 in. (46 cm); V origin = 42 in. (107 cm)

H destination = 30 in. (76 cm); V destination = 50 in. (127 cm)

D = 8 in. (20 cm); F = four lifts per minute

F_{max} = 18 (from F_{max} table, NIOSH 1981)

$$AL \text{ (destination)} = 90 \times (6/30) \times [1 - (0.01 \ |50 - 30|)] \times [0.7 + (3/8)] \times [1 - (4/18)]$$
$$= 90 \times 0.2 \times 0.8 \times 1.075 \times 0.78$$
$$= 12 \text{ lb } (5.4 \text{ kg})$$

The calculations using the 1991 lifting formula are as follows:

RWL (destination) = 51 × (10/H) × [1 − (0.0075 |V − 30|)] × [0.82 + (1.8/D)] ×
(1 − 0.0032 A) × FM × CM

H origin = 18 in. (46 cm); V origin = 30 in. (76 cm)
H destination = 30 in. (76 cm); V destination = 50 in. (127 cm)
D = 8 in. (20 cm); A = 0

FM = 0.84 (from table; using the criteria of four lifts per minute, duration
of ≤ 1 hour, V ≥ 30 in. [76 cm])
CM = 1.0 (from table; using the criteria of good coupling and V ≥ 30 in.
[76 cm])

RWL = 51 × (10/30) × [1 − (0.0075 |50 − 30|)] × [0.82 + (1.8/8)] × 1 × 0.84 × 1
= 51 × 0.33 × 0.85 × 1.045 × 0.84
= 12.56 lb (5.7 kg)

Discussion

The actual weight of the object being lifted is 2.3 kg (5 lb), well below the
5.4 kg (12-lb) AL calculated by the 1981 formula and the 5.7-kg (12.56-lb)
RWL calculated by the 1991 formula. Clearly, more risk factors are present for Harold than just lifting food trays. For someone with Harold's
diagnosis, activities that involve repetitive forward flexion should be
avoided. This example demonstrates an important concept for evaluators
of work sites. The NIOSH formula was designed to be used as a guideline
only and is not the only factor to be considered in the evaluation of a
workstation. The lifting formula does, however, provide a way to break
the lifting task into components. Analysis of the task variables of both
calculations shows that the horizontal multiplier causes the greatest
reduction in each LC (0.2 in the 1981 formula and 0.33 in the 1991 formula). Figure 9.6 shows that the horizontal reach of the job is of primary
importance.

This lifting task can be analyzed with the 1981 formula because no
asymmetric twisting is involved in the lift. When the 1991 formula is used,
the asymmetric and coupling multipliers are not a factor (A = 0; CM = 1).
For this job, the difference between the 1981 AL (12 lb [5.4 kg]) and the
1991 RWL (12.56 lb [5.7 kg]) is negligible.

Harold was never successfully returned to work as a fast-food employee.
He did benefit from education in proper body mechanics and learned how
to stabilize his back when performing the tray-lifting job. However, Harold
could not tolerate the constant standing and repetitive movements
involved in all aspects of fast-food work. He moved from a cold to a warm

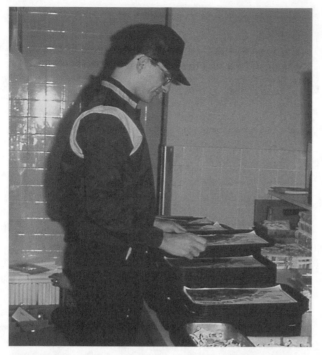

FIGURE 9.6.   Fast-food worker handing food tray to customer.

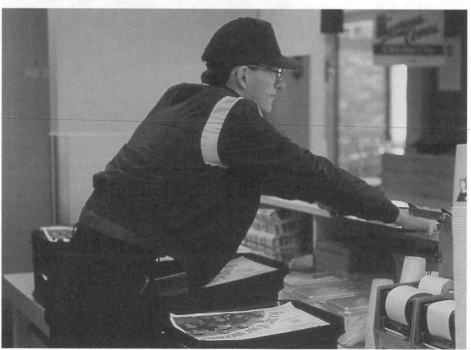

climate and assumed a job as a bookstore manager. He reported that he finds the warm climate better for his back.

Case Study 2

Job Description

Bob is a 32-year-old worker at a large medical center. His job in the linen service department was evaluated after he sustained a work-related back injury. The most essential job task requires him to load bags of wet laundry from the bottom of several laundry chutes into a linen cart. The revised NIOSH lifting formula was selected during the task analysis because asymmetric lifting was observed on the job (Figure 9.7).

Job Analysis

H origin = 20 in. (51 cm); V origin = 18 in. (46 cm)

H destination = 20 in. (51 cm); V destination = 52 in. (132 cm)

D = 34 in. (86 cm); A = 50 degrees

FM = 0.13 (from table; frequency = 10 lifts per minute;

   duration = 6 hours/day)

CM = 1.0 (good coupling)

Actual weight of the linen bags = 30 lb (13.6 kg)

$$
\begin{aligned}
RWL\,(org) &= 51 \times (10/H) \times [1 - (0.0075 \, |V - 30|)] \times [0.82 + (1.8/D)] \times \\
&\quad (1 - 0.0032\,A) \times FM \times CM \\
&= 51 \times (10/20) \times [1 - (0.0075 \, |52 - 30|)] \times [0.82 + (1.8/34)] \times \\
&\quad [1 - (0.0032 \, |0|)] \times 0.13 \times 1 \\
&= 51 \times 0.5 \times 0.91 \times 0.87 \times 1 \times 0.13 \times 1 \\
&= 2.6 \text{ lb } (1.2 \text{ kg})
\end{aligned}
$$

$$
\begin{aligned}
RWL\,(dest) &= 51 \times (10/H) \times [1 - (0.0075 \, |V - 30|)] \times [0.82 + (1.8/D)] \times \\
&\quad (1 - 0.0032\,A) \times FM \times CM \\
&= 51 \times (10/20) \times [1 - (0.0075 \, |18 - 30|)] \times [0.82 + (1.8/34)] \times [1 - \\
&\quad (0.0032 \, |50|)] \times 0.13 \times 1 \\
&= 51 \times 0.5 \times 0.84 \times 0.87 \times 0.84 \times 0.13 \\
&= 2 \text{ lb } (0.9 \text{ kg})
\end{aligned}
$$

LI (origin) = L/RWL = 30/2.6 = 11.5

LI (destination) = L/RWL = 30/2 = 15

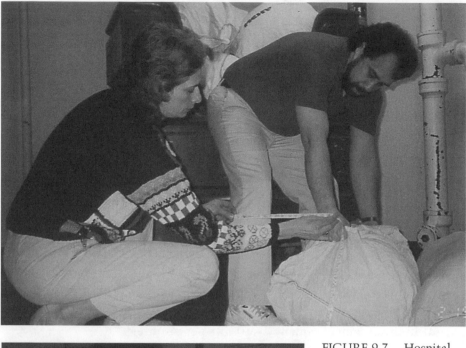

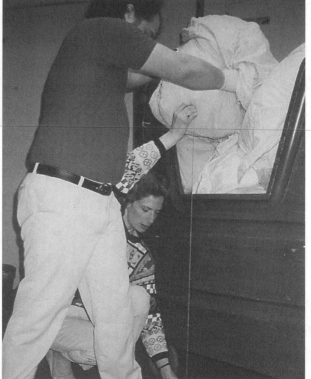

FIGURE 9.7.   Hospital laundry worker performing asymmetric lift.

Discussion

The LI reveals that performing repetitive lifting jobs has a high risk for injury. In this case, the worker lifts 12–15 times the RWL. In the analysis of the task variables, the factor that reduces the LC the most is the frequency multiplier (0.13). Adding another worker to help perform this job in addition to slowing the frequency of lifting would raise the frequency multiplier and allow overworked muscles a chance to rest between repetitive lifts. The horizontal factor of 0.5 reduces the LC and could be increased by asking workers to hold the linen bags closer to the body. The workers are reluctant to do so because the bags are wet and sometimes bloody. Providing full-cover body aprons would provide the protection necessary and encourage the workers to hold the soft linen bags closer to the body. The asymmetry variable could be eliminated with education in proper body mechanics. Twisting is not essential to performing the job.

Bloswick Measure of Compressive Forces

Neither of the two NIOSH lifting formulas was designed to calculate spinal compression forces for people-moving tasks, thus limiting their applicability in many work settings. The introduction of Bloswick's formula for spinal compression forces provided the opportunity to be more objective with these work activities, as the formula does not focus solely on lifting inanimate objects.

Bloswick (1993) devised a simplified version of a computer biomechanical model he obtained from the University of Michigan. Therapists should be aware that the Bloswick formula provides an estimation of back compression forces. If precision is desired, the computer biomechanical model should be used.

As with the NIOSH lift formula, the Bloswick formula estimates spinal compression forces mathematically by breaking down task variables into component parts. It focuses on the contribution of the weight of the worker's body to spinal compression forces and de-emphasizes the impact of repetition and coupling. Bloswick suggests using the NIOSH compressive limit of 770 lb or 3,400 N as the outside safe limit for young, healthy workers. This amount of compressive force may be unrealistic and therefore unsafe for older workers or workers recovering from an injury.

The following measurements should be taken at the workplace:

BW = Body weight of the lifter

L = Weight of the load being lifted

HB = Horizontal distance of the load being lifted, measured in inches from the hand to the lower back

Cos (theta) = Cosine of torso angle with horizontal (Figure 9.8)

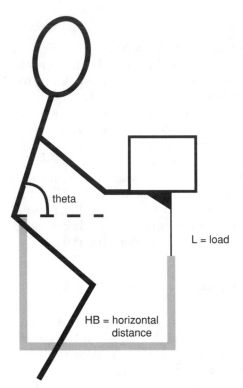

FIGURE 9.8.   Bloswick estimate of back compressive force.

If torso is vertical, use cos (theta) = 0
If torso is bent ¼, use cos (theta) = 0.38
If torso is bent ½, use cos (theta) = 0.71
If torso is bent ¾, use cos (theta) = 1

Bloswick's formula calculates back compressive forces as follows:

$F = A + B + C$

A = 3 (BW) cos (theta) = Back muscle force reacting to the upper body weight of the lifter as a result of posture during the lift

B = 0.5 (L × HB) = Back muscle force resulting from the weight being lifted and the distance away from the lifter's body

C = 0.8 [(BW/2 + L)] = Direct compressive contribution of load and upper body weight

The Bloswick formula can be used to calculate the spinal compression forces that occur when Harold hands trays of food to customers (Case Study 1):

BW = 230 lb

L = 5 lb

HB = 30 in.

Cos (theta) = 0.71 (torso bent 1/2)

F = A + B + C = 3 [(BW) cos (theta)] + 0.5 (L × HB) + 0.8 [(BW)/2 + L]

F = 3 (230 × 0.71) + 0.5 (5 × 30) + 0.8 [230/2 + 5]

F = 489.9 + 75 + 96

F = 660.9 lb of compressive force

Although the compressive force calculated is lower than the 770 lb recommended by NIOSH, it is too much for Harold because he is injured. As shown by the component parts of the task, the back angle required to accomplish the long horizontal reach of this task and the contribution of the worker's upper body weight are the most significant factors.

Conclusion

Therapists involved with injury prevention and injury management need to be familiar with the reasons that lifting injuries occur and the methods of successfully incorporating lifting assessments into a therapy program while considering the personal risk factors of each individual. Any educational program should include teaching a variety of lifting techniques, with specific emphasis on the technique that is safest for each specific lifting situation.

Therapists who perform work-site evaluations typically find that the revised NIOSH lift formula has more applicability to industrial work settings than its predecessor. Because the formula is a guideline and usually describes only one part of a worker's job, however, therapists should be conservative in the degree of importance they place on the formula's results. The NIOSH lift formula is an objective evaluation tool that should be combined with careful observation of the worker's postures and positions while working. In addition, NIOSH warns that the revised lifting formula needs to be validated through research before implementation of the formula's guidelines can be assumed to reduce the risk of injuries to the lower back (Waters et al. 1994). Therapists are encouraged, however, to use the formula when working with companies, to help facilitate research.

The Bloswick formula allows the objective work-site evaluator to assess spinal compression forces by focusing on other contributing factors important in lifting and lowering objects. In addition, it should be the formula of choice for client-moving tasks. The formula is an estimation of a computer biomechanical model, however, and is perhaps not as precise as the NIOSH lift formula.

References

Anderson GBJ (1985). Possible loads: biomechanical considerations. Ergonomics 28: 323–326.

Ayoub MM (1991). Psychophysical Basis for Manual Lifting Guidelines. In Scientific Support Documentation for the Revised 1991 NIOSH Lifting Equation: Technical Contract Reports. NIOSH Technical Report PB91226274. Washington, DC: NIOSH.

Batti'e MC, Bigos SJ, Fisher LD, et al. (1989). Isometric lifting strength as a predictor of industrial back pain reports. Spine 14:851–856.

Blankenship KL (1986). Functional Capacity Evaluation/Work Hardening. Portland, ME: American Therapeutics.

Bloswick D (1993). Ergonomics and the Rehabilitated Worker. Presented at Center for the Advancement of Industrial Rehabilitation and Evaluation conference. February. New Orleans.

Brooks J (1995). Lifting Testing and Analysis. In K Jacobs, CM Bettencourt (eds), Ergonomics for Therapists. Boston: Butterworth–Heinemann.

Carlton RS (1987). The effects of body mechanics instruction on work performance. Am J Occup Ther 41:1.

Chaffin DB (1975). Ergonomics guide for the assessment of human strength. Am Indust Hygiene Assoc J 1:505–511.

Chaffin DB, Anderson GB (1984). Occupational Biomechanics. London: Wiley.

Cholewicki J, McGill SM, Norman RW (1990). Lumbar spine loads during the lifting of extremely heavy weights. Med Sci Sports Exer 23:1179–1186.

Delitto RS, Rose SJ, Apts DW (1987). Electromyographic analysis of two techniques for squat lifting. Phys Ther 67:9.

Department of Labor Bureau of Labor and Statistics (1982). Back Injuries Associated with Lifting. Bulletin No. 2144. Washington, DC: U.S. Department of Labor.

Drury CG, Deeb JM, Hartman B, et al. (1989). Symmetric and asymmetric manual materials handling. 1. Physiology and psychophysics. Ergonomics 32:467–489.

Dueker JA, Ritchie SM, Know TJ, Rose SJ (1994). Isokinetic trunk testing and employment. J Occup Med 36:1.

Frymoyer JW, Pope MH, Clements JH, et al. (1983). Risk factors in low back pain. J Bone Joint Surg Am 65:213–218.

Frymoyer JW, Cats-Baril W (1987). Predictors of low back pain disability. Clin Orthoped 221:89–98.

Garg A (1989). An evaluation of the NIOSH guidelines for manual lifting with specific reference to horizontal distance. Am Indust Hygiene Assoc J 50:157–164.

Garg A (1991a). Biomechanical Basis for Manual Lifting Guidelines. In Scientific Support Documentation for the Revised 1991 NIOSH Lifting Equation: Technical Contract Reports. NIOSH Technical Report PB91226274. Washington, DC: NIOSH.

Garg A (1991b). Epidemiological Basis for Manual Lifting Guidelines. In Scientific Support Documentation for the Revised 1991 NIOSH Lifting Equation: Technical Contract Reports. NIOSH Technical Report PB91226274. Washington, DC: NIOSH.

Garg A, Badger D (1986) Maximum acceptable weights and maximum voluntary strength for asymmetric lifting. Ergonomics 29:879–892.

Garg A, Banaag J (1988). Maximum acceptable weights, heart rates, and RPEs for one hour's repetitive asymmetric lifting. Ergonomics 31:77–96.

Garg A, Chaffin DB, Herrin GD (1978). Prediction of metabolic rates for manual materials handling jobs. Am Indust Hygiene J 39:661–674.

Garg A, Hagglund G, Mericle K (1983). Physical fatigue and stresses in warehouse operations. U.S. Department of Health and Human Services, NIOSH Contract No. 210816008, Technical Report. Cincinnati: NIOSH.

Garg A, Rodgers SH, Yates JW (1990). Scientific Support Documentation for the Revised 1991 NIOSH Lifting Equation: Technical Contract Supports. Washington, DC: NIOSH.

Garg A, Saxena U (1980). Container characteristics and maximum acceptable weight of lift. Hum Factors 22:48–495.

Genaidy AM, Waly SM, Khalil TM, Higalgo J (1993). Spinal compression tolerance limits for the design of manual material handling operations in the workplace. Ergonomics 39:407–419.

Grandjean E (1988). Fitting the Task to the Man (4th ed). London: Taylor & Francis.

Hasue M, Fujiwara M, Kikuchi S (1980). A new method of quantitative measurement of abdominal and back muscle strength. Spine 5:2.

Hogan JC (1980). The State of the Art of Strength Testing. In DC Walsh, RH Egdahl (eds), Women, Work and Health: Challenges to Corporate Policy. New York. Springer-Verlag, 75–98.

Hsiang SM, McGorry RW (1997). Three different lifting strategies for controlling the motion patterns of the external load. Ergonomics 40:928–939.

Keyserling WM, Herrin GD, Chaffin DB (1978). An Analysis of Selected Work Muscle Strength. In Proceedings of Human Factors Society 22nd Annual Meeting. Detroit.

Keyserling WM, Herrin GD, Chaffin DB (1980). Isometric strength testing as a means of controlling medical incidents on strenuous jobs. J Occup Biomechanics 22:332–336.

King PM, Fisher JC, Garg A (1997). Evaluation of the impact of employee ergonomics training in industry. Appl Ergonomics 28:249–256.

Kroemer CH (1983). An isoinertial technique to assess individual lifting capability. Hum Factors 25:493–506.

Laflin K, Aja D (1995). Health care concerns related to lifting: an inside look at intervention strategies. Am J Occup Ther 49:63–72.

Laflin K, Aja D, Banasiak N (1997). Development of a post-offer screening tool for patient support services. Am J Occup Ther 51:10.

Langrana N, Lee C (1984). Isokinetic evaluation of trunk muscles. Spine 9:2.

Liles DH, Mahajan P (1985). Using NIOSH lifting guide decreases risks of back injuries. Occup Health Safety 2:5–60.

Marras WS, Mirka GA (1989). Trunk strength during asymmetric trunk motion. Hum Factors 31:36.

Matheson LN, Ogden LD, Schultz K (1985). Work hardening: occupational therapy in industrial rehabilitation. Am J Occup Ther 39:314–321.

Matheson LN, Moonley B, Grant JE, et al. (1995). A test to measure lift capacity of physically impaired adults. Part 1: development and reliability testing. Spine 20:2119–2129.

Mayer TG, Barnes D, Kishino ND, et al. (1988a). Progressive isoinertial lifting evaluation. 1. A standardized protocol and normative database. Spine 13:993–997.

McCauley M (1990). The effect of body mechanics instruction on work performance among young workers. Am J Occup Ther 44:5.

Mitral A, Fard HF (1986). Psychophysical and physiological responses to lifting symmetrically and asymmetrically. Ergonomics 29:1263–1272.

Nachemson AL (1992). Newest knowledge of low back pain: a critical look. Clin Orthopedics Rel Res 279:8–9.

National Safety Council (1988). Accident Facts. Chicago: National Safety Council.

NIOSH (1981). Work practices guide for manual lifting. U.S. Department of Health and Human Services. NIOSH Technical Report No. 81122. Cincinnati: NIOSH.

NIOSH (1986). Proposed National Strategy for the Prevention of Musculoskeletal Injuries. U.S. Department of Health and Human Services. Cincinnati: NIOSH.

NIOSH (1991). Scientific Support Documentation for the Revised 1991 NIOSH Lifting Equation: Technical Contract Reports. Springfield, VA: U.S. Department of Commerce, Technical Information Service.

Perrin DH (1993). Isokinetic Exercise and Assessment. Champaign, IL: Human Kinetics Publishers.

Perry L, Palmer J, Weyrich B, Guo L (1994). An effective preemployment screening protocol. Work 4:285–292.

Peterson JA (1990). Back pain in corporate America. Fitness Manage 9:36–38.

Punnett L, Fine LJ, Keyserling WM, et al. (1987). A Case-Referent Study of Back Disorders in Automobile Assembly Workers: The Health Effects of Nonneutral Trunk Postures. Ann Arbor, MI: University of Michigan Center for Ergonomics.

Putz-Anderson V, Waters TR (1991). Revisions in the NIOSH Guide to Manual Lifting. Presented at the National Conference for a National Strategy for Occupational Musculoskeletal Injury Prevention: Implementation Issues and Research Needs. April. Ann Arbor, MI.

Rodgers SH, Yates JW (1991). Physiological Basis for Manual Lifting Guidelines. In Scientific Support Documentation for the Revised 1991 NIOSH Lifting Equation: Technical Contract Reports. NIOSH Technical Report PB91226274. Washington, DC: NIOSH.

Ruhmann H, Schmidtke H (1989). Human strength: measurements of maximum isometric forces in industry. Ergonomics 32:865–879.

St. Vincent M, Tellier C, Lortie M (1989). Training in handling: an evaluative study. Ergonomics 32(2):191–210.

Smith JL, Jiang BC (1984). A manual materials handling study of bag lifting. Am Ind Hyg Assoc J 45:505–508.

Snook SH, Ciriello VM (1991). The design of manual handling tasks: revised tables. Ergonomics 34:1197–1213.

Waters TR, Putz-Anderson V, Garg A (1994). Application Manual for the Revised NIOSH Lifting Equation. Cincinnati: U.S. Department of Health and Human Services.

Webster BS, Snook S (1990). The cost of compensable low back pain. J Occup Med 32:13–15.

Wilson DJ, Hickey KM, Gorham JL, Childers MK (1997). Lumbar spinal moments in chronic back pain during supported lifting: a dynamic analysis. Arch Physical Med Rehabil 78:967–972.

Review Questions

(Answers are found in Appendix D.)

1. Which of the following structures is most likely to be stressed by over-head lifting?
   (a) Back
   (b) Neck
   (c) Shoulders
   (d) Wrists
   (e) All of the above

2. Overhead lifting causes the most stress to which of the following low back structures?
   (a) Disc
   (b) Vertebral body
   (c) Facet joint
   (d) Muscles

3. Which two reasons most accurately represent the cause of overexertion injuries?
   (a) The task exceeds the strength of the worker.
   (b) The workers did not get their 15-minute breaks in the morning and afternoon.
   (c) The task exceeds the strength of the physiologic structure.
   (d) The workers work the night shift.

4. Which of the following variables is *not* in the NIOSH lifting formula?
   (a) Horizontal reach
   (b) Coefficient of friction
   (c) Vertical reach
   (d) Travel distance

5. Which of the following are personal or physiologic risk factors that increase stress on the back?
   (a) Amount of muscular effort
   (b) Physical fitness
   (c) Medical history
   (d) Age
   (e) Race

CHAPTER 10
Seating

Diane C. Hermenau

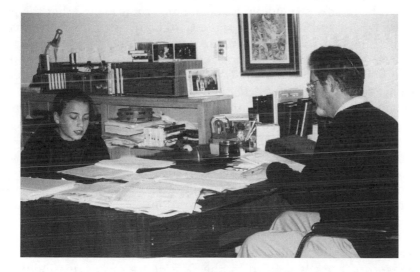

ABSTRACT

As computer use in offices and factories increases, jobs are evolving from multidimensional to unidimensional, often requiring workers to sit for long periods. Seating has become critical at the workplace, because a poorly designed computer workstation puts the user at risk for back, neck, shoulder, elbow, forearm, wrist, hand, and leg injuries. Therapists with expertise in seating and ergonomic workplace design are working increasingly as industrial consultants for seating issues. This chapter discusses the biomechanics of sitting; the risks related to prolonged sitting and poor posture; the features of ergonomic chair design; how to properly fit worker and workstation; indications for seated work; and special considerations, including use of a computer, the sit-stand position, kneeling chairs, and lumbar supports.

Research reveals that disc pressures are greater when a person is sitting than when he or she is standing. Radiographic studies show that the pelvis rotates backward and the lumbar spine flattens in sitting. Electromyography (EMG) supports the finding that sitting in a slouched or reclined position relaxes the trunk muscles and requires minimal muscle activity to hold the body weight in balance. However, disc pressures are greatest when a person sits with a slouched posture. Prolonged sitting in poor posture puts workers at risk for injuries. A good ergonomic chair design provides easily adjustable seat height and backrest, seat support, and inclination for correct posture. High backrests, armrests, and footrests are optional features; the need for these must be determined after tasks are analyzed to ensure compatibility between the chair selected and the tasks performed. A wide variety of seating options exist, including the saddle seat, kneeling chair, and sit-stand workstations, as well as supplemental devices such as lumbar supports, wedges, and back slings. These options are focused on promoting correct posture and worker comfort while increasing productivity and reducing risk of injuries.

Sedentary work is defined by the *Dictionary of Occupational Titles* as "exerting up to 10 pounds of force occasionally and/or a negligible amount of force frequently or constantly to lift, carry, push and pull, or otherwise move objects, including the human body. Sedentary work involves sitting most of the time, but may involve walking or standing for brief periods of time. Jobs are sedentary if walking and standing are required only occasionally and all other sedentary criteria are met" (U.S. Department of Labor 1991, p. 1013). Seated tasks require or feature the following characteristics: visual acuity; repetitive movements, particularly fine manipulation of the forearms and hands; and sitting for more than 4 hours (Eastman Kodak 1983).

Jobs that once involved a variety of tasks (allowing workers to move about their work areas) now require sitting for prolonged periods. This contrast is apparent in industries such as banking, insurance, publishing, and air travel. Computers are now used in nearly all work settings, and workers are spending greater periods in fixed postures at computer terminals. Thus, the chair used has increased importance.

Considerations of Sitting

Researchers began studying the effects of the seated position in the 1940s. *Sitting* has been defined as a position in which the weight of the body is transferred to a supporting area, mainly by the ischial tuberosities of the pelvis and their surrounding soft tissues (Schoberth 1962). In sitting, most of the body weight is on the buttocks, back, and feet.

A brief review of anatomy is helpful to fully appreciate the biomechanics of sitting. Thirty-three vertebrae compose the spine, including the cervical, thoracic, and lumbar vertebrae; the sacrum; and the coccyx. In standing, the spine forms three natural curves: (1) The cervical curve is inward (lordosis), (2) the thoracic curve is outward (kyphosis), and (3) the lumbar curve is inward (lordosis) The cervical and lumbar portions of the spine are mobile in relation to the thoracic spine. The intervertebral discs are located between the vertebrae. These act as shock absorbers between the vertebrae and provide flexibility to the spine. A disc is made up of viscous fluid contained by a tough, fibrous outside wall. Ligaments provide stability to the vertebrae and are located on the anterior and posterior walls of the spine. Muscles along the spine maintain posture and provide stability to the trunk. The nerves that compose the spinal cord are protected by the vertebrae and pass to the extremities, allowing motor and sensory information to pass to and from the brain. Blood flows along the spine, but the blood supply to the discs is limited.

The sacrum is essentially fixed and moves in relation to the pelvis; therefore, pelvic movement affects the shape of the lumbar spine. A forward or anterior rotation of the pelvis causes the lumbar spine to move toward increased lordosis to maintain an upright trunk. When the pelvis is tilted backward, the lumbar spine tends to flatten, sometimes causing kyphosis. Radiographic studies have verified that the pelvis rotates backward and the lumbar spine flattens during sitting (Åkerblom 1948; Andersson et al. 1979; Burandt 1969; Carlsoo 1972; Keegan 1953; Rosemeyer 1972; Schoberth 1962; Umezawa 1971). Disc pressures also change dramatically when a person moves from standing to sitting upright to sitting slouched. Nachemson and Elfstrom (1970) and Andersson and Ortengren (1974) developed methods to measure disc pressure. They found that disc pressure is greater during sitting than during standing. Nachemson and Morris (1964) published data on in vivo disc pressure measurements in people who stood and sat without support. The pressures measured when the subjects were standing were approximately 35% lower than those measured when the subjects were sitting. Research also demonstrates that increased disc pressure means that the discs are being overloaded and will wear out more quickly (Grandjean 1988).

Disc pressures drop with inclination of the backrest of a chair, especially when the backrest is tilted from vertical to 110 degrees (Andersson and Ortengren 1974). The backrest inclination is the angle between the seat and the backrest. Disc pressures are lower when a person is sitting and leaning back 110–120 degrees while using a 50-mm lumbar pad than when the person is standing in normal lumbar lordosis (Andersson and Ortengren 1974).

Muscle activity has been extensively researched through EMG of the back muscles during standing and sitting. Studies by Lundervold (1951a, 1951b, 1958) and Floyd and Roberts (1958) found that myoelectric activity decreased when the back support was located in the lumbar region rather than in the thoracic region. This confirmed a finding by Åkerblom (1948) that a support in the lumbar region is as effective as a full back support. Research has revealed a dichotomy: Disc pressures are reduced when a person sits in erect posture and maintains the three natural spinal curves, and the trunk muscles exert less energy when a person sits in a slightly flexed or slouched position.

Zacharokow (1988) has done extensive research to support the theory that supporting the sacrum and the lower thoracic spine is necessary to achieve proper sitting posture. The rationale behind sacral–lower thoracic support when sitting is that the proper axial relation between the thorax and the pelvis must be restored by bringing the upper trunk over the hips.

Zacharokow pointed out that sitting is a dynamic activity. People sit on their ischial tuberosities, causing the pelvis to rock. Without sacral support to produce an anterior tilt to the pelvis, the sacrum rotates posteriorly, bringing the lumbar spine into a flattened or kyphotic position. Zacharokow suggested that the use of a lumbar support with a seat backrest inclination of 110–120 degrees causes the worker doing close work to be too far from the surface. This requires flexion of the neck and upper body to compensate, increasing stress to these areas. Many therapists agree. Zacharokow designed a seating system—the Zack Back Posture Chair—to alleviate this problem.

A lumbar support may not be effective when the task involves writing or close work at a table top or bench. A study by Stewart and McQuilton (1987) found that a position of balanced pelvic muscle groups allows the body to be positioned over the ischial tuberosities (as in horseback riding) and not behind the seat base. This balance promotes greater accuracy in hand function and preservation of the lumbar curve.

Cervical Spine and Shoulders

The line of vision dictates head and neck posture. If the work surface is too low or the computer screen is too far away from the user, the result is neck and trunk flexion. If the head is held forward, increased cervical muscle activity is required to support the weight of the head and results in increased muscle fatigue. With increased use of computers, more workers are complaining of neck and shoulder pain. The complaints are becoming as common as complaints of low back pain (LBP). Diagnoses related to such injuries include shoulder and neck muscle strain, degenerative disc disease, and overuse syndrome. In Japan, these conditions are considered occupational diseases because they are often seen in typists, telephone and cash register operators, and assembly plant workers (Grandjean 1988).

Studies of VDT operators reveal that although the small muscles of the forearms and hands undergo almost constant dynamic contractions, the proximal muscles of the shoulders and neck provide postural support through static contraction. Prolonged static muscle contraction can cause considerable fatigue. Onishi et al. (1982) studied the EMG activity of the trapezius muscle during keyboard operations and found that when activity was present, the static loading of the trapezius muscle reached 20–30% of the level of maximum contraction.

Because the keyboard is the primary piece of equipment in the worker-machine interface, the correct relationship is of primary importance. Keyboard height is directly related to static loading of the trapezius muscle. Shoulder strain in keyboard workers is also related to forearm angle. Erdelyi et al. (1988) found a reduction in the static load of the trapezius muscle when the forearms were at an angle of at least 100 degrees. A properly adjusted armrest can provide the arm support necessary to reduce the level of myoelectric activity in the neck and shoulder muscles. Andersson et al (1974) found that the myoelectric activity was reduced in the lumbar region and the cervical and thoracic regions with a backrest inclination of 110–120 degrees.

Proper work surface height is important. If the work surface is too high, elbow flexion and shoulder abduction and elevation occur. This puts stress on the shoulder joints and increases the fatigue of the neck and shoulder muscles. The recommended position for desk work is shoulder abduction of 15–20 degrees or less and shoulder flexion of 25 degrees or less (Engdahl 1978).

Legs

Legs increase in volume by 4% over a workday (Winkel 1978, 1981). A chair that is too high or a seat pan that is too deep places pressure on the thighs and the back of the knees and can cause compression of the sciatic nerve. This increases the tendency toward swelling in the legs, ankles, and feet. A chair that is too high causes the worker to lean forward to support the feet on the floor. Consequently, the back of the chair is not used, and the individual sits in an unsupported position. A chair that is too low causes the hips and knees to flex beyond 90 degrees, resulting in a posterior pelvic tilt and lumbar flattening as well as a decrease in diaphragmatic breathing, which reduces energy.

The best way to avoid problems is to adjust the seat height so that the feet rest firmly on the floor or on a footrest. There should be 2.5 cm (1 in.) of space between the seat edge and the back of the knees. A worker can avoid swelling in the feet by taking frequent breaks; movement every 15 minutes can reduce swelling up to 2.3% (Winkel 1978, 1981).

Ergonomics of Sitting

People who sit for prolonged periods are at risk for back injury for the following reasons:

- Strained ligaments and stretching of muscles over time cause LBP.
- Approximately 60% of adults have a backache at least once in their lives; the most common cause is disc trouble (Grandjean 1988).
- Flattening of the lumbar spine during sitting causes disc herniation.

Therapists must emphasize to managers in industry that, although workers reduce the static muscular activity required on their hips, knees, ankles, and feet when sitting as opposed to standing, they put more strain on their backs, especially the lower part, when sitting. Therapists should promote the use of correct sitting posture and emphasize the health benefits of good posture. Good posture

- Decreases ligamentous strain to prevent overstretching
- Decreases muscular strain and overstretching of the back muscles, which causes muscle imbalances
- Decreases intradiscal pressure
- Helps provide a healthy spine along the whole kinetic chain caused by a reduction in stress on the thoracic and cervical spine and shoulder girdle
- Helps create more efficient muscle work and a reduction in fatigue because muscles are at a mechanical advantage; the postural muscles are used to support the spine and rib cage while the extremities are used to conduct work
- Provides a greater range of motion of the upper extremities when the worker reaches to shoulder level and overhead because the upper body is not flexed
- Assists in efficient diaphragmatic breathing because a greater distance is formed between the sternum and pelvis

- Helps in more efficient breathing, which provides oxygenated blood to vital organs (including the brain), resulting in increased productivity and diminished fatigue
- Provides improved lower-extremity circulation with proper seat tilt and depth
- Promotes a positive self-image

Therapists should have a thorough understanding of the biomechanics of sitting to assist industrial managers with workstation design. Therapists must be keenly aware of the type of tasks being performed by the worker. For example, writing at a desk and keying data into a computer may require different seating solutions. Variations in workers' body sizes and dimensions and individual personal sitting habits and movement patterns should also be taken into consideration. Each of these factors influences the selection of the chair and other equipment.

The components of most office or industrial chairs are as follows:

- Seat (width and depth)
- Backrest
- Pedestal base (seat height)
- Five-prong base (with or without casters)
- Tension adjustment for forward and backward inclination of tilted backrest
- Armrests and/or foot ring (optional)

Common Problems with the Typical Office or Industrial Chair

- The backrest is not easily adjustable and offers limited range of adjustment to provide adequate support to the lower part of the back. Often, the industrial chair is not padded, and sharp edges may come in contact with the worker.
- The seat height adjustment is often controlled by spinning the seat clockwise to raise it or counterclockwise to lower it. The worker must be out of the chair to do this.
- The tension control knob is often difficult to reach because it is under or behind the seat. Most workers are unfamiliar with the purpose of this tension control knob and rarely use it.
- If the chair has armrests, they are often too wide, too low, or too high to be used while the worker is at a work surface. If the armrests are too high, they can interfere with the ability to pull the chair under the work surface. This forces the worker to sit forward on the seat. Consequently, the backrest is not used, and the worker sits unsupported.

- The seat may be too deep for shorter people, causing their feet to dangle and failing to support their backs.

Good Ergonomic Chair Design

In the selection of an ergonomically appropriate chair, the most important feature to assess is adjustability. The adjustments must be easy to make and the controls must be accessible to the worker while he or she is seated. The purchaser must be aware that some manufacturers advertise a chair as "ergonomic" simply because it has pneumatic seat-height adjustment. These chairs may not meet the other criteria for an ergonomically correct chair. Even if a chair is labeled ergonomic and meets the American National Standards Institute/Human Factors Society standards, it may not be comfortable for all workers. These standards are minimal and do not apply to 10% of the population, because they pertain to the fifth to ninety-fifth (smallest to largest) percentile of the population according to anthropometric data. Therefore, a company that wants uniformity should select a chair that comes in more than one size.

A number of recommendations have been published with regard to anthropometric data related to seating design (i.e., dimensions, backrest, and seat-height adjustability) (Chaffin and Andersson 1984; Eastman Kodak 1983, 1986). The data differ from country to country because of the physical dimensions of individuals within a population.

Dynamic, a term used to describe an ergonomic chair, indicates that the chair is capable of leaning forward and backward and that the backrest inclination can be easily adjusted. Beyond this requirement, chairs differ widely. Some feature a "dynamic" forward tilt of the seat pan and backrest inclination as a unit; others feature an adjustable backrest inclination with seat tilt; still others feature a backrest and seat that adjust independently of each other. Some chairs allow the user to lock into a preferred position by means of static posture settings. Other chairs have a free-flowing (dynamic-motion) design that continuously moves with the user. Consideration must be given to the nature of the tasks done while sitting and the personal habits and preferences of the user. People sit in different postures to perform different tasks. Therefore, an ergonomic chair should fit comfortably while the worker performs various tasks.

In the budgets of most companies, chairs are capital equipment. An ergonomically correct office or industrial chair can cost as much $1,200. However, a good chair with pneumatic seat-height adjustment, an adjustable backrest, and a tilting seat pan costs approximately $250. Costs increase depending on the number of adjustable features and the fabric selected. The therapist may consider having various office or industrial chairs available in the clinic or workplace for workers to try. People need time to get used to different chairs that promote correct posture, especially if they have been sitting with poor posture for a long time.

The therapist can influence industry practices by educating managers, supervisors, purchasing agents, and employees about evaluating and selecting new chairs. Therapists should encourage employers to involve their employees in the evaluation and selection process. The features of an ergonomically well-designed chair are as follows:

- The seat height is easily adjustable, with a pneumatic pedestal base.
- The backrest is easily adjustable to support the lumbar spine vertically (height) and horizontally (forward and backward) and is narrow enough so that the worker's arms or torso do not strike it if rotation is required.
- The seat tilts forward and backward independently of the backrest. This feature is useful with fine detail work or office work.
- The seat edge is curved to reduce pressure behind the knees.
- Enough space is provided between the back of the chair and the seat to accommodate the buttocks.
- The adjustable armrests (optional) are small and low enough to fit under the work surface and to support the back when the worker works close to the work surface.
- The base has five points to prevent the chair from tipping.
- The worker can make adjustments easily with one hand while seated.
- The upholstery fabric is comfortable, reduces heat transfer in warm climates and static electricity in cold weather, and is stain resistant or easily cleaned.
- Training should be provided to ensure that workers are familiar with the features and adjustments of an optimally fitting chair.

A chair assessment is helpful to allow employers and employees to evaluate various chairs. An example of one such assessment is provided in Appendix 10.1. The guidelines for an ergonomically well-designed chair are specified in Figure 10.1.

An ergonomic chair, as with all ergonomic equipment, will not be effective unless it fits the worker properly. Workers must be trained to adjust the chair or equipment for proper fit and use. An excellent role for therapists who consult in industry is to help educate purchasing agents, managers, and chief executives about the medical cost savings of purchasing adjustable equipment and teaching employees how to use it.

Work Height

Employers frequently ask, "What is the proper desktop height?" This question is critical when an employer is designing new workstations. Information regarding recommended work surface heights has been provided by

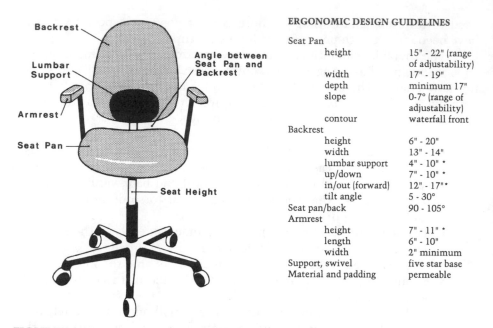

ERGONOMIC DESIGN GUIDELINES

Seat Pan		
	height	15" - 22" (range of adjustability)
	width	17" - 19"
	depth	minimum 17"
	slope	0-7° (range of adjustability)
	contour	waterfall front
Backrest		
	height	6" - 20"
	width	13" - 14"
	lumbar support	4" - 10" *
	up/down	7" - 10" *
	in/out (forward)	12" - 17" *
	tilt angle	5 - 30°
Seat pan/back		90 - 105°
Armrest		
	height	7" - 11" *
	length	6" - 10"
	width	2" minimum
Support, swivel		five star base
Material and padding		permeable

FIGURE 10.1.   Ergonomic design guidelines for a chair. (*Measured relative to chair seat.)

Eastman Kodak (1983). These recommendations are specified in Figure 10.2. In many situations, the workstation is fixed; for example, desks are permanent or countertops and shelves are built in. In these situations, the chair is the most flexible and usually the most critical piece of equipment to provide adjustability for a better worker-to-workstation fit. The working height depends on the nature of the tasks performed. Tasks such as writing or light assembly are most easily performed if the work is at elbow height. If the job requires fine detail and visual acuity, it may be necessary to raise the work to bring it closer to the eyes (Eastman Kodak 1983).

Consideration must be given to the layout of the workstation. Items at the workstation should be within comfortable reaching distance. A good rule is to place items within an arm's length or within the radius of both arms. Therefore, frequently used items, such as a telephone, dictation equipment, computer and keyboard, calculator, reference materials, or files, should be situated to achieve such proximity. Removing clutter by installing overhead shelves or additional file cabinets is recommended.

Armrests

Armrests are recommended for assembly or repair tasks in which the arm has to be held away from the body and is not moved extensively during the work cycle (Eastman Kodak 1983). EMG studies substantiate lowered

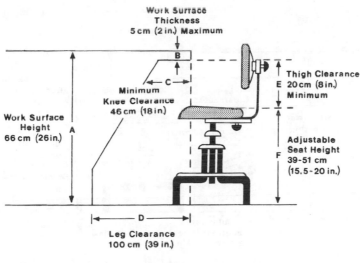

Work Surface
Thickness
5 cm (2 in.) Maximum

B

↑
C
Minimum
Knee Clearance
46 cm (18 in.)

Thigh Clearance
E 20 cm (8 in.)
Minimum

Work Surface
Height
66 cm (26 in.)
A

Adjustable
Seat Height
F 39–51 cm
(15.5–20 in.)

|← D →|

Leg Clearance
100 cm (39 in.)

Side View

FIGURE 10.2.   Recommended dimensions for a seated workstation without a footrest. (Reprinted courtesy of Eastman Kodak Company.)

trapezius muscle activity when armrest support is used. Disc pressure is reduced when armrests are used, provided the backrest-to-seat angle is not too large (Andersson and Ortengren 1974).

Nonadjustable armrests are often too wide for the average person and too high for a person with long arms, causing increased shoulder elevation. Armrests should be near the front of the work surface, should tilt without having to be readjusted manually, and should be cushioned to eliminate sharp edges.

In the textile industry, where sewing machine operators sit for prolonged periods, researchers are experimenting with specialized armrests to support the upper extremities. Some computer operators use elbow or forearm rests to support their upper arms while their wrists and hands are free to move.

Footrests

To accommodate variations in workers' heights, a workstation should include an adjustable footrest. Footrests come in a variety of styles: fixed or portable; horizontal, as in a platform; or tilted. Chairs with a foot ring may not be satisfactory, because the ring is often close to the floor and fixed. If a short person were to raise the chair, he or she would be unable to reach the foot ring. Some chairs are manufactured with foot rings that move with the seat as it is adjusted, and others have foot rings that can be adjusted independently. Portable footrests must be large enough to support the soles of both feet. A footrest of 30 cm × 41 cm (12 in. × 16 in.) with an angle of

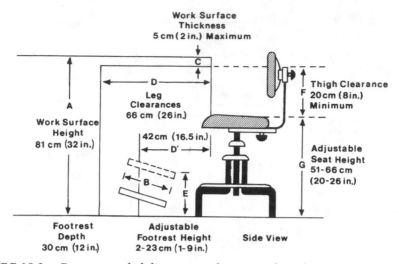

FIGURE 10.3. Recommended dimensions for a seated workstation with a footrest. (Reprinted courtesy of Eastman Kodak Company.)

25–30 degrees and a nonskid surface is recommended (Roebuck et al. 1975). If the footrest is built into the workstation, it should be 30 cm (12 in.) deep and wide enough to reach across the width of the seat. Built-in footrests in a workstation where the board can be varied in 5-cm (2-in.) increments (like a bookshelf) are recommended (Eastman Kodak 1983). These recommendations are specified in Figure 10.3.

A variety of footrests are available and may be found in many office and industrial supply catalogs. Telephone books or footrests built from wood scraps are inexpensive solutions. Workers often say footrests help remind them to sit up straighter. This is a tactile reminder to use better posture, regardless of the chair.

Special Considerations: Workstation Design for Seated Workers

Workers Who Use Computers

Poorly designed computer workstations put workers at risk not only for back injuries but also for neck, shoulder, forearm, wrist and hand, and leg problems. Vision problems are also widely reported.

The ergonomic chair has become the primary solution to office workplace problems. A poorly fitting chair affects all other aspects of the worker-to-workstation match. A correctly fitted chair affects the relation between the worker and the workstation, and all other components should be evaluated after the chair-to-worker fit is completed. Employers should be encouraged to invest in better-quality, user-friendly, adjustable chairs as a first step toward improving the workplace. Modular workstations and computer stands are more common in workplaces today. Studies confirm that worktables with an adjustable height and desktop inclination, along with ergonomic chairs, increase worker comfort and productivity.

Hunting and Grandjean (1976) conducted a study of office chairs. They compared three chairs: (1) a tiltable chair with a high backrest, (2) a similar model with a fixed seat, and (3) a traditional chair with an adjustable but short backrest. Their survey results indicated that after using each of the three chairs for 2 weeks, office workers preferred the two chairs with high backrests. A high backrest allows the user to lean back and supports the body's weight. The tilting feature was also noted to be undesirable because most users wanted a fixed position once they found a position of comfort. This research supports the findings of studies that suggest reduced disc pressure and reduced muscle strain with backrest inclination. For example, when driving a car for several hours, one would rather sit back slightly than in an upright position.

Finding the Fit Between Worker and Workstation

When determining the fit between a worker and a computer workstation, the best and easiest method to teach is a kinesthetic or tactile approach in which workers feel their body in relation to the machine (computer, keyboard, and terminal). The worker assumes the correct sitting posture: hip, knee, and ankle joints flexed to 90 degrees; feet firmly on floor; shoulder girdle over hip girdle; and head over shoulders to achieve the three natural spinal curves. The worker then adjusts the backrest or uses a lumbar cushion, towel roll, or seat wedge to achieve proper lumbosacral support. The distance from the worker to the screen dictates head position. The ergonomic literature suggests a viewing distance of 51–76 cm (20–30 in.) (Pinsky 1987). An arm's reach is an easy reference point.

Armrests or wrist rests are recommended to decrease shoulder muscle fatigue. A document holder attached to the screen allows lateral eye gaze as opposed to repetitive neck flexion and extension to look at work on a desktop surface. A footrest may be used either to support the feet of a short worker or to change leg position during prolonged sitting. Shoulders should be relaxed, flexed 25 degrees or less, and abducted 20–25 degrees or less. Elbows should be held comfortably by the sides and flexed to 90–100 degrees. Forearms and wrists should be in a neutral position, and the fingers and thumbs should be comfortably flexed.

Lighting, climate control, ventilation, work-space layout and storage, work breaks, and employee health and safety for computer operators are other important considerations in the analysis of an office (see Chapter 7).

A variety of educational sessions may be presented to workers to achieve worker compliance and follow-through. These sessions typically include a brief spinal anatomy lesson (including a discussion of disc pressure); the importance of proper sitting posture; the correct use of body mechanics while sitting, such as the avoidance of bending and twisting; and mechanisms of injury to the back, neck, shoulders, wrists, hands, and legs. The therapist must observe the work flow and work methods of the worker as well as individual habits, because these factors influence equipment recommendations. For example, if a worker uses a computer to access information, transfers the information into ledgers by hand, and uses a calculator intermittently, the chair requirements may be very different from those of a data processor who performs continuous keyboard work. The first worker may not need armrests or wrist rests at the workstation, and the second may benefit from one or both. People come in all shapes and sizes. Employers serve their employees best by providing options in chair selection and in the use and selection of adaptive equipment such as headsets, elbow supports, armrests, incline boards, split keyboards, wrist rests, footrests, antiglare screens, and screen hoods.

Sit-Stand Position

Sit-stand workstations should be considered when the worker must repetitively reach forward more than 41 cm (16 in.) or reach up more than 15 cm (6 in.) (Eastman Kodak 1983). A very high chair with a forward-sloping seat can be used for a semisitting posture. This posture provides torso support with lumbar lordosis for work that requires mobility and reach. Most of the weight is on the buttocks and the feet when the worker uses this kind of chair. Jobs such as graphic design and drafting, which require large work surfaces, are best suited for sit-stand workstations.

Computer work has traditionally been done while sitting. Given the long hours spent by some workers in front of a computer terminal and the wider acceptance of ergonomics in the office workplace, however, sit-stand computer workstations are becoming more common. Simply by pushing a button or switch, a worker can change from a sitting to a standing position. The manufacturer advertises that it accommodates user sizes from a fifth-percentile woman seated to a ninety-fifth–percentile man standing. Of course, such adjustability is expensive.

Kneeling Chairs

The Balans chair from Norway is probably the most famous of the half-sitting, half-kneeling posture chairs. It features a forward-tilted seat and a knee support. This design results in a wider hip angle and maintains the three natural curves of the spine, thus preserving lumbar lordosis. Studies by Krueger (1984), however, found that the load on the knees and lower legs is too great and sitting becomes painful. Work surface height is also critical for proper fit. Common practice in offices that have a kneeling chair is to rotate the chair among workers, limiting each worker's use to approximately 2 hours. This system provides a change in posture for those who must sit to perform work.

Lumbar Support, Wedge, and Back Sling

A wide variety of lumbar supports are available and range from small, rounded, oblong pillows to full-length molded plastic frames that feature lower back and lateral support (e.g., Obus chair). Most medical supply catalogs contain an array of lumbar cushions, rolls, and half-rolls. Therapists must educate people in the correct support based on body type and the particular chair or seat (e.g., office, industrial, home, car) for which the cushion is intended.

The seat wedge, which comes in a number of formats, provides the user the ischial support to tip the pelvis anteriorly when used correctly. It encourages upward posture and may be the best adaptation for a user who must sit close to a work surface to write. The seat wedge is useful in a chair that lacks a forward tilting feature and thus gives the user more variety when seated for long periods. Another simple remedy to promote an anterior pelvic tilt is to place a small towel roll under the ischial tuberosities. As the body weight is shifted forward, the upper body comes closer to the work surface, and the towel prevents the worker from rocking back on the ischial tuberosities.

A back sling is a device that works independently of the chair. Through a strapping system that consists of a lower back cushion and slings that anchor at the knees, the lumbar spine is held in lordosis. The strapping around the knees is typically held in place with a buckle between the thighs. Consequently, female office workers are often reluctant to use it. However, this device has met with great success for workers with LBP who sit on industrial stools at assembly lines all day.

References

Åkerblom B (1948). Standing and Sitting Posture: With Special Reference to the Construction of Chairs. Stockholm: Nordiska Bokhandeln.

Andersson GBJ, Murphy RW, Ortengren R, Nachemson AL (1979). The influence of backrest inclination and lumbar support on the lumbar lordosis in sitting. Spine 4:52–58.

Andersson GBJ, Ortengren R (1974). Lumbar disc pressure and myoelectric back muscle activity during sitting. 1. Studies on an experimental chair. Scand J Rehabil Med 3:104–135.

Burandt U (1969). Rontgenuntersuchung uber die Stellung von Becken und Wirbelsaule beim Sitzen auf vorgeneirten Flachen. In E Grandjean (ed), Sitting Posture. London: Taylor & Francis, 242–250.

Carlsoo S (1972). How Man Moves. London: Heinemann.

Chaffin D, Andersson G (1984). Occupational Biomechanics. New York: Wiley.

Eastman Kodak (1983). Ergonomic Design for People at Work. Vol. 1. New York: Van Nostrand Reinhold.

Eastman Kodak (1986). Ergonomic Design for People at Work. Vol 2. New York: Van Nostrand Reinhold.

Engdahl S (1978). Specification for Office Furniture. In B Jonsson (ed), Sitting Work Postures. No. 12. Solna, Sweden: National Board of Occupational Safety and Health, 97–135.

Erdelyi A, Silhoven T, Helin P, et al. (1988). Shoulder strain in keyboard workers and its alleviation by arm supports. Int Arch Occup Environ Health 60:119–124.

Floyd WF, Roberts DF (1958). Anatomical and physiological principles in chair and table design. Ergonomics 2(2):1.

Grandjean E (1988). Fitting the Task to the Man (4th ed). London: Taylor & Francis.

Hunting W, Grandjean E (1976). Sitzverhalten und subjektives Wohlbefinden auf schwenkbaren und fixierten Formsitzen. Z Arbeitswissenschaft 30:161–164.

Keegan JJ (1953). Alterations of the lumbar curve related to posture and seating. J Bone Joint Surg Am 35:589–603.

Krueger H (1984). Zur Ergonomie von Balans-Sitzelementen im Hinblick auf ihre Verwendbarkeit als regulare Arbeitsstuhle. Report 8092. Zurich: Department of Ergonomics, Swiss Federal Institute of Technology.

Lundervold AJS (1951a). Electromyographic investigations of position and manner of working in typewriting. Acta Orthop Scand (suppl 84).

Lundervold AJS (1951b). Electromyographic investigations during sedentary work especially typewriting. Br J Phys Med 14:31.

Lundervold AJS (1958). Electromyographic investigations during typewriting. Ergonomics 1:226.

Nachemson A, Elfström G (1970). Intravital dynamic pressure measurements in lumbar discs. A study of common movements, maneuvers and exercises. Scand J Rehabil Med Suppl 1:1–40.

Nachemson A, Morris JM (1964.). In vivo measurements of intradiscal pressure. J Bone Joint Surg Am 46:1077–1092.

Onishi N, Sakai K, Kogi K (1982). Arm and shoulder muscle load in various keyboard operating jobs of women. J Hum Ergol 11:89–97.

Pinsky M (1987). The VDT Book: A Computer Users Guide to Health and Safety. New York: New York Committee for Occupational Safety and Health.

Roebuck JA Jr, Kroemer KHE, Thomson WC (1975). Engineering Anthropometry Methods. New York: Wiley.

Rosemeyer B (1972). Eine Methode zur Beckenfixierung im Arbeitssitz. Z Orthopa Ihre Grenzgeb 110:514–517.

Schoberth H (1962). Sitzhaltung, Sitzschaden, Sitzmobel. Berlin: Springer.

Stewart P, McQuilton G (1987). Straddle seating for the cerebral palsied child. Physiotherapy 73:204–206.

Umezawa F (1971). The study of comfortable sitting postures. J Japan Orthop Assoc 45:1015.

U.S. Department of Labor (1991). Dictionary of Occupational Titles (4th ed). Washington, DC: U.S. Government Printing Office.

Winkel J (1978). Leg Problems from Long-Lasting Sitting. In B Jonsson (ed), Sitting Work Postures. No. 12. Solna, Sweden: National Board of Occupational Safety and Health, 72–78 (in Swedish).

Winkel J (1981). Swelling of lower leg in sedentary work: a pilot study. J Hum Ergol 10:139–149.

Zacharkow D (1988). Posture: Sitting, Standing, Chair Design and Exercise. Springfield, IL: Charles C. Thomas.

Suggested Reading

American National Standard for Human Factors Engineering of Visual Display Terminal Workstations (1988). ANSI/HFS Standard No. 1001988. Santa Monica, CA: Human Factors Society.

Diffrient N, Tilley A, Bardagjy J (1974). Humanscale 1/2/3. Cambridge, MA: MIT Press.

Mandal AC (1976). The Seated Man. Klampenborg: Mandal.

National Institute for Occupational Health and Safety (1991). Publications on Video Display Terminals (Revised). ANSI/HFS #1001988. Cincinnati: NIOSH.

Pheasant S (1986). Bodyspace: Anthropometry, Ergonomics, and Design. London: Taylor & Francis.

Rodgers SH (1984). Working with Backache. New York: Perinton.

Tadano P (1990). A safety/prevention program for VDT operators: one company's approach. J Hand Ther 3:64–71.

Yu CY, Keyserling WM (1989). Evaluation of a new work seat for industrial sewing operations. Appl Ergonomics 20:17–25.

Review Questions

(Answers are found in Appendix D.)

1. What is the *most* important feature to look for in the selection of an ergonomically appropriate chair?
   (a) Five-pronged base
   (b) Backrest
   (c) Adjustability
   (d) Armrests
   (e) Reasonable price

2. Research has shown that reduced disc pressure and reduced muscle strain occur in which of the following situations?
   (a) Sitting forward slightly
   (b) Sitting in an upright position
   (c) Sitting back slightly

3. Radiographic studies show that the pelvis rotates backward and the lumbar spine _____ in sitting. This can cause disc herniation.
   (a) rotates forward
   (b) flattens
   (c) is stretched
   (d) is not affected

4. Which of the following should therapists consider when assisting in workstation design?
   (a) Type of task being performed
   (b) Body size and height of the worker
   (c) Sitting habits of the worker
   (d) Movement patterns of the work (workflow)
   (e) All of the above

5. What workstation option should be considered when the worker must repetitively reach forward more than 16 in. or reach up more than 6 in.?
   (a) Higher work surface
   (b) Sit-stand position
   (c) Kneeling chair
   (d) Lower work surface

Appendix 10.1

Ergonomic Chair Assessment

Manufacturer: _____   *Model:* _____

_____ Does the seat height adjust easily while you are seated?
_____ Does the seat height allow you to rest your feet on the floor?
_____ Does the seat pan easily tilt forward and backward while you are seated?
_____ Does the backrest height easily adjust up and down while you are seated?
_____ Does the backrest easily move forward and backward while you are seated?
_____ Does the backrest provide firm support to the lower part of your back?
_____ Can you make the adjustments easily without assuming awkward positions?
_____ Are the seat and back contoured and comfortable to adjust to your movements and body shape?
_____ Have you been instructed in how to adjust this chair to fit you properly?
_____ Does the seat support your thighs to a point just behind the back of the knee?
_____ Do you experience a shock when you touch the chair in cold weather?
_____ Do the seat and back dissipate body heat?
_____ Do you feel supported and comfortable in this chair? If not, why?
_____ Do you like the overall appearance of the chair?

If arms are featured on this chair:
_____ Are you able to get in close to your desk?
_____ Do the armrests allow your elbows to remain comfortably by your side with your shoulders relaxed?
_____ Are the armrests contoured and comfortable?
_____ Are the armrests adjustable in height and distance from your body?
_____ Can the armrests be removed easily without affecting the appearance of the chair?

Manager and purchaser:
_____ Does this chair come in a variety of models to accommodate variations in size of people, yet give a uniform look?

CHAPTER 11
Computers and Assistive Technology

Tamar (Patrice L.) Weiss and Chetwyn C. H. Chan

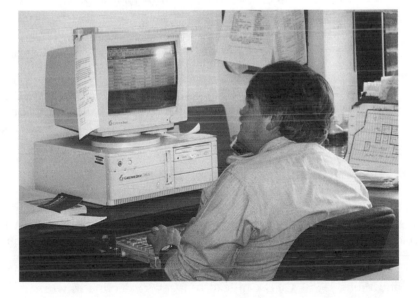

ABSTRACT

The computer workstation has become common both at work and at home and is now used routinely for many purposes, including data entry, word processing, telecommunications, web browsing, purchasing, inventory, designing, testing, and entertainment. Many computer operators type up to 60 words per minute (wpm) for more than 6 hours a day (i.e., more than 150,000 keystrokes per day). Workers commonly spend long periods sitting in a static posture at computer workstations, with only minimal need to reposition the trunk, neck, and arms.

Extensive evidence indicates that working with computer terminals and keyboards is associated with the development and exacerbation of a variety of work-related disorders involving the back, neck, and upper limbs (Armstrong et al. 1993). Such conditions, known as *cumulative trauma disorder* (CTD), are considered to be the "industrial injuries of the Information Age" (Doheny et al. 1995). Other terms for CTD include *repetitive strain injury, muscle tendon syndrome,* and *occupational overuse syndrome* (Frederick 1992). Medical problems commonly associated with CTD include tenosynovitis, wrist tendinitis, de Quervain's tenosynovitis, epicondylitis, carpal tunnel syndrome, and tension neck syndrome.

Epidemiology of Cumulative Trauma Disorder

The National Institute for Occupational Safety and Health (NIOSH) estimates that 15–20% of the work force in the United States is at risk for developing CTD. CTD costs industries in the United States $27 billion in 1989 (Mallory and Bradford 1989), and CTD claims made by workers in other developed countries, such as Australia and Canada, continue to escalate (Fast 1995; Hashemi et al. 1998). The number of computer keyboard workers with CTD is as much as 12 times the number of non-keyboard users with CTD (Fahrback and Chapman 1990; Oxenburgh 1984). Among keyboard users, the prevalence of CTD is as high as 60% (Schreuer et al. 1996). CTD is reported to be more than twice as common in women as in men in workers between 30 and 50 years old (Ballard 1993; Gun 1990; Leung and Wong 1995). CTD can lead to a severe decline in worker performance with serious consequences to the employee, to the employer, and to medical and social service resources (Vender et al. 1995).

A survey in Hong Kong examined musculoskeletal symptoms in office workers (Occupational Safety and Health Council 1997). A total of 688 workers in 96 companies were interviewed, 65% of whom were female and 68% of whom operated a computer keyboard for more than 4 hours daily. Workers reported a high incidence of musculoskeletal symptoms, particularly in the shoulder (42%), lower back (39%), neck (39%), and upper back (36%). Lower rates of incidence were reported in the elbow (6%), forearm (9%), and fingers (13%). Approximately 60% of the workers felt that the onset of discomfort began after the commencement of their present employment. Among the workers who reported musculoskeletal discomfort, approximately 44% experienced reduced capacities in lifting more than a 10-lb load, 42% in sports, 37% in child care, and 32% in housework. Results of the study also indicated that workplace design (e.g., desktop, chair height, leg room), job design (e.g., workload and work hours), and hours of computer operation were the most important risk factors contributing to symptoms.

The pathophysiology of CTD is not completely known. Epidemiologic and clinical studies suggest that causes of CTD consist of both intrinsic and extrinsic factors (Ballard 1993; Leung and Wong 1995). Studies have demonstrated that cumulative and repetitive force applied to the same muscle group, joint, or tendon causes soft-tissue microtears and trauma (Sjogaard 1990). The chronic soft-tissue condition is further aggravated by muscle exertion and excessive joint movements (Alqattan and Bowen 1993). Several risk factors, including repetitive motion, excessive force, and awkward working posture, are closely associated with CTD in keyboard operators (Yassi 1997). The risk of CTD is also associated with psychosocial factors such as role conflict or ambiguity, excessive workload and work stress, and negative social interaction (Alqattan and Bowen 1993; Doheny et al. 1995). The predictability and relative risk associated with these psychosocial factors have not been systematically studied, however.

Dose-Response Model

Armstrong et al. (1993) proposed a dose-response model for determining risk factors of CTD. The model has four interactive components: (1) exposure, (2) dose, (3) capacity, and (4) response. *Exposure* refers to the worker's external or work environment and includes physical characteristics of the job, including weight, size, and shape of tools, and psychological factors such as job security. *Dose* refers to the internal environment of an individual's body and includes mechanical forces acting on the body tissues, physiologic consumption of metabolic substrates, and production of metabolites within the tissues, as well as psychological disturbances, such as anxiety about work. These two factors are thought to act on every individual, in the workplace and at home.

Individuals react to these factors according to *capacity*, which is the physical and psychological ability to resist destabilization caused by one or more doses (Armstrong et al. 1993). An individual's reaction to exposure and dose, modified by his or her capacity, is a *response*. A vicious circle can occur in which responses elicit further disturbances within the body, often leading to severe tissue damage. CTD is the consequences of these responses when the body's capacity (e.g., a particular muscle or tendon) is incapable of resisting deleterious changes induced by the exposure (i.e., body tissues cannot repair the damage as fast as it occurs).

The dose-response model predicts that an individual's capacity can be reduced by continued mechanical, physiologic, and psychological events, such as muscle fatigue, minor injuries, and mental stress. CTD occurs when the exposure and doses exceed the capacity of an individual to respond in a healthy manner. The results of numerous experimental studies are consistent with the predictions of this model (Dobyns 1995; Lundborg and Dahlin 1995; Nathan et al. 1988; Wells 1993; Wieslander et al. 1989).

The dose-response model is also useful in explaining interventions that may prevent or reduce CTD. For example, interactions between an individual's capacity, dose, and response suggest that mobilization exercises, including stretching and strengthening of the body, can be beneficial in improving capacity by restoring weak and injured muscles (Taylor and Braun 1988). Regular mobilization exercise of the involved body parts reduces the discrepancy between the dose and capacity of an individual, decreasing the effects of a deleterious response and the probability of developing a CTD.

Risk Factors of Cumulative Trauma Disorder: Exacerbation and Reduction

Many investigators have identified risk factors that are closely associated with upper extremity CTD, including repetitive motion, excessive force, maintenance of awkward or constrained postures for prolonged periods, mechanical stress via direct pressure, vibration, and extreme temperatures (Armstrong 1990; Kierklo and Jones 1994; Stetson et al. 1991). These factors are not equally relevant for all tasks, however.

According to the dose-response model, the probability of developing CTD can be reduced by minimizing the exposure, and thus the dose, to the task and the work environment. An effective job modification program reduces the frequency with which a worker is exposed to one or more risk factors (Ballard 1993; Kierklo and Jones 1994; Wells 1993).

For most risk factors, exposure time is critical. Winkel and Westgaard (1992) recommended reducing exposure to less than 4 hours per day. Exposure time should be further reduced when the task is monotonous, the work environment is impoverished from a psychosocial viewpoint, an especially high demand is required for productivity, or rest breaks are infrequent. Varying the type of tasks in a work shift is advisable to ensure that the worker is not exposed to any single risk factor for an extended period. Although regular or frequent rest breaks are also recommended (Dul et al. 1994), rest breaks do not always prove to be beneficial (Feely et al. 1995; Henning et al. 1997; Wood et al. 1997).

A number of studies suggest that keyboard tasks entail exposure to a number of risk factors and are prime factors in the development of CTD. Not only are keyboard tasks performed for extended periods, but the tasks also usually involve the simultaneous presence of two or more risk factors, further increasing the risk of developing CTD (Rizzo et al. 1997; Rossignol et al. 1998). The combined effect of excessive force and repetitive movement has been suggested to be considerably more injurious than either factor alone (Rossignol et al. 1998; Silverstein et al. 1986; Sommerich et al. 1996). The relevance of working at a computer workstation to each of the major CTD risk factors is described in the following sections.

Repetitive Motion

Little doubt exists that high repetition is typical of the performance of many keyboard operators, who often type at rates of 10,000 to 25,000 keystrokes per hour (Rempel et al. 1991; Sommerich et al. 1996). Pan and Schleifer (1996) observed that subjects with higher ratings of upper extremity discomfort during a data-entry task had lower keystroke rates.

Forceful Motion

Keyboard operators exert peak forces in the range of 2–3 N, approximately three to five times more than the force actually required to activate the key (Armstrong et al. 1994; Feuerstein et al. 1997; Loeb 1983; Rempel et al. 1991; Sommerich et al. 1996; Weiss 1990). The use of this amount of force means that keyboard keys are moved downward to their limit (Armstrong et al. 1994; Radwin 1997). Not only does this result in greater travel than required to activate the keys, but the user may also encounter additional force by hitting down to the bottom of the key.

Whether the forces generated during each keystroke can be considered to be sufficiently high to be injurious is unclear, especially when their magnitude is compared to those generated during other manual jobs categorized as low (29 N) to high (125 N) force. Nevertheless, Feuerstein et al. (1997) found that office workers who reported upper extremity musculoskeletal symptoms with greater frequency and severity exerted higher levels of key force while typing than office workers who reported fewer and less severe symptoms. In contrast, Pan and Schleifer (1996) observed that subjects who had higher ratings of upper extremity discomfort during a data-entry task exerted *lower* key force. The two studies differed in several respects, however, including the exact nature and duration of the tasks

and whether the subjects reported previous symptoms. In tasks such as
typing, which are performed for extended periods, the cumulative typing
force, rather than the peak forces measured above, is highly likely to be
more important (Sommerich et al. 1996). Overall, the user's susceptibility
to injury is affected by typing speed, the forces exerted on each key, total
typing time, and the amount of time spent on each key.

With the surge in use of Windows-based software, menu-driven interfaces, and graphical user interfaces, manipulating a standard mouse now
accounts for as much as 65% of the time spent at some computer tasks
(Johnson et al. 1993). Certain mouse tasks, such as dragging, impose sustained loading on the finger flexor muscles.

Awkward Postures and Constrained Positions

Typing is a composite task in which the arms, shoulders, and trunk provide a static support base while the digits engage primarily in dynamic
work. In some cases, the same muscle alternately engages in both types of
work. For example, the extensor digitorum communis provides both static
wrist support and dynamic finger joint control (Sommerich et al. 1995). In
the classic typing position, elevated muscle activity has been found in the
proximal musculature including the muscles responsible for shoulder elevation and abduction, forearm pronation, and ulnar deviation (Nakaseko et
al. 1985; Zipp et al. 1983). Pascarelli and Kella (1993) observed a number of
postures used by keyboard operators who suffered from serious upper
extremity symptoms. These postures included the "alienated thumb" and
the hyperextended fifth digit, both of which induce users to access the keyboard at potentially injurious joint angles and muscle lengths.

Ulnar deviation of the wrist in excess of 20 degrees has frequently
been observed (Hunting et al. 1981; Pascarelli and Kella 1993) and has been
associated with elevated pressure in the carpal tunnel (Weiss et al. 1995).
Direct measurement of carpal tunnel pressure via a flexible catheter pressure transducer has shown that pressure is lowest when the wrist is
slightly extended and slightly ulnar deviated (Weiss et al. 1995).

Sauter et al. (1991) analyzed self-report data from several hundred
computer users and found a number of posture-related factors associated
with the presence of musculoskeletal discomfort. In particular, low and soft
seat surfaces were associated with leg discomfort, and keyboards placed
above elbow level were associated with arm discomfort, as well as high levels of neck and shoulder girdle discomfort. In one of the many studies that
have documented the relationship between user posture and CTD symptoms, Faucett and Rempel (1994) showed that keyboard height was significantly related to severe pain and stiffness in the shoulders, neck, and upper
back in a group of 150 computer operators working in a newsroom.

Awkward and constrained postures also typify use of a standard
mouse. Computer operators tend to maintain their shoulders in excessive
external rotation and keep their wrists in extreme ulnar deviation for pro-

longed periods (Karlqvist and Hagberg 1996). They also experience discomfort at the shoulder, elbow, and wrist. Significant increases in muscle activity levels and amount of perceived effort are related to the position of the arm and forearm during manipulation of the mouse and to users' anthropometric characteristics (Karlqvist et al. 1994, 1998). Less-than-optimal placement of the mouse was associated with a prevalence of upper-limb symptoms (Karlqvist and Hagberg 1996). Aaras (1994) concluded that the load on the trapezius muscle and pain intensity and duration were significantly reduced among computer operators when the workstation layout was adjusted by providing more work surface at the table top for operating the keyboard and mouse and an adjustable table and chair.

Although awkward and constrained postures undoubtedly contribute to the development of CTD, evidence exists that job design and work-style factors, such as task duration, are even more damaging (Matias et al. 1998).

Mechanical Stress Caused by Direct Pressure

Mechanical stress caused by direct pressure such as that exerted when objects press down on the base of the palm can contribute to the development of CTD. Feldman et al. (1983), for example, suggested that cubital tunnel syndrome with subsequent ulnar neuropathy is commonly caused by a worker's chronically leaning on his or her elbows on desks or armrests during typing. This results in disturbed sensation in the fourth and fifth fingers and lateral side of the hand and weakness of flexor carpi ulnaris, flexor digitorum profundus, and the interossei.

Vibration

Exposure to excessive vibration at the work site can lead to sensory impairments such as paresthesia and diminished tactility, reducing the worker's ability to determine or gauge the amount of force necessary to hold and manipulate objects (Armstrong et al. 1987). These individuals tend to exert too much force during repetitive manual tasks, causing soft-tissue damage. Although vibration is prevalent at many job sites, it rarely occurs during keyboard tasks.

Extreme Temperatures

Low temperature is another CTD risk factor. Low temperature (below 20°C) was found to reduce manual dexterity and to accentuate the symptoms of nerve impairment (Armstrong 1990).

Evaluation of the Impact of Exposure

The dose-response model emphasizes that exposure is a crucial factor in the occurrence of CTD. Methods commonly used to quantify the impact of exposure include self-report questionnaires, on-site observation, and electromyography (EMG). Self-report questionnaires are used to obtain information on workers' physical and psychological symptoms and focus on perceived job demands, subjective analysis of the workstation, parts of the body in which symptoms occur, the duration of symptoms over a particular period (e.g., the last 12 months, the previous 7 days), the effect of the symptoms on activities at work and during leisure time, and time off work. The standardized Nordic questionnaire is a well-known self-report form for the entire body (Kuorinka et al. 1987). Other questionnaires focus primarily on CTD in the neck and upper extremities (Ohlsson et al. 1994). Self-report questionnaires, many of which have been shown to be reliable and valid, provide valuable information about workers, their behavior, and their environment without being overly invasive and time-consuming. Nevertheless, this method is inherently subjective and often not sufficiently accurate.

On-site observation and measurement can provide more detailed information on the interactions between workers, work tasks, and workstations. Information is commonly recorded on video, which can be reviewed with behavioral checklists to quantify the content and duration of the relevant aspects of task performance (Leinonen and Kisko 1998). Metric measurement of the dimensions of the workstations and quantification of the job demands can be compared directly with the anthropometric database. The extent of the mismatch between workstation, task, and workers and its contribution to the occurrence of CTD can be estimated. Validity of on-site observation methods can be compromised, however, when tasks are variable and not well defined. Further, factors such as muscular load, angular velocity, and extent of fatigue cannot be addressed by observational methods (Juul Kristensen et al. 1997). The labor-intensive procedures of video analysis and the difficulty applying the results to other jobs when tasks are heterogeneous and work environments are atypical are also drawbacks of this method.

EMG evaluation of the magnitude and duration of muscle activity is another method commonly used to analyze the muscular work pattern at workstations (Veiersted et al. 1993). For example, EMG studies of the trapezius muscle under various load conditions revealed that workers who sat with the thoracolumbar spine slightly posteriorly inclined and with the cervical spine vertically aligned reported less strain on the muscle when compared with those who sat with whole spine straight and vertical or with the whole spine flexed (Schuldt et al. 1986). The occurrence of fatigue as shown by changes in the EMG spectral density can also be used to study the load on different muscles (Aaras 1994). EMG evaluation is accurate in isolating and quantifying the effect of the exposure on the worker's musculoskeletal capacity and responses. However, EMG is perceived by the workers as more invasive than either the questionnaire or the on-site observation approaches. Care must be taken to avoid disturbances (e.g., excessive movement of wires) when using EMG in the work environment to ensure that results are reliable.

Evaluation of Work Capacity of Keyboard Users

A functional capacity evaluation (FCE) can determine whether a worker has the attributes necessary for a specific job (Lechner et al. 1991). For the dose-response model, an FCE measures capacity in relationship to the exposure imposed by the performance of tasks. An FCE can also help clinicians monitor the progress of workers with injury undergoing rehabilitation programs and identify any need for specific clinical interventions to meet work demands.

A number of commercial or custom-made evaluation packages and instruments have been designed to implement an FCE. The most common approach for evaluating work capacity is the use of work samples. A work sample is a set of activities involving tasks, materials, and tools that are identical or similar to those in an actual job or job clusters (Malzahn et al. 1996). Because CTD has many causes, a number of work samples and actual tasks are more useful than single examples for evaluating computer and keyboard operators. The activities that are important to computer workers are those involving the upper extremities (fingering, reaching, and using manual dexterity); those concerning the head, neck, and back (sustained erect posture, prolonged sitting, and eye-hand coordination); and those requiring sustained attention, concentration, and memory. The work samples selected should evaluate these job demands.

Unfortunately, appropriate work samples for computer workers are uncommon. Valpar WorkSET components (available from Valpar International) include a few work sets that simulate the demands of sedentary work but are not specific to computer tasks. Other FCEs that simulate work tasks required in computer and keyboard operation include the BTE Primus (work simulator, available from Baltimore Therapeutic Equipment, Hanover, MD) and the LIDO Work Simulator (no longer available). The drawback of these computerized work simulators is that they involve the performance of isolated tasks in unnatural conditions, reducing the applicability of the results to real working environments. In addition to the work-sample approach, job-site evaluation, situational assessment, and psychometric instruments are used to address different clinical problems, leading to different strategies to improve work efficiency and minimize work-related injuries.

Solutions Related to Workstation Set-Up

Modifying the work environment to suit the worker's anthropometric characteristics and performance requirements is important in CTD intervention. Recommendations, ideally based on analysis of the specific job site, include providing adjustable tables and chairs that permit a more relaxed shoulder position and desktop surfaces large enough to accommodate a keyboard, a mouse, and adjustable computer mounts (Aaras 1994; Matias et al. 1998).

One of the greatest concerns in workstation design involves the need to accommodate varying task requirements and related postural requirements. For example, substantial differences exist between joint positions required when typing on a keyboard compared to those required when manipulating a pointing device. In some cases, the use of alternative devices, such as an ergonomic keyboard, require support surfaces that are larger than the standard keyboard tray (Wright and Wallach 1998). The larger size of some of the alternative "ergonomic" keyboards also forces users to make considerable changes in head, trunk, and upper extremity positions when switching between keyboard and mouse tasks (Wright and Wallach 1998).

Generally, users are advised to maintain their limbs in what is referred to as a *neutral posture* (Grandjean 1988; Wright and Wallach 1998). Neutral posture involves having

- Head, neck, and trunk aligned at mid-line
- Head upright (not too far forward)
- Shoulders retracted and relaxed
- Upper arms relaxed at side of body
- Elbows flexed to approximately 90 degrees
- Forearms not completely pronated, preferably close to mid-line
- Wrists aligned with forearms with minimal ulnar or radial deviation and minimal flexion or extension

Adjustment of keyboard height is one of the most frequently recommended changes in the computer workstation set-up. Support for the importance of this adjustment comes from studies, such as that of Sauter et al. (1991), in which several hundred computer users reported that arm discomfort increased as keyboard height was raised above elbow level. Although most investigators agree that correct keyboard height is important in achieving comfortable, safe, and efficient use during prolonged data-entry tasks, the range in the values recommended for the general population is extremely wide (Miller and Suther 1983; Nakaseko et al. 1985). This presumably reflects both a wide range of user preferences and significant variation in anthropometric characteristics.

Adjusting keyboard slope is another commonly recommended change. Almost all computer keyboards are constructed with a modest upward incline and have the option of achieving a small additional incline provided by two small pop-up support posts located beneath the keyboard. However, one study showed that subjects preferred typing on a keyboard that was declined by 12 degrees below the horizontal, essentially eliminating the built-in slope (Hedge and Powers 1995). The subjects in this study chose to sit approximately 10 cm farther from the computer screen when the keyboard angle was flattened.

Varying monitor height by 80–120 cm has been shown to have a significant effect on neck angle, thoracic bending, and vertical eye position (Villanueva 1996). In contrast, Kietrys et al. (1998) showed that raising the height of the computer monitor by approximately 13 cm, from an initial desktop height of 96.5 cm, had no significant effect on head and neck angle for a group of experienced computer users (at least not during the brief time they were monitored).

Hamilton (1996) found that source document position had a significant effect on muscle activity levels; the largest neck extensor and sternocleidomastoid EMGs were recorded when subjects read documents laid flat on a table. Placement of documents farther from the user's midline in either vertical or horizontal directions also increased EMG activity. Ideally, source documents should be placed so that the head and body remain symmetrically aligned in a middle position (Hamilton 1996).

Issues Related to Desktop and Laptop Computers

Compared to desktop computer users, laptop computer users are much more limited in their ability to adjust head and body posture to comfortable positions because the screen and keyboard of a laptop computer are joined. EMG and video studies have shown that laptop users have significantly more neck flexor activity and tilt their heads farther anteriorly than when they used a desktop computer (Saito et al. 1997; Straker et al. 1997). However, no other differences in body postures were observed, and users complained of more discomfort after their 20-minute session with the laptop than they experienced when using a desktop computer for the same amount of time. Whether and how much more habitual laptop users will suffer from CTD symptoms than desktop computer users remains to be determined. At the very least, users must be aware of the need to change their workstation support furniture when switching from a desktop to a laptop computer.

Issues Related to Keyboard Layout

Neither the layout nor the characteristics of individual keys in most standard computer keyboards take into account that fingers differ in strength, dexterity, and susceptibility to fatigue (Alden et al. 1972; Dvorak 1943; Kroemer 1972). For example, although the thumb possesses the greatest strength and agility, it is generally allocated the least amount of work (Dvorak 1943; Ferguson and Duncan 1974).

Over the years, the standard layout has been severely criticized. Ferguson and Duncan (1974) suggested that a more efficient layout would avoid the placement of commonly occurring letters in the front and back rows, unlike the standard QWERTY design, in which most of the typing is done on the back row. A major objective of Dvorak's (1943) alphanumeric layout was to diminish digit and hand movement. Indeed, this keyboard is considered by some to be an optimal layout because it permits the typing of an exceptionally large number of commonly used words exclusively with home row characters (Cooper 1983). Despite the considerable interest in Dvorak's and other layouts over the years, the standard layout dominates the market. Although some studies have reported that the Dvorak layout is easier to learn and enables its users to achieve greater speed and accuracy (Dvorak 1943; Yamada 1980), others dispute these findings (Kinkead 1975) and suggest that improvements of less than 5–10% are more realistic. Indeed, a critical examination of the evidence for and against the two keyboard layouts has shown that little, if any, advantage accompanies the Dvorak layout (Liebowitz and Margolis 1990). To date, no reliable evidence demonstrates that the Dvorak layout results in less fatiguing or injurious keyboard usage.

Solutions Related to Keyboard Structure

Variations in keyboard structure have been the subject of fairly intensive study over the years, with the objective of providing faster, more accurate, less fatiguing, and more comfortable keyboard access (Kroemer 1972). Splitting the keyboard into symmetric half-keyboards provides the possibility of tremendous flexibility in hand and digit position. Each half-keyboard can be tilted laterally, enabling the typist to rotate the forearm from prone to a middle position. In some models, the angle between each half can also be enlarged, enabling greater flexibility of the wrist.

In an early study, lateral tilt appeared to increase key press rate and decrease errors but did not alter users' perceived fatigue (Creamer and Trumbo 1960). In contrast, neither experienced nor inexperienced typists in Kroemer's (1972) study of a split keyboard demonstrated any significant improvements in typing speed or accuracy, although they did claim to feel more comfortable with the split, tilted keyboard. Lateral tilts in the range of 10–30 degrees combined with a modest opening angle decreased muscle activity in the shoulder girdle and arm region, suggesting more comfortable keying (Nakaseko et al. 1985). The latter study also showed that, in comparison to a standard keyboard, the split, open-angled keyboard greatly decreased ulnar deviation.

A survey of more than 400 alternative keyboard users found that 81% were satisfied with their keyboard, noting improvements in posture and comfort and reduction in pain (Wright and Andre 1996). A more recent study, however, did not demonstrate any significant difference in discomfort and fatigue reported by subjects who used both a standard and a split keyboard (over the 2-day period examined in the study) (Swanson et al. 1997). Another study showed that the Comfort keyboard (adjusted to a lateral slope of 30 degrees and a horizontal split of 20 degrees) enabled subjects to type with less ulnar deviation and wrist extension (Ro and Jacobs 1997). In the same study, the Tru-Form keyboard also reduced ulnar deviation but caused subjects to type with wrist extension beyond accepted safe wrist-extension values (15 degrees). Long-term data examining the ability of split keyboards to reduce CTD incidence or to reduce symptoms in those who have been injured while using a traditional keyboard are unavailable, however.

Despite mixed evidence concerning their effectiveness in CTD reduction, a number of split keyboards that cater primarily to computer users who have an existing injury or wish to avoid a potential injury are available (Wright and Andre 1996). Given the relatively low cost of many of these alternatives, typists should consider trying one or more of these keyboards, making sure to monitor productivity and comfort. The trial period should be long enough to ensure that the new keyboard is used in an automatic and natural way (Wright and Wallach 1998).

Fixed split keyboards, the most common and usually the least expensive of the alternative keyboards (Wright and Wallach 1998), have a fixed lateral split angle and, sometimes, a slightly raised center. Some of the more popular brands are listed in Table 11.1. Some models are larger than the standard keyboard, forcing the user to reach an additional 5–7 cm to operate the mouse (Wright and Wallach 1998). With adjustable split keyboards, the lateral angle and, in some models, the vertical angle can be varied.

Some keyboards have sculpted keyboard and keys to facilitate natural postures and movement patterns of the fingers, hands, and arms. Examples of these contoured keyboards include the Kinesis and Maltron keyboards. Readers are advised to consult the Typing Injury Frequently Asked Questions web site (www.tifaq.com) and the Massachusetts Institute of Technology's Access Technology for Information and Computing web site (www.mit.edu/afs/athcna.mit.edu/project/atic/www/index.html) for a frequently updated list of ergonomic alternative keyboards.

Issues Related to Key Characteristics

Key activation forces should be kept low because the force exerted by typists increases by approximately 40% and finger flexor EMGs increase by approximately 20% when key activation force is increased from 0.47 to 1.02 N (Rempel et al. 1997). A reduction in key switch activation force levels to levels lower than those currently recommended by the American National Standard for Human Factors Engineering of Visual Display Termi-

TABLE 11.1
Keyboards

Keyboard	Description	Manufacturer	Estimated Cost (U.S. Dollars)
Acer Future	Fixed split keyboard with two keying fields that form a triangle; a touch pad is embedded in the center with four arrow keys surrounding it	Acer America Corporation (www.aopenusa.com)	$100
Cirque Wave	Fixed split keyboard with built-in wrist rest, adjustable "pop-out" legs, extra backspace and tab keys	Cirque Corporation (www.cirque.com)	$100
Comfort keyboard system	Three-piece folding keyboard with each section on a separate mount, permitting enormous adjustability	Health Care Keyboard Company (e-mail: cksystems@aol.com)	$495
DataHand Professional II	Each hand has its own "pod"; four fingers each operate five switches by moving forward, back, left, right, and down; thumbs also have a few switches; built-in finger-mouse provided	DataHand Systems (www.datahand.com)	$2,100
Ergo Plus	Variable split keyboard with integrated wrist supports; split adjustable from 0 to 30 degrees in 5-degree increments; lateral tenting can be set to 0, 5, and 10 degrees	Cherry Electrical Products (www.cherrycorp.com/index.htm)	$199
Floating Arm	Keyboard split into two independent sections; mounted onto arms of a chair	Workplace Designs (www.wpdesigns.com)	$499
Kinesis contoured ergonomic	Contoured keyboard with keys in curves suited to natural structure of hand and movement of the fingers; each hand has its own set of keys; thumb buttons handle many major functions	Kinesis Corporation (www.kinesis-ergo.com)	$225–335
Maltron	Contoured keyboard with split design, tilted keys and pads; thumb keys used for common function keys; palm resting pads	PCD Maltron Ltd. (www.maltron.com)	$295

Name	Description	Source	Price
MAXIM adjustable	Variable split keyboard with adjustable lateral tilt; removable palm supports	Kinesis Corporation (www.kinesis-ergo.com)	$179
MiniErgo	Fixed split keyboard with embedded numeric keypad	Marquardt Switches (phone: 315-655-8050; fax: 315-655-8042)	$179
MyKey	Fixed split keyboard with center peak and a V shape; built-in palm rests; front and rear elevators to customize hand and wrist position; circular function-key layout	ErgonomiXX (www.intr.net/mykey)	$275
Natural	Fixed split keyboard with built-in palm rest and adjustable wrist leveler; numeric keypad can be used to navigate pointer; IntelliType Manager provides software adjustability for keyboard and pointer control functions	Microsoft (www.microsoft.com/products)	$100
PACE adjustable	Two-section split; tented keyboard with easy adjustability	Pace Development (www.ids2.com/pace)	$279
PerfecTouch 101	Split with knob that allows horizontal angling; can also detach completely	BackCare Corporation (phone: 888-868-2448; fax: 312-258-0090)	$109
SmartBoard	Fixed split keyboard with layout that fans the keys out slightly to match a typical relaxed hand	Darwin Keyboards (www.darwinkeyboards.com)	$100
Tru-Form	Fixed split keyboard similar to Microsoft's Natural keyboard, but for Macintosh; some models have a built-in pointing device	Adesso (www.adessoinc.com)	$100

Sources: Massachusetts Institute of Technology. Access Technology for Information and Computing. http://web.mit.edu/afs/athena.mit.edu/project/atic/www/index.html; and KS Wright, DS Wallach. Alternative Keyboard FAQ. www.tifaq.com/keyboards.html. (These sources should be consulted before the purchase of any pointing devices to obtain further details and user feedback.)

nal Workstations (1988) would help decrease the biomechanical load on forearm tendons and muscles of keyboard users.

The most obvious method of reducing excessive force during keyboarding tasks is to decrease the magnitude of the force needed to activate keyboard keys. This solution is not easy to implement, however. Reducing key activation force could cause typists to inadvertently activate keys or require them to exert additional muscular effort to minimize accidental activations through contraction of proximal agonist-antagonist pairs (Radwin 1997). Moreover, the results of several studies indicate that, in any case, users exert far more than the current key activation force, surpassing the activation value by as much as five times (Feuerstein et al. 1997). Thus, although the majority of manufactured keyboards comply with key switch standards published by organizations such as the American National Standards Institute, most typists continue to exert far more force than is actually needed.

An alternative approach to reducing keyboard force has been proposed by Radwin (1997). Radwin had subjects tap repeatedly on a single key in a keyboard mock-up, and found that the peak activation force could be lowered by approximately 24% simply by increasing the over travel (the displacement until a key hits bottom) from 0 to 3 mm. He suggested that the activation force was reduced because the additional over travel facilitated finger deceleration. He further suggested that the increased over travel may provide increased proprioceptive feedback, possibly giving typists better control over the force they exert.

Software Solutions

The ergonomic solutions described exemplify the more traditional approach of attempting to reconfigure standard data-entry devices. An alternative approach is to use computer management procedures to improve the efficiency of the typist and decrease the workload. Examples of these techniques include automation of computer start-up procedures, use of macros that store frequently used sequences of commands and phrases that can then be activated by one- or two-character commands, and command menus that minimize the number of key presses required to execute elaborate routines.

Another way to enhance the data-entry input-to-output ratio is word prediction. Often recommended for typists with severe motor disabilities (Anson 1993), this technique involves the use of software that presents a list of plausible completions to the initially typed characters from which the user selects the desired word. For example, subsequent to entering the initial characters *ex*, the words *exaggerate*, *except*, *explore*, and *extra* are listed. The appropriate word can then be selected by a single keystroke, reducing the total number of key-presses (Smith et al. 1989; Vanderheiden

1981). User performance with word-prediction software increases when more completions are presented (Venkatagiri 1994) and when the choices are ordered by word length rather than alphabetically (Lanspa et al. 1997). Research has focused on which systems and usage strategies are best for which types of users and tasks (Koester and Levine 1998), and considerable debate exists concerning the method's relative advantages and disadvantages. For words longer than three letters, word prediction can result in a considerable savings in keystrokes per word. Such savings may simply mean, however, that the users can complete a longer document in the same amount of time as a shorter one with no reduction of workload.

One-handed typing techniques in which the left half of the standard keyboard is mapped onto the right half (or vice versa) are a solution for users with good skill in only one hand (Matias et al. 1996). The user types those characters that normally appear on the left half of the keyboard with his or her right hand. Characters from the left half of the keyboard are mapped to the right side when the user presses the space bar. With this method, subjects can achieve 83% of their two-handed typing speed and reach speeds as high as 60 wpm. CTD sufferers would type with the non-symptomatic hand at times when the other hand is stricken with particularly severe symptoms.

Austin et al. (1997) proposed that programmers consider ways to alleviate the stress placed on typists who use standard or alternative keyboard layouts when designing their software. They recommend that, where possible, computer programs should be designed to avoid the use of keys that appear to be implicated in injurious typing and that frequently used commands should be allocated to keys that are more optimally placed.

Solutions Related to Alternate Input Methods

Speech Recognition

Speech recognition is a computer input method in which the user's voice is used to enter all alphanumeric data and commands. Speech recognition has evolved from programs with a very limited vocabulary to those containing more than 100,000 words and from programs that recognize only isolated letters to those that recognize free-flowing speech without pauses. Such systems allow for freer flow of thought and greater speed, theoretically as fast as natural speech rates (150–175 wpm) (Kraat 1987). Accuracy rates are also expected to improve, especially when systems become available that use context to recognize words and distinguish between homonyms.

Speech recognition is intensely marketed as a way to avoid typing-induced CTD of the neck, back, and upper extremities. Ironically, some users who use speech recognition as their primary typing method have subsequently developed CTD in their vocal chords (Arnaught 1995; Gooderham 1995; Kambeyanda et al. 1997), because some speech recognition systems require the user to speak in a monotonous tone and maintain a reasonably constant pitch and inflection. Such speech-recognition systems placed extended stress on the vocal cords, leading to swelling, hoarseness, and even complete loss of voice. The extent to which newer, continuous-speech systems may alleviate these problems has yet to be determined. The continuous-speech systems offer the advantage of greater voice modulation but may strain the vocal apparatus even more by allowing the user to speak faster and more continuously. Although avoiding use of the speech-recognition system for extended periods is one way to reduce vocal fatigue and the risk of CTD, such a precaution could significantly mitigate the successful integration of its users into the vocational environment.

Mouse Pointing Devices and Mouse Alternatives

Ergonomics literature has begun to address ways to alleviate problems caused by the rapidly increasing use of the mouse and other pointing devices (Fogelman and Brogman 1995; Hamilton 1996; Karlqvist et al. 1994, 1998). A number of variations in the design of the standard mouse have been proposed. Reductions in mouse size and modification of shape to fit the contours of a typical user's hand have been frequently advocated (Table 11.2). Even more interesting are devices that let the operator interact with graphical user interfaces by means quite different than those used to maneuver the standard mouse (Table 11.3). Users today can acquire pointing devices that incorporate different manipulation styles (e.g., push, roll, glide), control variables (e.g., position, force), and activation limbs (e.g., finger, hand, head, foot).

Different pointing devices must be evaluated for performance qualities, such as speed, accuracy, and endurance, and tendency to cause the user to develop CTD. Not all pointing devices are equal in terms of speed and accuracy and thus are not equally suitable to the operation of all software. In a study of pointing accuracy and speed, Albert (1982) compared the standard keyboard to five of the major cursor control methods. The trackball was considerably more accurate than all other devices, whereas the touch screen was the least. However, the touch screen was the fastest control method, and the keyboard was the slowest. The trade-off between performance and safety should also be taken into consideration, as some devices provide excellent speed and accuracy but produce a significant load on the hand and forearm soft tissues.

As for keyboard users, certain arm positions are more comfortable for mouse users. Karlqvist et al. (1998) found that users preferred manipulating a standard mouse when they had arm support and were able to maintain the forearm in a middle position. The user's body dimensions had a significant effect on preferred mouse location.

TABLE 11.2
Mouse Pointing Devices

Mouse	Description	Manufacturer	Estimated Cost (U.S. Dollars)
Alps Adjustable	Expands and contracts to fit each hand (see also Alps Professional Mouse, designed to fit right- or left-handed people)	Alps Electric (www.alpsusa.com)	$35
Anir (basic two-button and pro versions)	Designed like a pilot stick; promotes positioning of the supported forearm in midposition; switches activated by thumb	AnimaX International AS (www.animax.no)	$100
Contour	Contoured; both left- (2 sizes) and right- (5 sizes) handed versions; sculpted, elevated buttons; programmable software; thumb support; tilted palm support; elevated wrist support	Contour Design (www.contourdes.com)	$80–90
Digitus Magic Click	Finger and thumb grooves sculpted into rounded surface activated by thumb and middle finger	Assmann Data Products (www.usa-assmann.com/)	$35
Goldtouch	Designed to support the hand in relaxed, neutral posture; has button-activated scrolling and panning capabilities	Goldtouch Technologies (www.goldtouch.com)	$60
IntelliMouse	Provides scrolling, zooming, and navigating; comes with programmable IntelliPoint software	Microscft (www.microsoft.com/products/hardware/inputdev.htm)	$80
MouseMan+	Contoured surface; conveniently located thumb and wheel buttons; programmable software	Logitech (www.logitech.com)	$50–60
Thinking Mouse	Asymmetric shape narrower in the front and wider in the back; sides made of rubberized EasyGrip material; four easy-to-click buttons; programmable software	Kensington Microware (www.kensington.com/products)	$55

Sources: D Carroll. Ergonomic, Adaptive and Alternative Pointing Devices. www.setbc.org/mouse.ist/; Massachusetts Institute of Technology. Access Technology for Information and Computing. web.mit.edu/afs/athena.mit.edu/project/atic/www/index.html; Mouse-Group Home Page. www.ami.dk/mousegroup; and KS Wright, DS Wallach. Pointing Device FAQ. www.tifaq.com. (These sources should be consulted before the purchase of any pointing devices to obtain further detail and user feedback.)

TABLE 11.3
Alternatives to Mouse Pointing Devices

Product	Description	Manufacturer	Estimated Cost (U.S. Dollars)
A3 trackball	Programmable, medium-sized trackball with a button on either side and one below; large base to rest hand	Mouse Systems (www. mousesystems.com)	$40–50
EasyBall	Very large plastic ball (originally designed for use by children but also useful for those with limited range of motion or problems with fine-motor skills)	Microsoft (www. microsoft.com/products)	$50
Glidepoint/ Power Cat	Finger moves over small, touch-sensitive pad to control cursor position; available in several sizes	Cirque Corporation (www.glidepoint.com)	$30–90
HeadMouse	Tracks a small reflective dot placed on the user's forehead: head movement is translated into cursor movement; portable version has much smaller tracker unit; button clicks are through an adaptive switch or by dwelling on an image	Origin Instruments (www.orin.com)	$1,300
Jouse	Designed for the user with severe physical limitations; on the end of an adjustable arm that can be clamped to table; mouth or chin controls cursor; sip, puff, and bite switches are used for mouse clicks	Prentke Romich (www.prentrom.com)	$2,000
MicroTrac	Miniature trackball with 3 buttons: one on each side, one above; small enough to hold in hand	MicroSpeed (www.microspeed.com)	$75
Mouse Pen, Computer Crayon, Mouse Pen Pro	All shaped like a pen; pointer control in contact with a surface (e.g., desk, paper, hand); 2 buttons located near the tip for access by index finger; some models have variable pointer acceleration	Questec (www.questecmall.com/ Body.htm)	Mouse Pen: $20 Computer Crayon: $13–20 Mouse Pen Pro: $30–40 (cordless $80)

Mouse-Trak	Large trackball with button on each side, 1 large button below; speed and acceleration control; large padded base on which to rest hand	ITAC Systems (www.mousetrak.com)	$89–295
NoHands Mouse	Operated with the feet: 1 pedal moves the cursor, the other is used for clicking	Hunter Digital (www.footmouse.com)	$250
Orbit, Turbo/ Expert Mouse	Orbit: small programmable trackball with a large button on each side Turbo/Expert Mouse: large programmable trackball with a large button on each side	Kensington (www.kensington.com/products)	Orbit : $60 Turbo/Expert: $90–125
Trackman Portable, Trackman Marble	Trackman Portable: small programmable trackball; hand rests over the main button; thumb controls other buttons and cursor movement Trackman Marble: programmable trackball with a base to rest hard flat; index, middle, and ring fingers each rest on buttons; thumb controls cursor movement	Logitech (www.logitech.com)	Trackman Portable: $50 Trackman Marble: $80

Sources: D Carroll. Ergonomic, The Mouse List: Adaptive and Alternative Pointing Devices. www.setbc.org/mouselist/; Massachusetts Institute of Technology. Access Technology for Information and Computing. web.mit.edu/afs/athena.mit.edu/project/atic/www/index.html; Mouse-group Home Page. www.ami.dk/mousegroup; and KS Wright, DS Wallach. Pointing Device FAQ. www.tifaq.com/mice.html. (These sources should be consulted before the purchase of any pointing devices to obtain further details and user feedback.)

Certain mouse tasks, such as dragging, can be particularly taxing, causing sustained loading of the finger flexor muscles. Pointing-device manufacturers sometimes provide ways to carry out dragging without keeping the mouse button pressed. For example, the drag function can be locked by a third switch on some trackball devices or by some mouse driver programs. The user simply locks the cursor into drag mode and then proceeds to move the mouse as in other mouse tasks. Releasing the switch returns the mouse to regular operation.

Researchers active in ergonomics continually explore innovative methods of cursor position manipulation. Devices should provide high performance but not expose the user to harmful positions or forces. The Anir mouse (Aaras et al. 1997), for example, allows users to manipulate cursor position by lightly gripping an upright stick. The mouse is operated with the forearm in a middle position instead of the usual pronated position, and the mouse buttons are activated by slight movements of the thumb. Subjects exhibited lower EMGs in the extensor digitorum communis, extensor carpi ulnaris, and trapezius muscle when using the Anir mouse than with a standard mouse, even when the standard mouse was accompanied by forearm support (Aaras et al. 1997). Another novel mouse alternative is based on a finger-motion recognition system in which finger position and shape are recorded and recognized (Ko and Yang 1997). This technique allows for direct manipulation of the cursor without exposure to potentially dangerous positions or external forces.

Conclusion

Various solutions to CTD modify user comfort, increase efficiency, and reduce susceptibility. However, adjusting furniture, using alternative keyboards and pointing devices, and adopting various software solutions are only partial solutions to CTD. Many computer workstation users, particularly those who are highly motivated and who are working to meet one deadline after another, may need more than hardware and software solutions. Such users not only need to learn to use the equipment properly; they must learn to recognize the positions, postures, and working styles that place them at risk. Keeping workers aware of a taxonomy of injurious keyboard techniques serves to focus attention on technique errors that can be corrected with sufficient instruction (Pascarelli and Kella 1993).

A number of studies have examined the efficacy of educating workers to recognize, report, and seek intervention for CTD. Training programs of differing lengths and styles have aimed to teach workers to analyze their workstations, recognize hazards, and make appropriate changes (King et al. 1997). Addressing specific habits that the worker has developed is often useful. For example, observing a typist for the amount of force exerted in keystrokes could lead to individual recommendations to correct injurious work styles (Feuerstein et al. 1997). A lack of synchrony between the internal physiologic rhythms of a worker and the rhythm set by the work has also been noted to be a potentially significant source of stress in tasks that are inherently repetitive, such as keyboarding (Henning et al. 1992). Giving a worker greater control over his or her own work rhythm may help reduce this source of stress.

References

Aaras A (1994). Relationship between trapezius load and the incidence of musculoskeletal illness in the neck and shoulder. Int J Ind Ergonomics 14:341–348.

Aaras A, Westgaard RH, Stranden E, Larsen S (1997). Postural Load and the Incidence of Musculoskeletal Illness. In Proceedings from the NIOSH Workshop: Promoting Health and Productivity in the Computerized Office. New York: Taylor & Francis, 68–93.

Albert A (1982). The Effect of Graphic Input Devices on Performance in a Cursor Positioning Task. Proceedings of the Human Factors Society 26th Annual Meeting. Santa Monica, CA: Human Factors Society.

Alden DA, Daniels RW, Kanarick AF (1972). Keyboard design and operation: a review of the major issues. Hum Factors 14:275–293.

Alqattan MM, Bowen V (1993). Cumulative trauma disorders of the hand and wrist. Curr Opin Orthop 4:68–71.

American National Standards Institute (1988). American National Standard for Human Factors Engineering of Visual Display Terminal Workstations. ANSI/-HFS 100.

Anson D (1993). The effect of word prediction on typing speed. Am J Occup Ther 47:1039–1042.

Armstrong TJ (1990). Ergonomics and Cumulative Trauma Disorders of the Hand and Wrist. In JM Hunter, LH Schneider, EJ Mackin, AD Callahan (eds), Rehabilitation of the Hand: Surgery and Therapy (3rd ed). St. Louis: Mosby.

Armstrong TJ, Buckle P, Fine LJ, et al. (1993). A conceptual model for work-related neck and upper-limb musculoskeletal disorders. Scand J Work Environ Health 19:73–84.

Armstrong TJ, Fine LJ, Radwin RG, Silverstein BS (1987). Ergonomics and the effects of vibration in hand-intensive work. Scand J Work Environ Health 13:286–289.

Armstrong TJ, Foulke JA, Martin BJ, et al. (1994). Investigation of applied forces in alphanumeric keyboard work. Am Ind Hyg Assoc J 55:30–35.

Arnaught G (1995). Talking to computers has its hazards. Globe and Mail (online: www.theglobeandmail.com), September 15.

Austin H, Johnson M, Moras R (1997). Keyboard or Software Design? Norcross, GA: IIE Solutions.

Ballard J (1993). Work related upper limb disorders. Occup Health Rev 46:9–14.

Cooper WE (1983). Cognitive Aspects of Skilled Typewriting. New York: Springer-Verlag.

Creamer LR, Trumbo DA (1960). Multifinger tapping performance as a function of the direction of tapping movements. J Appl Psychol 44:376–380.

Dobyns JH (1995). Balancing Psyche, Soma and Society in Overuse Syndromes. In M Vastasmaki (ed), Current Trends in Hand Surgery. Amsterdam: Elsevier.

Doheny M, Linden P, Sedlak C (1995). Reducing orthopaedic hazards of the computer work environment. Orthop Nurs 14:7–15.

Dul J, Douwes M, Smitt P (1994). Ergonomic guidelines for the prevention of discomfort of static postures based on endurance data. Ergonomics 37:807–815.

Dvorak A (1943). There is a better typewriter keyboard. Natl Business Educ Q 12:51–58.

Fahrback PA, Chapman LJ (1990). VDT work duration and musculoskeletal discomfort. Am Assoc Occup Health Nurses J 38:32–36.

Fast C (1995). Repetitive strain injury: an overview of the condition and its implications for occupational therapy practice. Can J Occup Ther 62:119–126.

Faucett J, Rempel DM (1994). VDT-related musculoskeletal symptoms: interactions between work posture and psychosocial work factors. Am J Ind Med 26:597–612.

Feely CA, Seaton MK, Arfken CL, et al. (1995). Effects of work and rest on upper extremity signs and symptoms of workers performing repetitive tasks. J Occup Rehabil 5:145–156.

Ferguson D, Duncan J (1974). Keyboard design and operating postures. Ergonomics 17:731–744.

Feuerstein M, Armstrong T, Hickey P, Lincoln A (1997). Computer keyboard force and upper extremity symptoms. J Occup Environ Med 12:1144–1153.

Fogelman M, Brogmas G (1995). Computer mouse use and cumulative trauma disorders of the upper extremities. Ergonomics 38:2465–2475.

Frederick L (1992). Cumulative trauma disorders. Am Assoc Occup Health Nurses J 40:113–116.

Gooderham, M. (1995). High-tech RSI aid creates new problem. Globe and Mail (online: www.theglobeandmail.com), September 4.

Grandjean E (1988). Fitting the Task to the Man. A Textbook of Occupational Ergonomics (4th ed). London: Taylor & Francis.

Gun RT (1990). The incidence and distribution of RSI in South Australia 1980–1981 and 1986–1987. Med J Aust 153:376–380.

Hamilton N (1996). Source document position as it affects head position and neck muscle tension. Ergonomics 39:593–610.

Hashemi L, Webster BS, Clancy EA, Courtney TK (1998). Length of disability and cost of work-related musculoskeletal disorders of the upper extremity. J Occup Environ Med 40:261–269.

Hedge A, Powers JR (1995). Wrist postures while keyboarding: effects of a negative slope keyboard system and full motion forearm supports. Ergonomics 38: 508–517.

Henning RA, Sauter SL, Krieg EF (1992). Work rhythm and physiological rhythms in repetitive computer work: effects of synchronization on well-being. Int J Hum Comput Interact 4:233–243.

Henning RA, Jacques P, Kissel GV, et al. (1997). Frequent short rest breaks from computer work: effects on productivity and well-being at two field sites. Ergonomics 40:78–91.

Hunting W, Laubli T, Grandjean F (1981). Postural and visual loads at VDT workplaces. I. Constrained postures. Ergonomics 24:917–931.

Johnson P, Dropkin J, Hewes J, Rempel D (1993). Office Ergonomics: Motion Analysis of Computer Mouse Usage. In Proceedings of the American Industrial Hygiene Conference and Exposition. Fairfax, VA: American Industrial Hygiene Association.

Juul Kristensen B, Fallentin N, Ekdahl C (1997). Criteria for classification of posture in repetitive work by observation methods: a review. Int J Indust Ergonomics 19:397–411.

Kambeyanda D, Singer L, Cronk S (1997). Potential problems associated with use of speech recognition products. Assist Technol 9:95–101.

Karlqvist LK, Hagberg M (1996). Musculoskeletal symptoms among computer-assisted design (CAD) operators and evaluation of a self-assessment questionnaire. Int J Occup Environ Health 2:185–194.

Karlqvist LK, Hagberg M, Selin K (1994). Variation in upper limb posture and movement during word processing with and without mouse use. Ergonomics 37: 1261–1267.

Karlqvist LK, Bernmark E, Ekenvall L, et al. (1998). Computer mouse position as a determinant of posture, muscular load and perceived exertion. Scand J Work Environ Health 24:62–73.

Kierklo E, Jones S (1994). Stop repetitive injuries before they start. Safety Health 150:68–69.

Kietrys DM, McClure PW, Fitzgerald GK (1998). The relationship between head and neck posture and VDT screen height in keyboard operators. Phys Ther 78:395–403.

King PM, Fisher JC, Garg A (1997). Evaluation of the impact of employee ergonomics training in industry. Appl Ergonomics 28:249–256.

Kinkead R (1975). Typing speed, keying rates, and optimal keyboard layout. Proceedings of the Human Factors Society Nineteenth Annual Meeting. Dallas, TX. 159–161.

Ko BK, Yang HS (1997). Finger mouse and gesture recognition system as a new human computer interface. Comput Graphics 21:555–561.

Kraat A (1987). Communication Interaction between Aided and Natural Speakers. Madison, WI: Trace Research and Development Center.

Kroemer KH (1972). Human engineering the keyboard. Hum Factors 14:51–63.

Kuorinka I, Johnsson B, Kilbom A, et al. (1987). Standardized Nordic questionnaire for the analysis of musculoskeletal symptoms. Appl Ergonomics 18: 233–237.

Lanspa A, Wood LA, Beukelman DR (1997). Efficiency with which disabled and nondisabled students locate words in cue windows: study of three organizational strategies—frequency of word use, word length and alphabetic order. Augmentative Alternative Comm 13:117–124.

Lechner D, Roth D, Straaton X (1991). Functional capacity evaluation in work disability. Work 1:37–47.

Leinonen T, Kisko K (1998). A new method for work analysis. Int J Indust Ergonomics 21:361–367.

Leung PC, Wong SKM (1995). Extensor Origin Tendinitis around the Elbow: Its Relationship with Occupation. In M Vastasmaki (ed), Current Trends in Hand Surgery. Amsterdam: Elsevier.

Liebowitz SJ, Margolis SE (1990). The fable of the keys. J Law Econ 33:1–25.

Loeb KM (1983). Membrane keyboards and human performance. Bell System Tech J 62:1773–1748.

Lundborg G, Dahlin LB (1995). Vibration-Induced Hand Problems. In M Vastasmaki (ed), Current Trends in Hand Surgery. Amsterdam: Elsevier.

Mallory M, Bradford H (1989). An invisible work place hazard gets harder to ignore. Business Week (January 30):92–93.

Malzahn DE, Fernandez JE, Kattel BP (1996). Design-oriented functional capacity evaluation: the available motion inventory—a review. Disabil Rehabil 18:382–395.

Matias E, MacKenzie IS, Buxton W (1996). One-handed touch typing on a QWERTY keyboard. Hum Comp Interact 11:1–27.

Matias AC, Salvendy G, Kuczek T (1998). Predictive models of carpal tunnel syndrome causation among VDT operators. Ergonomics 41:213–226.

Miller W, Suther TW (1983). Display station and anthropometrics: preferred height and angle settings of CRT and keyboard. Hum Factors 25:401–408.

Nakaseko E, Grandjean E, Hunting W, Gierer R (1985). Studies on ergonomically designed alphanumeric keyboards. Hum Factors 27:175–187.

Nathan PA, Meadows KD, Doyle LS (1988). J Hand Surg 13:167–170.

Occupational Safety and Health Council (1997). Report on Survey of Office Environment and the Occupational Health of Visual Display Terminals (VDT) Users. Hong Kong: Occupational Safety and Health Council.

Ohlsson K, Attewell RG, Johnsson B, et al. (1994). An assessment of neck and upper extremity disorders by questionnaire and clinical evaluation. Ergonomics 37:891–897.

Oxenburgh M (1984). Musculoskeletal Injuries Occurring in Word Processor Operators. In A Adams, M Stevenson (eds), Ergonomics and Technological Change: Proceedings of the 21st Annual Conference of the Ergonomics Society of Australia and New Zealand. Sydney. November 28–30. Victoria, Australia: Ergonomics Society of Australia and New Zealand, 137–143.

Pan CS, Schleifer LM (1996). An exploratory study of the relationship between biomechanical factors and right-arm musculoskeletal discomfort and fatigue in a VDT data entry task. Appl Ergonomics 26:195–200.

Pascarelli EF, Kella JJ (1993). Soft-tissue injuries related to use of the computer keyboard. J Occup Med 35:522–531.

Radwin RG (1997). Activation force and travel effects on overexertion in repetitive key tapping. Hum Factors 39:130–140.

Rempel DM, Harrison RJ, Barnhart S (1991). Work-related cumulative trauma disorders of the upper extremity. JAMA 267:838–839.

Rempel DM, Serina E, Kinenberg E, et al. (1997). The effect of keyboard keyswitch make force on applied force and finger flexor muscle activity. Ergonomics 40:800–808.

Ro J, Jacobs K (1997). Wrist postures in video display terminal operators (VDT) using different keyboards. Work 9:155–166.

Rossignol M, Patry L, Sacks S (1998). Carpal tunnel syndrome: validation of an interview questionnaire on occupational exposure. Am J Ind Med 33:224–231.

Saito S, Miyao M, Kondo T, et al. (1997). Ergonomic evaluation of working posture of VDT operation using personal computer with flat panel display. Ind Health 35:264–270.

Sauter SL, Schleifer LM, Knutson SJ (1991). Work posture, workstation design, and musculoskeletal discomfort in a VDT data entry task. Hum Factors 33: 151–167.

Schreuer N, Lifshitz Y, Weiss PL (1996). The effect of typing frequency and speed on the incidence of upper extremity cumulative trauma disorder. Work 6:87–95.

Schuldt K, Ekholm J, Harms-Ringdahl K, et al. (1986). Effects of changes in sitting work posture on static neck and shoulder muscle activity. Ergonomics 12: 1525–1537.

Sjogaard J (1990). Work Induced Muscle Fatigue and Its Relation to Muscle Pain. In Conference Proceedings: Occupational Disorders of the Upper Extremity. Ann Arbor, MI: University of Michigan. March 29–30.

Smith RO, Christiaasen R, Borden B, et al. (1989). Effectiveness of a writing system using a computerized long-range optical pointer 10-branch abbreviation expansion. J Rehabil Res Dev 26:51–62.

Sommerich CM, Marras WS, Parnianpour M (1996). Activity of Index Finger Muscles during Typing. In Proceeding of the Human Factors and Ergonomics Society 39th Annual Meeting. 620–624.

Stetson DS, Keyserling WM, Silverstein BA, Leonard JA (1991). Observational analysis of the hand and wrist: a pilot study. J Appl Occup Environ Hyg 6:927–937.

Straker L, Jones KJ, Miller J (1997). A comparison of the postures assumed when using laptop computers and desktop computers. Appl Ergonomics 28:263–268.

Taylor PM, Braun KA (1988). Stretching Exercise. In PM Taylor, DK Taylor (eds), Conquering Athletic Injuries. Champaign, IL: Leisure Press.

Vanderheiden GC (1981). The practical use of microcomputers in rehabilitation. Rehabil Lit 44:66–70.

Veiersted KB, Westgaard RH, Andersen P (1993). Electromyographic evaluation of muscular work pattern as a predictor of trapezius myalgia. Scand J Work Environ Health 19:284–290.

Vender MI, Kasdan ML, Truppa KL (1995). Upper extremity disorders: a literature review to determine work-relatedness. J Hand Surg 20:534–541.

Venkatagiri HS (1994). Effect of window size on rate of communication in a lexical prediction AAC system. Augmented Alternative Commun 10:105–112.

Villanueva MB, Sotoyama M, Jonai H, et al. (1996). Adjustments of posture and viewing parameters of the eye to changes in the screen height of the visual display terminal. Ergonomics 39:933–945.

Weiss ND, Gordon L, Bloom T, et al. (1995). Position of the wrist associated with the lowest carpal-tunnel pressure: implications for splint design. J Bone Joint Surg Am 77:1695–1699.

Weiss PL (1990). Mechanical characteristics of microswitches adapted for the physically disabled. J Biomed Eng 12:398–402.

Wells R (1993). Job modification—check out challenge. Occup Health Safety Can 9:62–64.

Wieslander G, Norback D, Gothe CJ, Juhlin L (1989). Carpal tunnel syndrome (CTS) and exposure to vibration, repetitive wrist movements, and heavy manual work: a case-referent study. Br J Ind Med 46:43–47.

Winkel J, Westgaard R (1992). Occupational and individual risk factors for shoulder-neck complaints. Part I—guidelines for the practitioner. Int J Ind Ergonomics 10:79–83.

Wood DD, Fisher DL, Andres RO (1997). Minimizing fatigue during repetitive jobs: optimal work-rest schedules. Hum Factors 39:83–101.

Wright KS, Andre AD (1996). Alternative Keyboard Characteristics: A Survey Study. In Conference Proceedings: ErgoCon 1996. San Jose, CA: Silicon Valley Ergonomics Institute, 148–157.

Wright KS, Wallach DS (1998). CTD Resource Network (www.tifaq.com).

Yamada H (1980). A historical study of typewriters and typing methods: from the position of planning Japanese parallels. J Inform Process 2:177–202.

Yassi A (1997). Repetitive strain injuries. Lancet 349:943–947.

Zipp P, Haider E, Halpern N, Rohmert W (1981). Keyboard design through physiological strain measurements. Appl Ergonomics 14:117–122.

Review Questions

(Answers are found in Appendix D.)

1. Which of the following risk factors appear to contribute to the pathophysiology of CTD?
   (a) Repetitive motion
   (b) Excessive force
   (c) Awkward working posture
   (d) Excessive vibration
   (e) a, b, and c

2. In the dose-response model of CTD, *dose* refers to
   (a) mechanical forces acting on the body tissues, physiologic consumption of metabolic substrates, and production of metabolites within the tissues, as well as psychological disturbances such as anxiety about work
   (b) physical characteristics of the job, including the weight, size, and shape of tools, and psychological factors such as job security
   (c) physical and psychological ability to resist destabilization
   (d) an individual's reaction to exposure, modified by his or her capacity
   (e) none of the above

3. For most risk factors, exposure time is critical, thus
   (a) exposure should be reduced to less than 2 hours per day
   (b) exposure time should be reduced where the work environment is impoverished from a psychosocial viewpoint
   (c) varying the type of work tasks performed in a work shift such that the worker is not exposed to any single risk factor for an extended period is advisable
   (d) rest breaks are not always beneficial
   (e) b, c, and d

4. EMG evaluation is used to analyze the muscular work pattern of workers at their workstations. This technique
   (a) reveals how a muscle responds to varying load conditions
   (b) shows when a muscle becomes fatigued
   (c) can identify which muscles are used to carry out specific tasks
   (d) is easy to use in all work environments
   (e) a, b, and c

5. A keyboard user's susceptibility to injury will not be affected by
   (a) typing accuracy
   (b) force exerted on each key
   (c) total typing time
   (d) amount of time spent on each key
   (e) all of the above

6. Computer users are advised to maintain their limbs in a neutral posture, which includes
   (a) tilting the head anterior approximately 20 degrees
   (b) aligning the head, neck, and trunk midline
   (c) protracting the shoulders
   (d) pronating the forearms completely
   (e) all of the above

7. In comparison to desktop computers, laptop computers
   (a) limit the user's ability to adjust head and body posture to comfortable positions
   (b) cause users to generate significantly more neck flexor activity and tilt their heads anteriorly
   (c) cause greater discomfort to the user
   (d) both a and b
   (e) a, b, and c

8. Compared to the standard QWERTY keyboard layout, the Dvorak layout is
   (a) much easier to learn
   (b) enables its users to achieve greater speed and accuracy
   (c) less fatiguing to use
   (d) less injurious
   (e) none of the above

9. Word prediction
   (a) does not necessarily help the typist with CTD, because he or she is now able to complete a longer document in the same amount of time with no reduction of workload
   (b) was originally developed for users with severe motor disabilities to enhance their input and output efficiency
   (c) only provides considerable savings in keystrokes per word for words longer than six characters
   (d) both a and b
   (e) a, b, and c

10. Mouse and mouse-alternative pointing devices differ in
   (a) manipulation styles (e.g., push, roll, glide)
   (b) control variables (e.g., position, force)
   (c) activation limbs (e.g., finger, hand, head, foot)
   (d) performance characteristics (e.g., speed, accuracy, endurance)
   (e) all of the above

PART IV

Application Process

CHAPTER 12
Applied Ergonomics in Injury Prevention and Disability Management

Debbie Holmes-Enix and Marilyn Wright

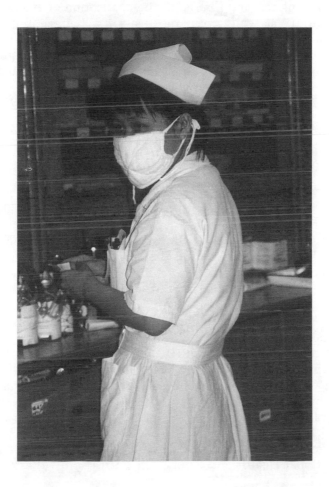

ABSTRACT

Financial and legislative incentives have encouraged the development of prevention and disability management programs in industry. Ergonomics plays an important role in preventing work-related injuries and helping successful return-to-work efforts. This chapter discusses Occupational Safety and Health Administration (OSHA) guidelines for program development, as well as ergonomic injury prevention teams; vital considerations in program development; and the roles of the employer, injury prevention and disability management teams, and the consulting therapist.

The adage "an ounce of prevention is worth a pound of cure" alludes to the reasons employers are seeking prevention strategies that decrease or eliminate workplace injuries and illnesses. The application of ergonomic principles before injury as well as during disability management and early-return-to-work (ERTW) processes has been highly effective. The development of a prevention and disability management program requires special considerations, commitment, detailed preparation, and planning. The program should be a process of growth and education administered by an ergonomics team or an individual consultant.

Incentives for Ergonomics and Injury Prevention Programs

Employers are looking for ways to manage and decrease escalating costs related to cumulative trauma disorder (CTD). CTD accounted for almost 60% of all recorded work-related illnesses in 1993 (Carson 1994), and the Bureau of Labor Statistics reported that this figure increased by 10% in 1994. Data collected from records of Liberty Mutual Insurance Company from 45 states during 1989 estimated the costs for treatment of upper extremity CTD in the United States to be $563 million (Zabel and McGrew 1997). This statistic included all injuries, although carpal tunnel syndrome and upper extremity tendinitis were most frequently noted.

The illnesses most frequently reported to OSHA are related to repeated trauma (Hansen 1993). CTD comprises physical ailments and injuries caused by repeated mechanical stresses or strains that wear and tear on the body. These stresses, combined with forceful exertions, awkward postures, and high repetitions, greatly increase a worker's risk of developing CTD (Karwowski and Marras 1997).

Employers are also required to maintain a safe work environment. The Occupational Health and Safety Act (1970) states that a duty of all employers is to furnish a workplace "free from recognized hazards that are causing or are likely to cause death or serious physical harm" (Heck-Edwards 1990). In 1990, OSHA developed ergonomic guidelines for the meat-packing industry, precipitating a model for ergonomic safety and health management standards. California adopted an abbreviated standard for repetitive strain injuries in 1997.

Employer and Employee Commitment

The full commitment of the employer and the complete involvement of employees are important initial factors that enable a successful prevention program. In many industries, upper-level management establishes goals and influences the climate and direction of the workplace. Decision makers of a company must be seriously committed to injury prevention and initiate a specific program for eliminating and controlling ergonomic hazards (Bragg 1996). The commitment level of safety should match that of production (Jacobs 1995).

The commitment of the employer should be demonstrated in a clearly written policy and a program that documents the goals and plans for job safety, health, and ergonomics. Specific goals for the program should be clearly stated to address areas such as injury reduction, lost time containment, liability reduction, increased productivity, decreased turnover, and increased employee morale, as well as workforce health and safety improvement and maintenance (Schwartz 1991). These goals and objectives should be suitable for the size, culture, and complexity of workplace operations. All personnel should be involved in the program, although programs can be applied to individual company sites.

After identifying injury prevention as a priority, the employer must demonstrate support of the program by providing resources and incentives to ensure employee involvement. A reactive organization builds a health and safety culture based on external pressures, such as the fear of prosecution, trade union pressures, external authority inspections, or standards modified by enforcement notices. A proactive organization develops a health and safety culture based on positive total quality management and motivational factors (Deith 1995).

Because one person alone may not be able to effectively change workplace attitudes, behaviors, design, tools, equipment, productivity standards, policies, or practices, companies should consider external and internal resource consultants. External resource consultants can include occupational and physical therapists, engineers, occupational health nurses, physicians, chiropractors, exercise physiologists, psychologists, equipment vendors, insurance experts, and loss-control specialists. These individuals may not be directly involved in the daily operations of the business; internal resource consultants, however, should be familiar with the company and can include management, supervisors, employees, union representatives, members of risk management or human resources departments, controllers, health and safety officers, workers in the tool and die department, industrial engineers, on-site or designated consultants, medical staff, and maintenance department workers (Melnik 1997). Management may designate an individual with a background in participatory ergonomics and program administration to coordinate program development.

Participatory Ergonomics Teams

Participatory ergonomics is not novel. The success of the formal and informal team approaches for solving ergonomic problems in the workplace is well documented (Bohr et al. 1997; Guinter et al. 1995; MacLeod 1993; Melnik 1995; Moore and Garg 1996, 1997; Owen and Garg 1994). Participatory ergonomics can involve focus group activity, total quality management, or task force procedures outside of health and safety. Working as a group promotes higher levels of individual and group achievement, increased productivity, a higher frequency of fresh ideas, the use of better reasoning strategies, and more frequent transfer of learning (King 1994). *Participatory ergonomics* in the context of an ergonomics program has been defined as "the involvement of people in planning and controlling a significant amount of their own work activities, with sufficient knowledge and power to influence both processes and outcomes to achieve desirable goals" (Wilson and Haines 1997). The type and form of participation in decision making has a marked effect on the outcome of a proposed intervention. Employee involvement in decision making can range from the employee's having no prior information about the decision to be implemented to being completely responsible for making and implementing the decision (author unknown 1992; King 1994). Other aspects of participation that should be considered include formal versus informal involvement; policy issues versus specific task performance issues; direct versus indirect involvement; management control versus employee control, which fosters increased productivity and receptive response to intervention; and short versus long duration (King 1995). The goals, mindset, needs, and size of the company determine the combination of properties that characterize a participatory team. Ergonomics consultants have found that informal and direct programs of long duration have been most effective in making and maintaining ergonomic changes.

Program Versus Process

Although the term *injury prevention program* has been used to identify interventions, it is a misnomer. A *program* is "a plan or procedure for dealing with some matter," whereas a *process* is "a continuing development involving many changes; the course of being done" (Guralnik 1982). Injury prevention and management is a process.

Injury Prevention Teams

Some smaller companies do not have internal resources for intervention and may contract an external consultant to lead the ergonomics program. The team may include the ergonomics consultant and either a human resources director, a risk manager, or a safety coordinator. An informal team can be assembled and used as needed and can include workers from target areas, foremen, or other professionals whose services are on retainer with the company. These team members should remain connected through periodic project progress updates from the ergonomics consultant.

A well-constructed injury surveillance program is also a valuable source of data. However, injury prevention should be both proactive and reactive; injury surveillance is reactive and should be only one of several approaches used by the team. The injury prevention team should also have a close relationship with the person or committee responsible for disability management and Americans with Disabilities Act (ADA) compliance.

The injury prevention team members should have a basic knowledge of ergonomic principles and an awareness of federal and state OSHA laws, state workers' compensation laws, labor relations, and any other professional, trade, or industrial standards related to the company. The team's education is a continuous process.

Team Leader

The team leader should be able to recognize and maximize each team member's strengths. He or she should meet with management to clarify goals and objectives of the injury prevention program, discuss financial and human resources, and review past and present prevention programs.

Elements of a Prevention Program

Based on OSHA's guidelines for meat-packing plants, a basic injury prevention program should include risk assessment, work-site analysis, hazard prevention and control, training and education, and medical management (Jacobs 1995).

Risk Assessment

Management or the injury prevention team should perform a thorough risk assessment that includes evaluating the frequency and severity of CTD cases. It should also examine the incidence of CTD for the past several years, the number of work days lost because of CTD, the costs of existing cases, projected costs at case closure, estimated numbers and costs of anticipated cases, and impact of CTD on the company (Ross 1994). OSHA logs and workers' compensation records are useful resources. Frequency and severity should be included in the analysis. Frequency is the number of injuries in a department or job classification. Severity can be interpreted several ways and developed as a weighted number. It should include direct financial losses incurred, as well as lost work days. Risk identification can be facilitated through interviews, brainstorming sessions, or focus groups; symptom surveys; job-risk rating questionnaires; standardized observation techniques; and videotaping (Karwowski and Marras 1997; Zabel and McGrew 1997).

The injury prevention team should consider only those cases in which ergonomics is a suspected factor. Data that are not ergonomic should be provided to the safety team for follow-up. The team analyzes the injury data and targets areas that exceed established levels. Including a statistician or person with a background in statistical analysis can be useful.

Jobs identified in the high-risk category should undergo more detailed ergonomic job analyses. Keyserling recommends the use of ergonomics checklists to facilitate the collection of ergonomic data. The two major factors that determine checklist design are the level of user expertise and the intended use of the collected data (Keyserling et al. 1992). Posture analysis coupled with a biomechanical model was shown to provide a workable analysis system application (Lee and Chiou 1995). Areas to focus on in assessing for risks include the following (Ayoub et al. 1997; Karwowski and Marras 1997; Zabel and McGrew 1997):

- Forceful exertions
- Workstation or tool design
- Extreme or awkward postures (static and during task performance)
- Lifting techniques
- Vibration
- Temperature
- Work intensity and duration
- Repetitions per minute or shift
- Mechanical stress
- Work organization
- Task invariability
- Cognitive demands
- Duration of exertions, motions, or postures
- Use of gloves
- Insufficient rest or break time

High-risk departments often stand out. Although insurance adjusters can identify high-risk areas without having to examine details, analysis can show the degree of the problems and the financial impact of the injuries caused by insurance reserves and medical costs. As the team identifies and remedies injury risks through ergonomic solutions, incidence statistics change. A formerly trouble-free department can suddenly appear at the top of an "at-risk" list because of misguided cost-cutting measures or restructuring instigated by a detached management system. An example would be a department with increased workloads or staff cuts. The administrator who focuses on short-term cost savings needs to realize the greater potential cost from workers' compensation claims or lost productivity. This realization must include the costs associated with recruiting, hiring, and training new workers when a worker with an injury does not return to that job.

Heads of departments with elevated injury statistics can provide valuable information to the team. The injury prevention team can request a formal presentation from the department head involving internal insights about the data. The team's approach in contacting department heads, supervisors, or management helps determine future rapport and results from ergonomic control efforts.

Work-Site Analysis

Work-site analysis involves evaluating risk factors in the environment, tasks, or worker practices to eliminate or limit potentially harmful stressors. Preparation requires a risk assessment that includes evaluation of employee data related to past and present injuries, an objective job analysis, and employee interviews. Work-site analysis is designed to recognize, identify, and correct ergonomic hazards. Reasons for conducting a work-site analysis include

- Preparing for education and training
- Continuing an ergonomics process
- Evaluating a job in relationship to a worker who is experiencing a problem or returning to work after injury (Melnik 1997)

An ergonomics consultant outside the company can request a walk-through in which he or she becomes oriented to the plant's processes and product development. During this period, the consultant should also define potential ergonomic problems. The consultant can also gain insight into the plant's atmosphere and operation by talking to workers. However, the walk-through is not sufficient to determine the magnitude, frequency, and duration of exposures to risk factors. This process can be enhanced when combined with worker and supervisor interviews or risk factor checklists (Karwowski and Marras 1997).

The following are basic guidelines for performing an ergonomic work-site analysis:

1. Obtain general information about the job in question via job description or job analysis on file with the company, the *Dictionary of Occu-*

pational Titles (U.S. Department of Labor 1991), and employee interviews. Obtain clearance for photography or videotaping.
2. Contact the manager or supervisor in the area of analysis.
3. Request an interview with a skilled, uninjured worker in the job position in question. This is particularly important if the analysis is for ergonomic intervention for a worker with an injury. Compare the work practices of workers in the same position (Anderson 1995).
4. Observe the job for several work cycles if possible and document frequency of specific task performance.
5. Take measurements of the workstation and of the worker as applicable for workstation-to-worker fit recommendations.
6. Weigh and measure tools, equipment, work aids, and products that the worker handles.
7. Document workstation layout (by photographing, drawing, etc.).
8. Document relevant heights and distances.
9. Identify risk factors associated with tasks. Solutions should be developed with input from individuals who have the greatest knowledge about the job.
10. Make recommendations for possible ergonomic interventions.
11. Plan follow-up meeting(s) with management, area supervisors, and workers affected by interventions to present findings and recommendations, time lines, costs, and so forth.

Hazard Prevention and Control

Hazard prevention and control involves applying ergonomic principles to specific work settings. Ergonomic intervention can initially increase reports of CTD as employees realize the importance of early identification of musculoskeletal symptoms.

Repetitive motions of the hands, wrists, shoulders, and neck are common in the workplace. Lack of recovery time causes inflammation. Too many forceful exertions of the muscles can cause corresponding tendons to stretch, which compresses microstructures of the tendons, causes ischemia and microscopic tears in the tendons, and causes inflammation. Mechanical stress is a result of tendon, nerve, or other soft-tissue compression caused by contact between the body and another object (usually sharp, hard, or firm). An example is the stress placed on the soft tissues of the palm by hard, sharp, or short tool handles. Mechanical stress can also occur when the wrist rests against the sharp edge of a desk for an extended period. Mechanical stresses can lead to inflammations and nerve compression. Tasks performed in awkward or static postures increase the level of mechanical stress produced by the muscle contraction, leading to chronic localized pain and fatigue. Vibration transmitted to the upper extremities from impact or power tools, sanders, buffers, or grinders can cause damage to both the circulatory and nervous systems. Vibrating hand-held tools also require stronger grips for control and can cause sustained forceful exertions. Cold temperatures decrease circulation to tissue and slow muscle reaction time, reducing dexterity and efficiency of motion (Snook et al. 1988).

The back is also susceptible to overuse, sprain, and strain. Static postures lead to decreased nourishment of the intravertebral discs of the back, gradually causing disc deterioration and degeneration. Narrowed, undernourished discs put additional strain on the facet joints, causing subluxation and tearing of the surrounding tissues (Seymour 1995). Work-related low back disorders can be caused by cumulative exposures or isolated incidents of overexertion from lifting, lowering, carrying, pushing, pulling, or holding activities. Job dissatisfaction, social support, level of responsibility, and family problems have been identified as psychosocial factors that affect the incidence of low back strain (Ayoub et al. 1997). Work organization and psychosocial factors affect responses to work and the potential for work-related injury or illness. Productivity requirements, incentives or piecework systems, extended shifts, company cutbacks, and layoffs are a few such factors.

Prevention Controls

Occupational injury or illness affects both workers and the workplace. Techniques for preventing injury and illness involve engineering controls, administrative controls, and personal protective equipment. These are discussed in order of desired implementation.

Engineering controls change the workplace layout, environment, or production processes through modifications to workstations, tools, and machinery. Although they are frequently the best and most lasting interventions, engineering controls are usually the most costly (Snook et al. 1988; Zabel et al. 1997). An example is a workstation with a hydraulic-lift adjustment used to provide a sit/stand workstation for a worker with low back problems.

Administrative controls are decisions made by management intended to reduce the duration, frequency, and severity of exposure to existing hazards in an attempt to diminish the effects of the hazard on the worker. Examples include job rotation, job enlargement or enrichment, work scheduling, altering work methods, and automation (Jacobs 1995).

Personal protective equipment includes safety glasses; protective clothing; ear protection; head, hand, or foot coverings; and ventilation and respiration devices. Personal protective equipment lessens the likelihood or effect of exposure to harmful conditions.

Forceful Exertions

Most forceful exertions are related to lifting, lowering, pushing, pulling, or holding. A few techniques are used in teaching proper materials handling and tool use. General guidelines are as follows (Anderson 1995; Karwowski et al. 1997; Laing 1993; Pheasant 1991a):

1. Use mechanical aids.
2. Redesign the job to eliminate materials handling.
3. Train workers in proper materials handling techniques and ergonomic principles.
4. Provide good handholds (couplings) and good contact between shoes and floor surfaces.
5. Keep reach, push, pull, and lift distances to a minimum.
6. Raise the load height to avoid bending and lifting.
7. Minimize the required force by using mechanical devices, conveyors, wheel maintenance, altered floor surfaces, lighter container materials (e.g., plastic vs. wood), divided loads, and assistance when possible.
8. Maintain the natural curves of the spine.
9. Minimize weight-handling exposure by allowing proper breaks, providing adjustment time for extreme environment changes, or changing work methods.
10. Eliminate the need for pushing or pulling by using conveyors, slides, or chutes.
11. Locate handholds on carts between 35 and 50 in. from the floor (Laing 1993). Get a good grip on the load.
12. Keep arms close to the body.
13. Keep loads close to the body, have feet in stable base of support position, move feet in the direction of transport, and lift with legs.
14. Do not twist or bend laterally when lifting.
15. Decrease the need for undue forceful gripping or pinching by controlling friction through proper selection of tool handles, tool handle cleanliness (e.g., free of oil), size, length, and gloves (if gloves must be worn, note material and fit).
16. Limit torque or vibration with dampening devices, torque-reaction bars, lower settings, reduced speeds, suspension, machine maintenance and mounting, and decreased exposure times.
17. Use power tools to decrease force.
18. Provide tools that have nonslip, nonporous, and nonconductive handles.
19. Control friction by maintaining floor surfaces (e.g., repair cracks, deterioration) and using the appropriate type and size of casters on carts or devices with wheels.

Repetitive Work

Repetition is measured by number of repetitions per hour, day, or cycle time and number of cycles per hour or per day. Repetitious work multiplies the effects of all of the documented ergonomic risk factors (Anderson 1995). Considerations for intervention are as follows:

- Can mechanical aids or power tools decrease the frequency or duration of repeated or sustained exertions?

- Can the work-to-worker exposure rate to a repetitive task be reduced by work enlargement, adding variety to tasks, work rotation, or increasing the number of workers assigned to the task?
- Are production quotas flexible? Can line or production speeds be reduced?

Workstation Design

Different types of work require different heights to minimize fatigue and injury. The height of the object being worked on is more important than the height of the workbench (Carson 1994). Precision work or writing tasks should be located a minimum of 2 in. above elbow level. Keyboard and mouse functions should be located at elbow level. Light assembly work should be located within several inches below elbow level. Heavy work should be at least 4 in. below elbow level.

The workstation should be designed for easy access to all frequently used tools and parts. Items used most should be located at or within several inches of the distance from the worker's elbow to the fingertips, within a 90-degree arc in front of the worker, and between elbow and shoulder level. The workstation should allow freedom of movement, support and maintenance of neutral trunk and upper extremity postures, and postural change.

Wrist postures should remain neutral and limit deviation to less than 15 degrees. Extreme forearm rotation or repetitive pronation or supination should be avoided. The elbows should move below chest level and as close to the body as possible. Frequent reaching above shoulder level and away from and behind the body is a risk factor, especially when arms are fully extended.

Seating should be adjustable to allow comfortable support of the trunk and legs, postural changes of seat pan to seat back angle, adequate lumbar support, seat-back height adjustment, and easy seat height adjustment. Optional features include a seat pan glide and three-way arm rest adjustments.

Cold and Hot Temperatures

Cold environments can decrease sensitivity, dexterity, and muscle strength (Anderson 1995). Hot environments can cause easy fatigue, muscle weakness, low visibility in eye wear, and poor hand grasp due to perspiration. Using proper personal protective equipment, decreasing exposure times, implementing job rotation, and providing proper ventilation are appropriate interventions.

Lighting

The design of the working environment and evaluation of tasks with visual components are important because

- Visual elements of task determine the posture of the head and neck
- Visually demanding work or adverse viewing conditions can result in visual fatigue and eyestrain
- Visibility, legibility, and clarity of visual displays can be critical to working efficiency and safety
- Aesthetics of the visual environment are important for the quality of working life (Pheasant 1991b)

Glare is usually assessed for computer workstations. Overhead light diffusers, glare screens, task lights, and change of position in relationship to windows are possible interventions.

Work Organization

Incentive payment structures, rigid break times, mandatory overtime, work overload, production lines, deadline-driven work projects, poorly trained or under-skilled workers, and other psychosocial factors can have a role in increasing work-related stress, muscle tension, fatigue, and physical discomforts (Williams 1993).

Training and Education

Training and education include providing training in all aspects of the ergonomic prevention and disability management program. Ergonomic method training should be provided to all new employees. Managers or supervisors are responsible for ensuring that workers follow healthy and safe work procedures and also must participate in risk assessment, work-site analysis, and return-to-work programs.

Education is a major prerequisite to a solid injury prevention and management program. Lines of communication are often confused or nonexistent between management and employees. Training programs must include basic ergonomic principles, interventions, techniques of job analysis, and redesign. Supervisors are responsible for ensuring that workers are following safe work practices and thus need instruction in sign and symptom recognition for CTD, return-to-work procedures, modified duty or transitional work programs, fitness-for-duty assessment, and ergonomic principles. A few tips for effectively educating workers include the following (adapted from Quinn 1988):

- Developing the program in the trainee's literal and technical language
- Defining specific and clearly stated goals
- Beginning each program with a brief overview and summarizing the most important facts
- Building an evaluation mechanism that is easily adapted for each program
- Using participatory teaching methods with the traditional lecture approach

Encourage participation through brainstorming, group discussions, experience sharing, small group exercises, problem solving, hands-on training, performing some of the ergonomic testing, role playing, or practicing new methods in a class.

Medical Management

Medical management requires choosing medical professionals to help the employer provide timely, cost-effective, and relevant prevention and therapeutic interventions. A prevention program should have a medical management system with a health care provider who is part of an ergonomic team (Jacobs 1995). The health care provider has the responsibility of providing early recognition, reporting, and possible treatment of complaints. They must be familiar with the industry, job requirements, and required worker capacities. The health care management program can include systematic evaluation procedures, conservative treatment protocols, ERTW programs, pre- and postinjury assessments, and treatment outcome data (Zabel et al. 1997).

Employers and medical professionals use simulated work experiences for prevention and disability management. The medical protocol at AT&T Bell Laboratories included a simulation of typical conditions in an ergonomics laboratory during the medical evaluation. An employee sets up the equipment in the laboratory to simulate his or her workstation and demonstrates typical activity (Guinter et al. 1995). The physician or health care professional can supervise the simulated work effort. Basic ergonomic training can take place with the employee during this period. Employers have realized greater success for prevention and early intervention through on-site rehabilitation programs that implement traditional clinical interventions at the workplace (Holmes-Enix and Lopez 1998).

The health care provider may offer a full selection of services, including prevention classes, pre-employment screening, preplacement physical demands testing, stretch and warm-up classes, job coaching, fitness-for-duty evaluations, acute therapy services, work hardening or work simulation, ergonomics consultation, and job analysis.

Program Evaluation

The prevention program documents program effectiveness or lack thereof. The company must develop a program evaluation protocol based on risk analysis data. Program evaluation is both qualitative and quantitative. The qualitative aspect considers the needs of the organization and the establishment of measurable prevention program goals. The quantitative aspect of program evaluation looks at numeric data, such as lost time, trends over time, types of injuries, and return-to-work statistics. An outcome evaluation must clearly define the goals of the prevention program. Identifying the indicators of a successful program is beneficial before program implementation. The team can consider including an individual trained in outcome and system evaluation (Schwartz 1997).

Injuries Can Still Occur

Even with an ergonomics program that emphasizes prevention, injuries can still occur. "In many organizations, cumulative trauma now is responsible for over half of occupational injuries including repetitive strain, carpal tunnel, certain types of back injuries, and a variety of other soft-tissue ailments" (Barge and Carlson 1993).

Ergonomics and Disability Management

Ergonomics extends beyond prevention, playing a key role in disability management after an injury or illness has occurred. "[E]rgonomics is the central scientific discipline in injury or disability management. It not only aims at preventing injuries in general, but also plays a key role in returning the injured worker, or workers with any other limitations, to work" (Shrey and Lacerte 1995).

Therapist as Consultant

In the employee with a disability, short-term or long-term physical, sensory, or cognitive limitations must be considered. These limitations can prevent return to the usual job either temporarily or permanently. When an employee has been injured, therapists trained in ergonomics can provide substantial assistance to the recovery and return of that employee. The consulting therapist can function as an advisor to the employer on suitable return-to-work procedures, workstation redesign, and long-term solutions for the worker. The worker can initially be placed in an ERTW program at a completely different location performing different tasks. "Changing the physical location of someone's work, access to the work, design of the workstation, and the like can make the difference between being able to return or remaining on disability" (Akabas et al. 1992).

A trained therapist is capable of providing internal or external ergonomics consulting services to employers. A therapist providing internal consulting is an employee of the organization, perhaps working for a self-insured and self-administered company (i.e., a company that maintains and administers its own workers' compensation and health and liability insurance). A therapist who functions as an external consultant can have a private practice and provide ergonomics assistance to several companies simultaneously. To perform competently, the therapist must obtain sufficient training and experience before promoting him- or herself as a consultant. A consulting therapist has obligations that are different from those of a treating therapist, and the consultant must be confident of his or her role before offering services.

As a member or chair of the ergonomics committee, a consulting therapist must consider many issues. Knowledge of current and future functional abilities and limitations based on various disease and injury processes allows unique insight into analysis of injury data. Familiarity with task analysis, ergonomic principles, and musculoskeletal and psychosocial processes helps provide unique insight on causality and remediation.

Barriers and Management

Barriers are often present in return-to-work processes after an industrial injury. Fear of retribution, job security concerns, fear of equipment that caused an injury, personnel conflicts, financial problems, deterioration of the worker's role, and bad feelings about how the employer treated the worker with an injury all factor into return-to-work potential. Persons with nonindustrial injuries have many of the same barriers. These issues are promptly dealt with by enlightened employers through a comprehensive disability management program. From the moment of injury, savvy employers provide emotional and financial support. In addition, the worker with an injury needs clear information about procedures and events that will take place.

Some employees experience symptoms for a long period (e.g., carpal tunnel syndrome) before filing a claim, whereas others sustain a sudden injury (e.g., crush injury). Both types can be caused by a poor worker-environment fit. Some employees have off-duty injuries that include both acute (broken arm) and chronic (arthritis) conditions. The purpose of the consulting therapist is to ensure a good fit between the work environment and the individual worker's capabilities. Having an employee return to the same activity that caused the injury is usually counterproductive. At this point, ergonomics moves from group to individual application. In a proactive mode, ergonomics is applied to groups to ensure the best possible fit for the greatest physical and psychological range of workers. When ergonomics is applied in a reactive mode (i.e., after an illness or injury), the therapist looks at the fit of the environment in comparison to the individual's limitations and abilities. The therapist can also look at the work environment not only for nonmaleficence but also for curative potential. Therapeutically graded activities include work.

Early-Return-to-Work Programs

A therapist skilled in ergonomics and industrial rehabilitation can also have a substantial impact on a company's bottom line by consulting as an ERTW program developer or specialist. This program helps injured or ill employees return to work as soon as possible, derailing secondary disabilities such as physical deconditioning and anger at the employer for perceived abandonment. "Workers, despite their impairments, must continue to perceive themselves as valued employees who remain attached to the workplace. Otherwise, the worker's disability will manifest itself in extended lost time and more severe occupational disability" (Shrey and Lacerte 1995). An ERTW program is a method of controlling employer costs while maximizing recovery when an employee has experienced an industrial injury or illness that might otherwise result in lost time, which is expensive. For instance, in California in 1997, the dollar amount for temporary total disability benefits through workers' compensation was $448 per week. Essentially, the employer pays the worker with an injury a substantial sum to sit at home. ERTW programs are a significant component of comprehensive disability management programs. The "principle of 'early return to work' is essentially the second half of the formula for achieving successful rehabilitation outcome" (Shrey and Lacerte 1995).

Developing and managing a successful ERTW program requires someone knowledgeable in the broad field of industrial rehabilitation. The program specialist needs to be familiar with a variety of topics, including

- Physical, environmental, and psychological causes of injury
- Relationships between insurer, employer, physician, treating therapist, and employee
- Task analysis and synthesis
- Principles and practical applications of ergonomics
- Theory and practice of preventing delayed recovery
- Nature and typical course of injury, illness, and recovery processes

In addition, the ERTW specialist should have good patient skills, be able to understand and communicate terminology of physicians and insurance carriers, and be able to persuade others to follow a program.

A ERTW specialist should consider medical restrictions; evaluate the required tasks; and upgrade, downgrade, or substitute the tasks to meet the abilities of the worker. Any ambiguities in the restrictions are clarified by communication with a physician. A preliminary work tolerance screening can provide precise data on the actual capabilities of an employee with an injury, if any doubt or concern exists. A skillful ERTW specialist structures the work tasks to improve tolerances over time, thereby achieving the goals of promptly returning the worker to duty, preventing secondary disabilities, and achieving improvement through occupational performance.

Three types of ERTW programs are prevalent:

1. Temporary work assignment (TWA): Workers with temporary limitations preventing performance of the usual and customary job are provided with temporary work within their stated restrictions.

2.   Modified work assignment: Workers with temporary limitations are
     provided with temporary work composed of parts of their regular job
     or modified methods of doing their regular job.
3.   Temporary reassignment: Workers with temporary limitations are
     reassigned to vacant temporary positions that are within their stated
     restrictions (Wright 1997).

The term *light duty* is often used to describe an ERTW program but
implies that the work done is less valued. *Early-return-to-work* is preferred
to *light duty*.

In each type of temporary activity, the worker is expected to return to
his or her job after recuperation and within a reasonable period. Programs
generally use either temporary work assignment or temporary reassignment, depending on corporate culture. When a worker is identified as permanently unable to return to his or her usual and customary job, the
ERTW program is no longer appropriate. The employee with an injury is
then potentially eligible for assistance under the ADA and possibly vocational rehabilitation services.

Of the three types of ERTW identified above, the type most useful as
a workers' compensation cost control device is TWA. TWA is based on created work (i.e., work assembled from component parts of different jobs).
TWA work is created specifically for the person involved and is not a regular job. After restrictions have been received from the worker's physician,
the job is assembled based on those restrictions, the worker's current
skills, the potential worker-workplace ergonomic fit, and the needs of the
organization. Tasks can be reselected as the worker's capabilities improve.
The TWA job ceases to exist after a set period.

An important aspect of TWA is that temporary created work is not
prone to entanglement with the ADA and associated regulations. The job
cannot be perceived as a reasonable accommodation under the ADA,
because it is artificial and temporary. A TWA program coordinator creates
temporary jobs by consulting a bank of tasks that need to be done.

Modified work assignment involves placing a worker in his or her regular job, modified to accommodate the employee's restrictions. Modifications can include changes to the ergonomics of the environment, adaptive
equipment, changes in schedules, deletion of key work tasks, or similar
adjustments. Should the job continue in this manner for a significant
period, however, the modified job could be considered a reasonable accommodation under the ADA. The employer is then obligated to consider it a
regular job. Modified work as a management tool is useful but should be
coordinated with an ADA specialist to minimize confusion with federal
and state disability laws.

Temporary reassignment occurs when a worker is placed in a vacant
temporary position that is ergonomically a better fit and less demanding
physically or mentally. The demands are within the limitations of the

worker with a disability. As with modified work, care must be taken to keep this form of ERTW from entanglement with the ADA. The ADA maintains that when a worker is not able to perform his or her regular job, with or without reasonable accommodation, an employer is obligated to look for other work within the organization. For ERTW purposes, reassignment is to a temporary position. However, temporary reassignment can become confused with the requirement under the ADA for long-term reassignment. An aggressive ADA program emphasizing returning the worker with an injury to his or her usual job prevents much of this confusion.

Establishing an Early-Return-to-Work Program

A sequence of steps should be taken by an internal or external consulting therapist, in collaboration with others, to develop a successful ERTW program.

Identify True Costs of Workers' Compensation

The first step has already been defined: Identify direct and indirect costs for workers' compensation. Direct costs can be obtained from data gathered either by a risk management department for self-insured, self-administered organizations or from a third-party administrator or the company's contracted insurance carrier. After direct costs are identified, indirect costs must also be analyzed. Remember to include the adjuster's time in these costs. Include all costs in the report to administration.

Study Models Available

An ERTW program begins with gathering and considering sample programs from other organizations. Seminars, journal articles, sample policies, and procedures should be obtained and reviewed.

The basic structure of the program should be identified. Which of the three types of temporary work will be offered? What are the arrangements to pay the worker? Some programs pay only a percentage of the full salary of the worker; others pay full salary. In the case of shift work, will payment be for night differential? What hours will ERTW work be performed? Structuring the work to occur only when ERTW personnel are available can be useful. The number of hours per week worked can have a large impact on the claim costs; close collaboration with the insurer is necessary. The physical location of the ERTW program can vary. Risk management centers, human resources management centers, and employee health clinics are potential sites. Placing the program specialist in the health clinic is helpful initially because the program specialist can work directly with the industrial physicians. Considerations in developing parts of the program include the following:

- An ERTW specialist needs to gain the trust of the physicians who see employees with new injuries. The best way may be to have the specialist work out of the same office as the doctors to allow opinions and questions to be exchanged immediately.
- Employees and managers who become involved with the ERTW need closer supervision, especially in the start up phase. Employees' work hours should perhaps be limited to the hours that the specialist is available.
- If employee physicians believe that night shift and 12-hour shifts are not conducive to healing, the program eliminates those hours.
- To motivate workers, the policy might allow workers to be paid their regular hourly rates.
- To motivate managers, workers can be provided without charge to the accepting department.

Each organization, based on its corporate culture, needs to customize the structure of its program. Unionized organizations need to work with unions within negotiated agreements.

Select the Manager for the Program

The nature of the organization to some degree dictates the individual selected to run the ERTW program. An experienced occupational or physical therapist can be selected to run the program, although the management of such a program is not limited to therapists. A rehabilitation counselor or rehabilitation nurse can also perform well as a program manager. Depending on the size of the organization, the human resources manager may want to begin the program, in consultation with therapists. An ERTW specialist who can interpret a physician's restrictions in terms of tasks to be done should be selected. An ERTW specialist should also have determination and excellent interpersonal skills.

Allowing labor organizations to have a say in the process is important. Although some labor organizations are skeptical, the unions of most companies that have engaged in temporary duty programs have found a generally cooperative atmosphere. Labor agreements about various trades can limit the flexibility of the program, but difficulties can be minimized by an innovative program manager.

Develop Policies and Procedures

Policy, procedures, and guidelines are most helpful when established from the outset. Review of pre-existing policies for areas of conflict with an ERTW program should occur at the same time as the development of an ERTW policy. The wage costs for the program can be substantial. An account should be set aside and decisions regarding cost allocation methods made. Some organizations bill the home department, whether the worker is based there or not. Other facilities allocate wage costs by the number or severity of injuries that have occurred recently in each department. Thus, if a department has a high number of injuries, that department bears a higher burden of the allocated cost for the ERTW program.

Under the Family Medical Leave Act (FMLA), an employer cannot make an ERTW program mandatory. If qualified, the employee can select instead to take up to 3 months of unpaid leave on FMLA. Existing human resources policies may need to be reworked for consistency between ERTW, FMLA, and ADA.

Analyze Jobs and Tasks

After the program has been planned and personnel recruited to implement it, job analysis should begin. Particularly for a program emphasizing TWA, a task bank should be established for a variety of jobs, if not all. A task bank identifies the various tasks required in each position. The first goal of task bank development is to emphasize to managers that jobs are composed of tasks. Managers may first report that no "light-duty" jobs are available. This may be true enough, but light-duty tasks almost always exist within any job. Additionally, ergonomic conditions of each task must be kept in mind. This necessitates an on-site visit to see the tasks being performed and the physical and psychological environment. Over time, the specialist should become familiar with sites and managers, which will reduce on-site visits. Even ERTW tasks can have ergonomic adjustments made to enable the worker with an injury to do the task safely. If the program tends toward modified work or temporary reassignment, an analysis of the environment, tasks, and ergonomics of the positions may still be necessary.

Managers need to be encouraged to think of jobs as a collection of tasks that may be divided—the foundation of an ERTW program. When tasks are identified, they can be reassembled into a temporary position and customized to the physical or mental restrictions of the worker with an injury. Often, these tasks are high-priority jobs that never seem to get done. If the program provides the wages of the worker, the specialist can emphasize the benefit of "free" workers available to managers.

Determine the Process for Program Performance and Evaluation

On-site visits and phone calls to and from the employee with an injury and the new supervisor are a form of process evaluation that allows changes to take place mid-course. An impact evaluation regarding the performance of the program also needs to be developed and applied. Outcome data can be in the form of changes in days lost, claims costs, reserves, litigation frequency, vocational rehabilitation expenditures, and so forth. Such data are valuable in justifying continuance of the ERTW program. The outcome evaluation should also include comments from managers and employees on how the program worked for them. Each manager should formally evaluate the worker with an injury they had in the ERTW program. Some of these evaluations prove most revealing. "Problem" employees for the home department may be "model" employees for a different manager.

Program Structure to Encourage Compliance

An ERTW program can only be successful when it motivates both the managers and the workers. Orchard Supply Hardware motivates managers through a bill-back system: "[W]orkers' compensation premiums are allocated to the various stores based on the frequency and severity of claims. The more claims a store has, the higher its share of the insurance bill" (Taylor 1992).

A subtler form of encouragement for workers with injuries can be successful. Recuperating employees can be paid a full salary (no night-shift or other special pay) to do assigned work while they heal. In comparison to temporary total disability pay, this approach preserves most of the worker's income, instantly motivating many workers. Unless the ERTW specialist is astute, however, high-end wage earners paid their full salary can generate excess cost over benefit. In this case, the key is to use expensive staff in positions where their skills are most needed. For low-end wage earners, the pay to work may be no more than the pay to stay home on total disability. The motivation here is that, should a worker choose not to work, total disability payments are not continued, because work was available. However, remember that ERTW cannot be mandatory, as an employee can choose to take unpaid family medical leave, perhaps supplementing with paid vacation time.

With motivated workers, the question becomes how to motivate managers to accept the workers. Initially, quite a bit of resistance can exist. Usually, enough managers are desperate for help to allow ERTW employees to work. If a home department supervisor reports no temporary work for an employee, the ERTW manager then works with other supervisors to find tasks for that employee. The supervisor who accepts the employee gets additional work done, whereas the home department supervisor does not. Such events, often spread by word of mouth, help increase the acceptability of ERTW programs.

Orient Workers to the Program

To successfully enroll workers in an ERTW program, the following steps should be taken:

1. Contact the department manager by phone to confirm that tasks are available.
2. Meet with and train the worker with an injury.

3.   Review the rules of the program and have employees and department managers sign the rules.
4.   Arrange for transfer of time clock reporting to the appropriate cost center.
5.   Have the ERTW manager make unexpected on-site visits to ensure the process is going smoothly.

Ergonomics and the Americans with Disabilities Act

The therapist consulting in ergonomics is a valuable resource for organizations addressing the requirements of the ADA. This federal law states that an employer is obligated to help qualified employees with disabilities (industrial and otherwise) stay on the job. Employers are also obligated to provide assistance (i.e., reasonable accommodation) for newly hired workers who need modifications to perform the essential functions of a job. Not all disabilities require accommodation. Sometimes, a limitation is too mild to require accommodation, and often a disability has nothing to do with job performance. As the workforce ages, more workers will have limitations on their performance due to disability.

The therapist consulting in ergonomics can provide employers with significant and cost-effective assistance regarding the ADA. The consultant can provide useful information regarding task and environment redesign, enhancing the opportunity for the employee with a disability to stay on the job. An assessment of the worker-workplace interface can help satisfy requirements for reasonable accommodation for return to the regular job under the ADA. Improving the ergonomics of the situation may be all the reasonable accommodations needed. Consulting therapists can suggest changes that have significant effects and cost very little.

Occasionally, the consultant may report that the job or environment cannot be modified. If the employee cannot return to the regular job, even with reasonable accommodations, the consultant can advise employers about the match between other positions available and the abilities of the worker. Simple changes in work method or environment can make the difference between return to work or long-term disability for workers with injuries. A therapist with a knowledge of ergonomics and rehabilitation is the ideal consultant for this area.

To avoid being confused with a permanent light-duty position, all ERTW programs should have a limited duration. The ADA does not require the creation of a light-duty position (Equal Employment Opportunity Commission [EEOC] 1992). ERTW programs are a cost control technique for management, not a benefit guaranteed to workers under federal or state law. Data have shown that workers on TWA more than approximately 6 weeks are less likely to return to their usual jobs.

If an organization decides to use temporary reassignment, a short job duration should be established and held without exception: "If a light duty job is a temporary job, reassignment to that job need only be for the temporary period of the job. An employer need not convert a temporary job into a permanent one" (Ogletree et al. 1995). The ERTW program specialist must take care to assign workers with injuries to positions that are recognized as temporary if the intent is to keep ERTW programs and ADA separate (a good idea). If the worker with an injury is assigned to a job on a temporary basis and cannot be accommodated in his or her usual job, the employer is obligated by the ADA to try to reassign the worker to a regular (permanent) position within permanent restrictions. The temporary job becomes an ADA reassignment.

Reassignment should never be used punitively, as this can open the organization to discrimination claims and destroy the program completely. Nothing is more detrimental than an angry worker who is forced to work for a supervisor or department he or she dislikes.

A review of what constitutes a temporary condition under the ADA is useful. The ERTW manager is usually among the first to notice a worker whose rate of improvement does not allow return to regular work within a short period: "A condition does not have to be permanent to qualify as a disability" (Ogletree et al. 1995). Temporary impairments usually include injuries and illnesses such as broken arms or legs, sprains, and chicken pox. The EEOC Technical Assistance Manual reports that on-the-job injuries causing impairments that heal within a short period with little long-term or permanent impact are not considered disabilities under the ADA (EEOC 1992). However, "the fact that in a *particular* case a physical or mental impairment was held in one or more cases *not* to rise to the level of 'handicap' under the Rehabilitation Act does not necessarily mean the particular physical or mental impairment never may constitute a 'handicap' under the Rehabilitation Act or 'disability' under the Americans with Disabilities Act" (Ogletree et al. 1995). The ERTW manager may also be the ADA specialist. If this is not the case, the two specialists should remain in close contact on cases that go on long enough, or are projected to go on long enough, to be considered a disability under the ADA.

"Selling" the Early-Return-to-Work Program

Internal Marketing

After a task bank is completed and a policy is developed, the internal marketing campaign must begin in earnest. Managers and employees need to be educated about the ERTW program. Employees frequently believe that any change in the workers' compensation benefit is for the worse. For some managers, any change is seen as "softening" on the workers, and the start of any insurance "bill-back" system may be greeted with dismay. Both management and employee groups must be taught that ERTW programs benefit all involved parties. Managers must also be informed of expectations the ERTW specialist has of them when they begin accepting program workers. Employees should be taught to expect to return to work promptly after an injury.

External Marketing

After the program begins, external marketing becomes important. Besides the regular employee health service provider, other area physicians should be informed of the employer's desire to get employees back to work as soon as possible. When an employee does not recover quickly, care can be transferred to a community-based physician. Meetings, phone calls, informational brochures, tours, or similar marketing techniques can be used to remind doctors of the ERTW program. A simple technique, such as stamping each piece of correspondence to a physician with "We will accommodate restrictions," may be successful.

The ERTW specialist should not hesitate to call and clarify any points concerning restrictions that may cause problems. If a worker protests that he or she cannot do a particular task, even if it is within the stated limitations, the ERTW specialist should contact the risk manager and physician immediately. In some cases, the ERTW specialist may go to the doctor's office with the employee. A videotape of the selected job tasks may be brought along for the doctor to ensure better communication. The physician and therapist working together can also develop additional modifications to the ergonomic environment to increase the comfort of the worker with an injury. Work tolerance screening can also be helpful.

Potential Problems

For every action, some sort of reaction usually occurs, sometimes completely out of proportion to the original action. Examples of potential problem are discussed in the following sections. Most of these situations can be avoided through prevention.

Chair Envy

After a workstation evaluation has been conducted, the evaluated worker, Sam, receives a change in his environment—a new chair. Instantly, other workers want the same thing. Sam, who is already anxious about how he will be accepted, suddenly finds himself the object of irritated stares and pithy comments from coworkers. Fellow workers demand to know why

Sam got a new chair and they did not. Medical information is confidential, and Sam's supervisor is not at liberty to discuss Sam's condition. Thus, little information is available, except that Sam received extra attention and now has a new cushy chair. A proactive approach to this type of problem is telling newly hired workers that everyone does not necessarily do the same job in the same way and that others may need different schedules, supplies, or equipment to accomplish work.

Insurer's Control Issues

As external and internal consultants, insurers may tell the consulting therapist to provide only information they want to know. For insurance companies, the costs of getting the employee recovered and back to work are very important. Some insurers limit the scope of an ergonomics consultation with instructions given before the evaluation. They do not want to provide "blank check" consultant evaluations. Examples of limitations include restrictions on what is to be evaluated, what can be said to the people in the environment being evaluated, and what can be written in the report. These limitations require careful consideration of the ethical, moral, and legal dimensions of such restrictions. Limitations on what should be evaluated can be phrased, "I want you to look at the desk and computer system—but don't tell me about the chair. We can't afford new chairs for the whole office." Limitations on conversations can be, "Don't talk to the person about your findings. We want to be first to know what you found." Restrictions on reporting can be, "Don't report on anything except what you were instructed to look at. If you see some problems elsewhere, just don't put it in the report."

A consultant's initial reaction to limitations may be resentment, but contractual relationships must be considered. Therapists traditionally treat patients/clients. Therapists establish relationships with patients/clients that require primary consideration of the welfare of the patient/client. The occupational therapy and physical therapy codes of ethics are clear about the therapist-patient/client relationship: The recipient is the therapist's patient. To do less than a complete job of evaluation might not fully address the welfare of the patient/client. The occupational therapy code of ethics requires that therapists collaborate with patients/clients, and the physical therapy code of ethics insists that the therapist should be guided by concerns for the welfare of "those individuals entrusted to their care" (Scott 1997).

When a therapist is retrained by an insurance company or employer, a question can arise: Is the person at the workstation in question actually a patient/client of the therapist? Consulting therapists often have worked years in clinical care. Although any professional action must follow the applicable code of ethics, consulting is not entirely the same as treating. If a therapist is required to appear as an expert witness in a trial, does the "treating therapist–recipient patient/client" relationship apply? Most would argue it does not. The job of the expert witness is to provide information to the court (the contracting agency). No patient/client relationship is established. Similarly, a consultant is contracted to an agency that pays the bill, usually the employer or the insurer. The consultant must discuss the costs, risks, and resources involved in the evaluation with the contracting agency (Bellman 1990): "The client and consultant need to be mutually clear about what each expects of the other and what each is going to provide the other" (Bellman 1990). To neglect this area of consulting can lead to unfortunate misunderstandings. Kornblau (1998) suggests that the "ergonomic consultant owes a duty to those with whom he or she establishes a professional relationship. Thus, the consultant owes a duty of care to the client company with who he or she consults, and probably to any reasonably foreseeable 'patient' or client worker affected where the company follows the consultant's advice. This duty of care also extends to the individual worker about whom the consultant provides case consultation." The matter of whether a worker incidentally encountered in the process of workstation evaluation for ergonomics is owed a duty of care is less than concrete. A consultant should determine clearly in his or her own mind what level of restriction on evaluations and findings is acceptable. In some situations, the therapist may have to explain to the worker that he or she is not the treating therapist or explain to the insurer that particular restrictions are unacceptable. The insurer knows the value of the therapist's findings and advice; otherwise, the insurer would not have contacted the therapist.

A consulting therapist should impose limitations on contractual relationships to meet professional ethics, legal requirements, and moral reasoning. The rehabilitation field is comparatively small, and therapists must believe that their reputations precede them: The most valued practitioners are those known to be ethical and unbiased.

Resistant Management and Employees

Managers often resent outsiders' making recommendations. Employees and managers misidentify therapists as "efficiency experts," who are almost universally disliked. Frequently, the consultant in ergonomics encounters employees and managers who consider any change to be detrimental. In disability management, an ergonomics consultant who helps an employee return to work often is viewed with suspicion by managers and employees. In the best of circumstances, employees see the logic of the modifications and welcome their coworker back. In the worst of circumstances, the ergonomics consultant is part of a team that supports the mandatory assignment of a worker with an injury to a vacant position in compliance with the ADA. The consultant's job in this case is to make modifications to the work environment that allow the person with a disability to be successful in the position. In this case, both managers and employees may see the consultant as evil. Negative feelings towards workers with disabilities by other workers and mangers can become significant. An ergonomics consultant who makes the worker's return to work possible can be on the receiving end of some of those negative feelings.

Conclusion

Ergonomic intervention is the principal component of a successful injury prevention and disability management process. Total commitment to training, education, communication, and program participation is essential. A thorough analysis of work sites, tools and equipment, work tasks, corporate culture, and work methods provides vital data for risk assessment, training, return-to-work programs, medical management, hazard prevention, and control. The policies and procedures for an injury prevention and disability management program must be tied to corporate goals and program outcome assessment.

The ergonomics team or consultant must carefully apply knowledge in ergonomic principles and interventions, participatory team concepts, workers' compensation guidelines, ADA, risk management, company and union policies on light-duty and modified work, professional ethics, and diplomacy.

References

Akabas SH, Gates LB, Galvin DE (1992). Disability Management: A Complete System to Reduce Costs, Increase Productivity, Meet Employee Needs and Ensure Legal Compliance. New York: Amacon.

Anderson MA (1995). Ergonomics: Analyzing Work from a Physiologic Perspective. In SJ Isernhagen (ed), The Comprehensive Guide to Work Injury Management. Gaithersburg, MD: Aspen.

Author unknown (1992). Participatory ergonomics. Work Injury Manage Dig 1(2):1, 3–4.

Ayoub MM, Dempsey PG, Karwowski W (1997). Manual Materials Handling. In G Salvendy (ed), Handbook of Human Factors and Ergonomics (2nd ed). New York: Wiley, 1085–1123.

Barge BN, Carlson JG (1993). The Executive's Guide to Controlling Health Care and Disability Costs: Strategy-Based Solutions. New York: Wiley, 298.

Bellman G (1990). The Consultant's Calling. San Francisco: Jossey-Bass, 90.

Bohr PC, Evanoff BA, Wolf LD (1997). Implementing participatory ergonomics teams among health care workers. Am J Ind Med 34:190–196.

Bragg TL (1996). An ergonomics program for the health care setting. Nurs Manage 27(7):58–62.

Carson R (1994). Reducing cumulative trauma disorders. AAOHN J 42(6):270–227.

Deith B (1995). Promoting health and safety programs in the workplace. Nurs Times 91(9):38–39.

EEOC (1992). Technical assistance manual on the employment provisions (Title 1) of the Americans with Disabilities Act. Section 9.4.

Guinter R, Eagels S, Haringer R, Trusewych T (1995). AT&T Bell lab's ergonomic program aims to cure VDT workstation ills. Occup Health Safety 64(2): 30–35.

Guralnik D (ed) (1982). Webster's New World Dictionary of the American Language (2nd ed). New York: Simon & Schuster.

Hansen JA (1993). OSHA regulation of ergonomic health. J Occup Med 1(35):42–46.

Heck-Edwards C (1991). Applied ergonomics. Work 9(1):27–37.

Holmes-Enix D, Lopez S (1998). How early is early? Onsite early return-to-work programs cut losses and costs. Rehabil Manage 11(2):28–35.

Jacobs K (1995). Injury prevention in the workplace. Rehabil Manage 8(3):119–121.

Karwowski W, Marras WS (1997). Work-Related Musculoskeletal Disorders of the Upper Extremities. In G Salvendy (ed), Handbook of Human Factors and Ergonomics. New York: Wiley, 1124–1173.

Keyserling WM, Brouwer M, Silverstein BA (1992). A checklist for evaluating ergonomic risk factors resulting from awkward postures of the legs, trunk and neck. Int J Ind Ergon 9:283–301.

King PM (1994). Participatory ergonomics: a group dynamics perspective. Work 4(3):195–200.

Kornblau B (1998). The Americans with Disabilities Act: Legal Ramifications of ADA Consultation. In VJB Rice (ed), Ergonomics in Health Care and Rehabilitation. Boston: Butterworth–Heinemann, 297.

Laing PM (ed) (1993). Ergonomics: A Practical Guide (2nd ed). Chicago: National Safety Council.

Lee YJ, Chiou WK (1995). Ergonomic analysis of working posture in nursing personnel: example of modified Ovako working analysis system application. Res Nurs Health 18:67–75.

MacLeod D (1993). What works to cut CTD risks, improve job productivity? CTD News 2(1):1–3.

Melnik MS (1997). Designing a Prevention Program. In MJ Sanders (ed), Managing Cumulative Trauma Disorders. Boston: Butterworth–Heinemann, 261–277.

Mook J (ed) (1995). Americans with Disabilities Act: Employee Rights and Employer Obligations. New York: Matthew Bender, 3–41.

Moore JS, Garg A (1996). Use of participatory ergonomics teams to address musculoskeletal hazards in the red meat packing industry. Am J Ind Med 29: 402–408.

Moore JS, Garg A (1997). Participatory ergonomics in a red meat packing plant. Part II: case studies. Am Ind Hyg Assoc J 58:498–508.

Ogletree, Deakins, Nash, et al. (1995). Americans with Disabilities Act: Employee Rights and Employer Obligations. New York: Matthew Bender, 3–41.

Owen BD, Garg A (1994). Reducing back stress through an ergonomic approach: weighing a patient. Int J Nurs Stud 31:511–519.

Pheasant S (1991a). Clinical Ergonomics. In Ergonomics, Work, and Health. Gaithersburg, MD: Aspen, 320–328.

Pheasant S (1991b). Visual Work. In Ergonomics, Work, and Health. Gaithersburg, MD: Aspen, 196–211.

Quinn MA (1988). Effectively Educating Workers. In BS Levy, DH Wegman (eds), Occupational Health: Recognizing and Preventing Work-Related Disease (2nd ed). Boston: Little, Brown, 47–48.

Ross P (1994). Ergonomic hazards in the workplace: assessment and prevention. AAOHN J 42(4):171–176.

Scott R (1997). Promoting Legal Awareness in Physical and Occupational Therapy. New York: Mosby.

Schwartz RK (1991). Preventing the incurable: proactive risk management. Work 1:12–26.

Schwartz RK (1997). Outcome Assessment of Prevention Programs. In MJ Sanders (ed), Management of Cumulative Trauma Disorders. Boston: Butterworth–Heinemann, 339–363.

Seymour MB (1995). The ergonomics of seating posture and chair adjustment. Nurs Times 91(9):35–37.

Shrey DE, Lacerte M (1995). Principles and Practices of Disability Management in Industry. Winter Park, FL: G. R. Press.

Snook SH, Fine LJ, Silverstein BA (1988). Musculoskeletal Disorders. In BS Levy, DH Wegman, (eds), Occupational Health: Recognizing and Preventing Work-Related Disease (2nd ed). Boston: Little, Brown, 345–370.

Taylor S (1992). Enhancing productivity with return-to-work programs. Risk Manage Mag 2:43–46.

U.S. Department of Labor (1991). Dictionary of Occupational Titles (4th ed). Indianapolis: JIST Works.

Williams N (1993). WRULDs: encouraging an ergonomic approach. Occup Health (London) 45:401–404.

Wilson JR, Haines HM (1997). Participatory Ergonomics. In G Salvendy (ed), Handbook of Human Factors and Ergonomics (2nd ed). New York: Wiley, 490–513.

Wright MC (1997). Early return to work and occupational therapy. Occup Ther Prac 2(5):36–42.

Zabel A, McGrew AB (1997). Ergonomics: a key component in a CTD control program. AAOHN J 45(7):350–360.

Review Questions

(Answers are found in Appendix D.)

1. What is the primary goal of a work-site analysis program?
   (a) Improve employee productivity and satisfaction
   (b) Develop an idea of time and motion processes
   (c) Identify and correct ergonomic hazards
   (d) Help employees respond to the psychosocial environment

2. Risk assessment of cumulative trauma cases should include
   (a) frequency and severity of cumulative trauma injuries
   (b) projected risk computations per capita
   (c) analysis of employee leisure occupations
   (d) cardiac status of all employees

3. Which of the following is identified as a psychosocial factor that has an impact on the incidence of low back strain?
   (a) Family problems
   (b) Use of antidepressants
   (c) Amount of vacation time taken in the last 6 months
   (d) History of military service
   (e) Number of children in the family

4. A formerly quiescent department appears at the top of the injury charts. Which factor(s) should you suspect regarding this change?
   (a) Sudden change in the amount of work expected from workers
   (b) Staff cutbacks
   (c) Poor morale
   (d) Change in management
   (e) All of the above

5. TWA is most useful as a cost control device for workers' compensation because
   (a) work is created, not pre-existing
   (b) the job cannot easily become entangled with the ADA
   (c) the work is always very easy
   (d) workers are always anxious to return to work immediately
   (e) both a and b
   (f) both a and c

CHAPTER 13
Evidence-Based Practice

*Chetwyn C. H. Chan, Tatia M. C. Lee, Cecilia Tsang-Li,
and Paul Chi-Wai Lam*

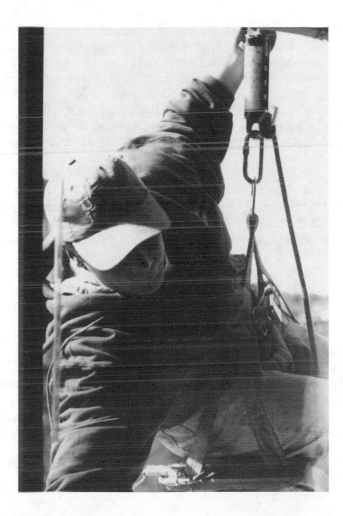

ABSTRACT

Evidence-based practice (EBP) began in the early 1980s and has since been adopted by many health care professionals, including occupational and physical therapists and nurses. EBP is believed to contribute significantly to improved clinical effectiveness, increased ability to provide clients access to information about services received, and increased success meeting administrators' target costs (Dowie 1994; Partridge 1996). This chapter discusses methods for establishing scientific evidence for work-related rehabilitation and explains relationships between EBP, clinical research, and practice guidelines. It also discusses difficulties that clinicians and researchers encounter in pursuing EBP in work rehabilitation.

Evidence-based medicine (EBM) was introduced in the 1980s at McMaster University in Canada for training medical practitioners (Deighan and Boyd 1996; Rosenberg and Donald 1995). In contrast to conventional curriculums, EBM introduced practitioners to problem-based learning and less structured tutorial groups. The EBM program helped McMaster graduates develop self-directed learning skills that enabled them to attain high levels of clinical competence years after their graduation. In comparison, the clinical competence of non-McMaster graduates tended to deteriorate progressively. The positive effect of self-directed learning among medical practitioners provided the impetus for the development of EBP. EBM is primarily associated with the practice of medicine, whereas EBP, or evidence-based health care, is used in many professional services (Deighan and Boyd 1996).

EBP involves the use of the best available evidence, preferably generated scientifically, to guide decisions on clinical diagnosis, treatment, and intervention (Sackett and Rosenberg 1995). At the operational level, EBP circumscribes different systems of reviewing and integrating clinical evidence through organizations such as the Cochrane Collaboration (Glanville 1994; Hayes and McGrath 1998) and the Journal Club (Partridge 1996). Reviewed evidence is disseminated through CD-ROMs and the Internet (Greengold and Weingarten 1996; Sharpe et al. 1996).

The process of EBP is complicated and multidimensional (Greenhalgh 1996; Greenhalgh and Macfarlane 1997). EBP begins with the identification of a problem and systematically reviews, analyzes, evaluates, and synthesizes existing published and unpublished evidence. Results of the review are then used to determine the most efficient and cost-effective interventions. Various methods are used to disseminate the results to clinicians, researchers, managers, and clients. Clinical experts use the reviewed evidence to develop practice guidelines. Different review groups update existing systems and establish new databases. Because results of EBP directly influence clinicians' decisions in practice, stringent and bias-free criteria are used to ensure the best quality information is gathered and disseminated.

Although discussion of EBP is abundant, information on EBP applied to rehabilitation is scarce. Issues identified in rehabilitation-related literature include advantages versus disadvantages of EBM in the clinical practice (Law and Baum 1998; Wallace et al. 1997), methods of establishing evidence (Haynes and McGrath 1998; van Tulder et al. 1997), and integration of evidence into clinical practice (Egan et al. 1998; Hunt 1997; Turner and Whitfield 1997). Various questions have been raised concerning whether EBP can be equally applied to ergonomic and work rehabilitation: What is the best evidence? How can the evidence be pooled? Is the evidence available? Can research evidence be realistically generalized to be incorporated in daily clinical practice?

Determining the Clinical Question

The process of gathering evidence in EBP requires a well-defined question relevant to day-to-day clinical practice rather than to theoretical or philosophical propositions, because evidence established through EBP is used by practitioners, administrators, and clients. Compared to clinical research, EBP involves several factors, such as theoretical work, empirical findings, and clinical applications. In contrast to a general question such as "What is the best treatment for clients with cumulative trauma disorders," a typical EBP clinical question is "Is the combined mobilization and work-hardening program increasing work endurance of clients with tennis elbow?" However, a question such as "Is Armstrong's dose and response model sufficient to explain the phenomenon of cumulative trauma disorders" is too theoretical.

Sources of Information and Evidence

After a clinical question is defined, the next step is to gather information and evidence relevant to the question. Assembling a group of practitioners and researchers is an efficient way to form a review group that can identify a number of sources for information before the search. In addition to being found in CD-ROMs, citation indices, and Internet searches, information can be requested from authors; relevant national and international agencies, foundations, associations, and content experts; and through bibliographic screening of all articles. The Cochrane Collaboration (http://www.nihs.go.jp/acc/cochrane/cc-broch.htm) has developed a system to coordinate activities and provide technical support for journal searches through a methods working group (Silagy 1995). Examples of search strategies are available in the abstracts of review of the Cochrane Library at the Cochrane Collaboration Internet site. When this chapter was written, the site contained a search field called "Cochrane Rehabilitation and Related Therapies," which was the closest search field for rehabilitation disciplines. No search field on ergonomic and work rehabilitation was available.

Randomized Clinical Trials

The quality of the evidence reviewed on a clinical question plays a significant role in EBP. Various organizations have established different criteria for evaluating evidence (Raphael and Marbach 1997; van Tulder et al. 1997). The Quality of Evidence Ratings used by the National Health and Medical Research Council (NHMRC) (1995) classify evidence into four categories according to quality: Category I indicates the best evidence, and category IV indicates less reliable evidence (Wallace et al. 1997) (Table 13.1). Category I identifies evidence completely generated by randomized controlled trials (RCTs), and category II includes evidence based primarily but not exclusively on RCTs. Evidence obtained from stringent study designs such as controlled trials without randomization, cohort or case-control analytic design, and multibaseline and time series is identified by category III. Category IV includes evidence generated from descriptive studies, respected authorities, and clinical experience.

The NHMRC ratings identify evidence gathered from RCTs as the best, based on internal validity and reliability. Another system, used by Raphael and Marbach (1997), also considers RCTs the best source of reliable data, primarily because of randomization. Clinical trials that are

TABLE 13.1
Rating of Evidence

Category	Criteria from Which Evidence Is Derived
I	Systematic review of all relevant randomized controlled trial
II	At least one properly designed randomized controlled trial
III-1	Well-designed controlled trial without randomization
III-2	Well-designed cohort or case-control analytic studies
III-3	Multiple time series with or without the intervention; dramatic results in uncontrolled experiments
IV	Opinions of respected authorities, based on clinical experience, or reports of expert committees

Source: Reprinted with permission from MC Wallace, A Shorten, KG Russell. Paving the way: stepping stones to evidence-based nursing. Int J Nurs Prac 1997;3:147–152.

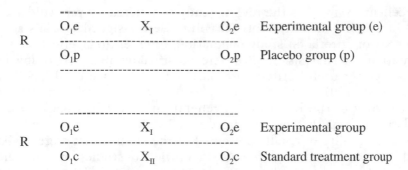

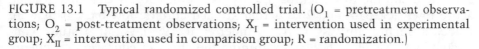

FIGURE 13.1   Typical randomized controlled trial. (O_1 = pretreatment observations; O_2 = post-treatment observations; X_I = intervention used in experimental group; X_{II} = intervention used in comparison group; R = randomization.)

uncontrolled or nonrandomized have an intermediate strength of inference. Case series or case studies involving prospective follow-up of clients have the weakest strength of inference.

Why do RCTs produce the best evidence? The answer is random assignment and control (Figure 13.1). RCTs require participants to be assigned randomly to two or more intervention groups. Randomization can eliminate potential biases attributable to differences (e.g., age, gender, ethnic backgrounds, severity of disability, and prior clinical interventions) that create nonequivalent baselines between the experiment and control groups. Randomization helps achieve a condition of equivalence for intervention and control groups.

The control in an RCT can be a placebo or a standard treatment group (see Figure 13.1). A controlled placebo group helps ensure that performance is solely caused by the intervention provided. Problems with natural changes in clients (maturation effect) or other environmental factors (history effect) ($O_2e - O_2p$ = effect due to X_I; where O_2e and O_2p are post-treatment observations of experimental and placebo groups, respectively) can be eliminated. In contrast, treatment comparison groups are less desirable because net gain in the experimental group can be caused by differences in the strength of interventions ($O_2e - O_2c$ = effect due to $X_I - X_{II}$; where O_2c and O_2c are post-treatment observations of experimental and standard treatment groups, respectively). Effects of the experimental intervention X_I therefore cannot be interpreted directly. The clinical trials most able to provide strong data are, in descending order, randomized placebo-controlled, randomized comparison-controlled, nonrandomized placebo, nonrandomized comparison, and uncontrolled single-group trials.

Results obtained by clinical trials are also evaluated for methodologic quality. EBP differentiates results generated by studies with higher internal validity from those produced from studies with lower standards.

An excellent example is the review study conducted by van Tulder et al. (1997) in which a maximum of 100 points were assigned to trials according to a set of criteria on study population, interventions, effect, and data presentation and analysis. Studies were classified by high (≥50) or low (<50) qualities. Other useful criteria are outlined by Wallace et al. (1997) and Raphael et al. (1997).

A review of the literature in rehabilitation for low back pain and cumulative trauma disorders revealed that RCTs are not commonly used. Further, the quality of results presented in the studies that were available ranged from moderately high to poor. In a review of studies on treatment of acute and chronic low back pain, only 34.6% of 150 articles that studied acute low back pain and 25.0% that studied chronic low back pain were graded as high-quality RCTs (van Tulder et al. 1997). Another study, conducted by Gross et al. (1998), examining the effect of education on clients with mechanical neck disorders, reported that the two RCTs related to the topic were rated moderately strong in terms of methodologic quality.

Amalgamation of Results

After the review and evaluation of methodologic quality, evidence is compared. This process involves pooling results of studies with similar characteristics, such as methodologic quality, demographics, diagnoses, and treatment interventions. The purpose of amalgamation is to increase the strength of the inference by increasing the total sample size and the number of observations contributed from individual studies, enabling conclusions drawn from reviews to be more objective and powerful compared with those based on single studies.

Different methods can be used to amalgamate results of various studies, ranging from simple frequency counts of studies for positive or negative effects to sophisticated meta-analytic procedures that consider mean differences, effect sizes, and sample sizes. The selection of a particular method is determined by the methodologic quality of studies reviewed and whether placebo groups and similar measures were used in the studies.

Meta-analysis is a statistical procedure that combines the effect size (ES) of different studies. ES is a scale-free index of effect magnitude, or the mean difference between experimental and control groups divided by the group's standard deviation (Glass et al. 1981). Effect sizes are estimated for each study in terms of either a d or g index (Hedges and Olkin 1985; Glass et al. 1981). The g index is a biased ES estimate that overestimates the population ES when sample size is small (Figure 13.2). The d index is an unbiased ES estimate derived for studies with small sample sizes. The mathematical expression of ES indicates that studies with placebo group design obtain the most information on the effects of the clinical intervention under investigation because the difference between experimental interventions (Me) and control

$$g = \frac{(Me - Mc)}{Sp}$$

where

Me = Post-test mean score of experimental group

Mc = Post-test mean score of control group

Sp = Pooled standard deviation

$$d = g \ \{1 - [3/(4N - 9)]\}$$

where

N = Ne + Nc

Ne = sample size of experimental group

Nc = sample size of control group

FIGURE 13.2   Mathematical expression of indices g and d. The g index is a biased ES estimate that overestimates the population ES when sample size is small. The d index is an unbiased ES estimate derived for studies with small sample sizes.

interventions (Mc) yields the treatment effect. This conclusion is substantially weakened if a comparison group is used. Pooling results becomes even less meaningful if the interventions used in control groups differ among studies. The estimated ESs are pooled by weighted integration methods that consider the sample size of each study. A mean ES and its 95% confidence interval (CI) are calculated. Positive effect of a particular intervention is indicated if the 95% CI of the ES is not 0. An overlap of the 95% CI of mean ES and 0 indicates that clinical intervention has no effect. Validity of the pooled ESs is tested by homogeneity statistics, which determine whether all ESs belong to the same population (Hedges and Olkin 1985).

An example of a descriptive method that integrates the results of review is found in the study conducted by van Tulder et al. (1997). Of 81 RCTs relevant to treatment for chronic low back pain clients, 10 studies employed back schools as the clinical intervention. Among the two studies that were regarded as having high methodologic quality, the effectiveness of back schools was positive in both studies when compared with no actual treatment. In the other four studies with low quality, three reported positive and one reported negative results. The conclusion of van Tulder et al. was as follows:

There is strong evidence (level 1) that an intensive back school program in an occupational setting is more effective than no actual treatment for chronic low back pain. There is limited evidence (level 3) that a back school is more effective than other conservative types of treatment for chronic low back pain. (p. 2135)

Gross et al. (1998) used a meta-analytic method to analyze the studies. Of three studies related to the use of education strategies to reduce pain for clients with mechanical neck disorders, two were rated moderately strong or better in methodologic quality. The study demonstrated that the use of neck school with exercise (standard mean difference [SMD] = 0.366; 95% CI [–0.951, 0.219]) or neck school with psychological counseling and exercise (SMD = 0.073; 95% CI [–0.513, 0.659]) did not reduce pain. Two other studies found that individualized teaching combined with medication and soft collar was not as effective as the controlled treatment (SMD = 0.233; 95% CI [–0.577, 1.065]) or placebo treatments (SMD = –0.617; 95% CI [–1.048, –0.186]). The conclusion drawn by Gross et al. was that

> [p]atient education utilizing individualized or group instructional strategies was not shown to be beneficial in reducing pain for mechanical neck disorders. Larger RCTs are needed to demonstrate lack of benefit conclusively. Future studies using sound research design and methodology are warranted. (http://www.nihs.go.jp/acc/cochrane/revabstr/ab000962.htm)

Review of the EBP materials in the field of ergonomics and work rehabilitation emphasizes the field's underdevelopment.

Results Integration and Dissemination

EBP is highly dependent on the dissemination of evidence to clinical communities. In the past, the flow of information relied heavily on professional journals, conferences, symposiums, seminars, workshops, and professional meetings. However, EBP entered a new era of information exchange with the establishment of the Cochrane Collaboration. The Cochrane Collaboration was founded in 1993 to help health care professionals "make well informed decisions about health care by preparing, maintaining and ensuring the accessibility of systematic reviews of the effects of health care interventions" (Cochrane Collaboration 1998). Core activities are carried out by the collaborative review groups. In 1997, more than 40 groups covered most of the important areas of health care. These groups consisted of researchers, health care professionals, consumers, and others who shared an interest in generating reliable, up-to-date evidence for clinical interventions. A full list of all review groups is available at Cochrane Collaboration Web sites (Table 13.2). Activities of the review groups are enhanced by Cochrane fields and Cochrane centers, which were established to coordinate the interests and review activities of the groups by fostering international and interdisciplinary collaboration, organizing workshops, and initiating and participating in exploratory discussions and meetings.

The back review group and rehabilitation and related therapies field are the Cochrane fields most closely associated with work rehabilitation

TABLE 13.2
Cochrane Internet Sites, Centers, and Review Groups Relevant
to Work Rehabilitation

Cochrane Internet sites
   http://www.nihs.go.jp/acc/cochrane/default.html
   http://hiru.mcmaster.ca/cochrane/
Cochrane centers
   Australasian Cochrane Centre:
      http://som.flinders.edu.au/fusa/cochrane/cochrane/accbroch.htm
   Baltimore Cochrane Center: http://www.cochrane.org
   Canadian Cochrane Center:
      http://hiru.mcmaster.ca/cochrane/centres/canadian/
   Nordic Cochrane Centre: http://www.cochrane.dk/ncc/home.htm
   UK Cochrane Centre: E-mail: general@cochrane.co.uk
Cochrane review groups
   Back review group: http://www.iwh.on.ca/cochrane/cochrane.htm
   Musculoskeletal injuries group: send e-mail to h.handoll@ed.ac.uk
   Rehabilitation and related therapies field:
      http://www.unimaas.nl/~epid/cochrane/field.htm

(see Table 13.2). The back review group is part of the Cochrane Collaboration's musculoskeletal review group, which has an international editorial board with members from the United States, the United Kingdom, the Netherlands, and France (Institute for Work and Health 1997). Approximately 40 members actively engage in conducting systematic reviews of interventions for back and neck pain. Interventions reviewed and under review include transcutaneous electrical nerve stimulation, acupuncture-like *transcutaneous electrical nerve stimulation, spinal manipulation,* client education, exercise therapy, back school, and behavioral therapy. Originally called the *rehabilitation and related therapies field,* the physical therapy and rehabilitation field (PTRF) was established in 1996 by de Vet and de Bie of the Department of Epidemiology of the University of Maastricht in the Netherlands (de Vet and de Bie 1998). PTRF has reviewed 3,400 articles related to rehabilitation and physical therapy, of which approximately 1,200 address RCTs. All articles are available in hard-copy and CD-ROM versions for members of PTRF and Cochrane Collaboration reviewers, and PTRF issues newsletters are available for all interested individuals. A large number of journals related to work rehabilitation are also surveyed for information, including the *British Journal of Occupational Therapy,* the *American Journal of Occupational Therapy, Physiotherapy Theory and Practice, Physiotherapy,* the *European Journal of Physical Medicine and Rehabilitation,* and the *Austrian Journal of Physical Medicine.*

    To disseminate results of various review groups, the Cochrane Collaboration has established a formal channel called the *Cochrane Library* that

TABLE 13.3
Databases Associated with the Cochrane Library

Database	Function
Cochrane database of systematic review	Contains Cochrane reviews, structured abstracts, reports of reviews, discussion of results, implications for practice and research, full citation reports
Cochrane controlled trials registers	Bibliographic database of controlled trials
Database of abstracts of reviews of effectiveness	Structured abstracts of systematic reviews critically appraised by reviewers at the National Health Service Centre for Reviews and Dissemination (e.g., from the American College of Physicians' Journal Club and the journal *Evidence-Based Medicine*)
Cochrane review methodology database	Bibliography of articles on the sciences of research synthesis
Software review manager (RevMan)	Used for preparing and maintaining reviews
Software modular manager (ModMan)	Used by editorial team to assemble protocols and complete reviews

assembles reviews in electronic formats. Several databases are included in the Cochrane Library (Table 13.3). Hayes and McGrath (1998) detail the purpose and format of each database. The Cochrane Library can be accessed by subscription through Update Software (e-mail: info@update.co.uk or updateinc@home.com) or through distribution partners (the American College of Physicians, the Australian Medical Association, the British Medical Journal Publication Group, and the Canadian Medical Association). The CD-ROM and online versions of the Cochrane Library are updated quarterly.

Evidence-Based Practice and Work Rehabilitation

Review of existing systems indicates that EBP is still underdeveloped in the areas of ergonomics and work rehabilitation. The back review group and rehabilitation and related therapies field are the two established groups closest to the subject of ergonomics and work rehabilitation. However, the abstracts published by these two groups do not seem to cover this aspect of rehabilitation. The various reasons that account for this phenomenon are discussed in the following sections.

Lack of Theoretical Background

Well-established theoretical backgrounds supporting the effectiveness of different rehabilitation interventions, such as ergonomics, are scarce.

According to Brandt and Pope (1997), little formal theory exists in rehabilitation to guide research and clinical decisions. The practice of clinicians is often based on experience (the lowest level of clinical evidence). The majority of evidence is accumulated for studying causes of impairments rather than their consequences or resulting disabilities, and advances in ergonomics and work rehabilitation are over-studied causes of the problems. For example, the study of cumulative trauma disorders has been dominated by exploring impacts of repetitive tasks (Veiersted and Westgaard 1993), predicting the model of carpal tunnel syndrome (Matias et al. 1998), and establishing relationships between trapezius load and incidence of musculoskeletal illness (Aaras 1994). Other important areas of focus are the development of instruments to measure muscle load (Aaras and Stranden 1998) and the establishment of the validity of functional capacity evaluations, such as the Baltimore Therapeutic Equipment (BTE) Work Simulator evaluation (Bhambhani et al. 1994) and the available motions inventory (Malzahn et al. 1996).

Outcomes of Ergonomic Interventions

Outcomes of ergonomic interventions for work rehabilitation are difficult to define, partly because they are multifaceted. Most studies emphasize the physical outcomes of different work health improvement programs, such as those that examine the incidence of trapezius myalgia (Veiersted et al. 1993) and those that involve statometric measurements obtained from inclinometer through subjective acceptability (Bendix 1984). In contrast, data of higher ecologic validity, such as long-term health, work style, and quality of life, are rather uncommon.

Method of Investigation

RCTs are seldom used as the primary method for investigation. Instead, most studies use quasi-experimental designs with or without comparison groups. A good example is the study by Schuldt et al. (1986) that adopted single-group pre- and post-test design and used electromyelography as the outcome parameter. Another example is from a study by Westgaard and Aaras (1985) in which the effectiveness of ergonomic factors for improving the health of workers was studied through single-group pre- and post-test design. The difficulties of using RCTs to test the effectiveness of ergonomic interventions are largely due to labor law protection and objections from employers and labor unions.

Technology

Technology is not transferred from research institutions to clinical practitioners, particularly in rehabilitation. According to Brandt and Pope (1997), some of the reasons for the failure of such information transfer are that clinical rehabilitation research lacks funds; little formal theory has emerged across the disciplines in rehabilitation; formal mechanisms for transferring knowledge are limited; and a market link that ties the products of research to the market economy, such as employers and workers' associations, is absent.

EBP in ergonomics and work rehabilitation should establish a theoretical framework for explaining the phenomenon of how tasks, the physical and psychological environment, and the worker's capacity impact work performance. Instead of solely focusing on the impact of a particular factor, studies should strive to be multidimensional to facilitate better understanding of ergonomic intervention's impact on long-term occupational health. More studies that use RCTs should be conducted to test the effectiveness of particular ergonomics and work interventions. The benefits of EBP to rehabilitation should be explained to clients, employers, and unions. More channels should be established to facilitate the transfer of knowledge, methodology, and results of clinical trials from researchers to clinicians. Both researchers and clinicians should be active in collaboration and sharing of knowledge.

Evidence-Based Practice and Clinical Guidelines

The development of clinical guidelines based on evidence is the goal of EBP. Systematic methods linking evidence to daily clinical practice are still in their infancy. Formulating clinical pathways using Clinical Pathway Constructor (CPC) computer software (Greengold and Weingarten 1996) demonstrates the potential of EBP. CPC computer software is equipped with a database that contains a large number of review abstracts on different clinical conditions and categories of care for acute medical and surgical conditions, such as total hip replacement and stroke. A typical clinical pathway is constructed as a computer grid consisting of standardized categories of care (e.g., diagnostic procedures and discharge planning) and a time line (in terms of postadmission days or phases) in which the care should be carried out. Clinicians should review all available evidence and determine guidelines to be encoded in different clinical pathways. These pathways can be printed, disseminated to all team members, and used as guidelines for service provision. The guidelines can also be submitted to quality assurance offices as targets for clinical audit.

Greengold and Weingarten's clinical pathway is inpatient acute care oriented, however. Clinicians working in different settings dealing with different clinical populations should be more innovative in designing their own systems using information (and evidence) resulting from the systematic reviews in EBP. More interinstitutional and multidisciplinary collaborations should also be developed to make this process an effective and efficient effort.

Conclusion

EBP is both an old and new concept in health care. The preference for RCTs, detailed review and evaluation of literature, collation, and amalgamation of evidence is not new in scientific and critical inquiry circles. However, the quality of evidence reviewed, the comprehensiveness of methods used, and collaboration between researchers and clinicians has distinguished EBP by improving quality of clinical decision making, clinical practices, professional accountability, and client choice. Although EBP has not been widely developed to facilitate clinical practices in ergonomics and work rehabilitation, the benefits and potential of its development are well recognized.

References

Aaras A (1994). Relationship between trapezius load and the incidence of musculoskeletal illness in the neck and shoulder. Int J Ind Ergonomics 14:341–348.

Aaras A, Stranden E (1998). Measurement of postural angles during work. Ergonomics 31:935–944.

Bhambhani Y, Esmail S, Brintnell S (1994). The Baltimore therapeutic equipment work simulator: biomechanical and physiological norms for three attachments in healthy men. Am J Occup Ther 48:19–25.

Bendix T (1984). Seated trunk posture at various seat inclinations, seat heights, and table heights. Hum Factors 26:695–703.

Brandt EN, Pope AM (eds) (1997). Enabling America. Assessing the Role of Rehabilitation Science and Engineering. Washington, DC: National Academy Press.

Cochrane Collaboration (1998). Cochrane Brochure. http://www.nihs.go.jp/acc/cochrane/cc-broch.htm.

Deighan M, Boyd K (1996). Defining evidence-based health care: a health-care learning strategy? NT Res 1:332–339.

de Vet R, de Bie R (1998). Rehabilitation and Related Therapies Field. http://www.unimaas.nl/~epid./cochrane/field.htm.

Dowie J (1994). The research practice gap and the role of decision analysis in closing it. Paper presented at European Medicine Decision Making conference. October. Lille, Norway.

Egan M, Dubouloz CJ, von Zweck C, Vallerand J (1998). The client-centred evidence-based practice of occupational therapy. Can J Occup Ther 65:136–143.

Glanville J (1994). Evidence-based practice: the role of NHS centres for reviews and dissemination. Health Libraries Rev 11:243–251.

Glass GV, McGaw B, Smith ML (1981). Meta-Analysis in Social Research. Newbury Park, CA: Sage Publications.

Greengold NL, Weingarten SR (1996). Developing evidence-based practice guidelines and pathways: the experience at the local hospital level. J Qual Improvement 22:391–402.

Greenhalgh T (1996). Is my practice evidence-based? (editorial). BMJ 313:957–958.

Greenhalgh T, Macfarlane F (1997). Towards a competency grid for evidence-based practice. J Eval Clin Prac 3:161–165.

Gross AR, Aker PD, Goldsmith CH, Peloso P (1998). Conservative Management of Mechanical Neck Disorders. Part IV: Patient Education. Abstract of Cochrane reviews. The Cochrane Library. Oxford, UK: The Cochrane Collaboration.

Hayes R, McGrath J (1998). Evidence-based practice: the Cochrane Collaboration, and occupational therapy. Can J Occup Ther 65:144–151.

Hedges LV, Olkin I (1985). Statistical Methods for Meta-Analysis. New York: Academic Press.

Hunt J (1997). Towards evidence based practice. Nurs Manage 4:14–17.

Institute for Work and Health (1997). The Cochrane Collaboration Back Review Group for Spinal Disorders. http://www.iwh.on.ca/cochrane/cochrane.htm.

Law M, Baum C (1998). Evidence-based occupational therapy. Can J Occup Ther 65:131–135.

Malzahn DE, Fernandez JE, Kattel BP (1996). Design-oriented functional capacity evaluation: the available motions inventory—a review. Disabil Rehabil 18:382–395.

Matias AC, Salvendy G, Kuczek T (1998). Predictive models of carpal tunnel syndrome causation among VDT operators. Ergonomics 41:213–226.

Partridge C (1996). Evidence-based medicine—implications for physiotherapy? Physiother Res Int 1:69–73.

Raphael K, Marbach J (1997). Evidence-based care of musculoskeletal facial pain: implications for the clinical science of dentistry. J Am Dent Assoc 128:73–79.

Rosenberg W, Donald A (1995). Evidence-based medicine: an approach to clinical problem solving. BMJ 310:1122–1126.

Sackett DL, Rosenberg WM (1995). The need for evidence based medicine. J Royal Soc Med 88:620–624.

Schuldt K, Ekholm J, Harms-Ringdahl K, et al. (1986). Effects of changes in sitting work posture on static neck and shoulder muscle activity. Ergonomics 29:1525–1537.

Sharpe M, Gill D, Strain J, Mayou R (1996). Psychosomatic medicine and evidence-based treatment. J Psychosomatic Res 41:101–107.

Silagy C (ed) (1995). Registering a Field. In Cochrane Collaboration Handbook. Vol. III. Representing the interests of fields. Oxford, UK: The Cochrane Collaboration [updated 14 July 1995].

Turner P, Whitfield TWA (1997). Physiotherapists' use of evidence based practice: a cross-national study. Physiother Res Int 2:17–29.

van Tulder MW, Koes BW, Bouter LM (1997). Conservative treatment of acute and chronic nonspecific low back pain. A systematic review of randomized controlled trials of the most common intervention. Spine 22:2128–2156.

Veiersted KB, Westgaard RH (1993). Development of trapezius myalgia among female workers performing light manual work. Scand J Work Environ Health 19:277–283.

Veiersted KB, Westgaard RH, Andersen P (1993). Electromyographic evaluation of muscular work pattern as a predictor of trapezius myalgia. Scand J Work Environ Health 19:284–290.

Wallace MC, Shorten A, Russell KG (1997). Paving the way: stepping stones to evidence-based nursing. Int J Nurs Prac 3:147–152.

Westgaard RH, Aaras A (1985). The effect of improved workplace design on the
development of work-related musculo-skeletal illnesses. Appl Ergonomics
16(2)91–97.

Review Questions

(Answers are found in Appendix D.)

1. The concept of EBP is *not* based on which one of the following state-
   ments?
   (a) Individuals are life-long learners.
   (b) Professionals should choose the best interventions.
   (c) Clients have the right to know what is best for them.
   (d) Health services are operated as a business that imposes quality control.

2. What is the relationship between EBP and RCTs?
   (a) EBP considers all results other than those obtained from RCTs.
   (b) EBP accepts the results obtained only from RCTs.
   (c) EBP prefers to gather the results obtained from RCTs.
   (d) EBP has no relationship to RCTs.

3. Methodologic quality of studies reviewed in EBP cannot be assessed on
   the
   (a) presence of control or placebo groups
   (b) equivalence among different comparison groups
   (c) factors related to internal validity
   (d) differences in scores on the outcome measures before and after the
   intervention

4. Which of the following methods is *not* relevant to the process of amal-
   gamating the results in EBP?
   (a) Determination of sample sizes
   (b) Combination of ES
   (c) Estimation of CI
   (d) Computation of standardized differences

5. Which of the following is *not* a reason for the underdevelopment of
   EBP in work rehabilitation?
   (a) Lack of well-defined outcome variables
   (b) More emphasis on workers' impairment than on disability and
   handicap
   (c) Lack of studies with high methodologic quality
   (d) Weak technological support from companies

CHAPTER 14
Certification in Ergonomics

Karen Jacobs

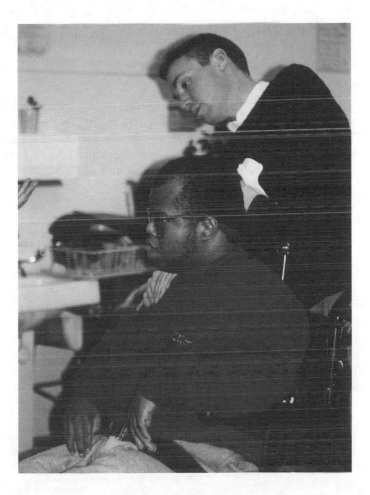

ABSTRACT

The Human Factors and Ergonomics Society has always been concerned about establishing some type of quality control or credentialing of ergonomists. The Board for Certification in Professional Ergonomics (BCPE) and Oxford Research Institute (ORI) are the two most prominent ergonomic certification boards in the United States. This chapter briefly describes the process of certification in ergonomics by each.

Board for Certification in Professional Ergonomics

Formed in October of 1990, BCPE, an independent, nonprofit certification organization (Rice 1994b), offers three designations of certifications in ergonomics or human factors:

1. Certified professional ergonomist (CPE) or certified human factors professional (CHFP)
2. Associate ergonomics professional (AEP)
3. Certified ergonomics associate (CEA)

The CPE or CHFP is involved in the full spectrum of ergonomics: analysis, design, and test and evaluation activities; the CEA is limited to system evaluation and intervention using well-established ergonomic principles, methods, and tools (BCPE 1998). The latter is a more recent certification program; the first examination was given in October 1998.

Certified Professional Ergonomist or Certified Human Factors Professional

The requirements for the designation of CPE or CHFP are as follows:

- Master's degree or equivalent in one of the correlative fields of ergonomics, such as biomechanics, human factors/ergonomics, industrial engineering, industrial hygiene, kinesiology, psychology, or systems engineering
- Four years of demonstrable experience in the practice of ergonomics
- Evidence of ergonomic contribution to design by submission of a work product to BCPE, such as a technical report, design paper, or patent application
- Receiving a passing score on the BCPE examination (BCPE 1998)

An individual meeting the minimum requirements can initiate the certification process by requesting an application and mailing $10 to

BCPE, P.O. Box 2811, Bellingham, WA 98227-2811. The BCPE can also be reached by phone at (206) 671-7601 or by fax at (206) 671-7681. The BCPE can be contacted by e-mail at BCPEHQ@aol.com, and additional information is available at the BCPE Internet site at http://www.bcpe.org.

After evaluating a completed application, a review panel makes recommendations to the BCPE regarding whether the applicant will be permitted to take the written examination.

Associate Ergonomics Professional

AEP certification is the precursor to CPE certification and is available to a person who

- Meets the education requirements for BCPE certification (master of science degree in human factors/ergonomics or related field)
- Has passed part I (basic knowledge of human factors/ergonomics) of the BCPE certification examination
- Is working toward fulfilling the BCPE requirement of 4 years of practical experience as a human factors and ergonomics professional (BCPE 1998)

As of August 1998, 741 CPEs or CHFPs and 59 AEPs have been registered. Of these, eight have educational degrees at some level of occupational therapy, and 12 have physical therapy degrees (K Jahns, personal communication, August 18, 1998).

Certified Ergonomics Associate

The expected requirements for designation as a CEA are as follows:

- Bachelor's degree from an accredited university
- At least 2 full-time years in the practice of ergonomics
- At least 200 contact hours of ergonomics training
- Obtaining a satisfactory grade on a 5-hour, two-part multiple-choice examination on ergonomic foundations and ergonomic practice (BCPE 1998)

If one of the three designations of CPE or CHFP, AEP, or CEA fit an applicant's area of expertise, taking the self-screening for BCPE certification is advised (Rice 1994a, 1994b; Appendix 14.1).

Because "the dynamics of technological and societal change make ergonomics a rapidly evolving career field . . . professional practice standards developed by the BCPE is a continuous improvement process. Issues such as 'speciality practice areas' within ergonomics based on diverse educational backgrounds; multilevel certifications conforming to ergonomics

skill levels of practitioners; CEU [Continuing Education Units] requirements for certification (and skill/knowledge) maintenance; and certificate
revocation criteria are being actively explored" (BCPE 1994, p. iii).

Oxford Research Institute

Since 1993, ORI has been certifying professionals as industrial ergonomists
(CIEs) or human factors engineering professionals (CHFEPs). Requirements
for certification are as follows:

1. Bachelor's degree, although preferably a master's degree
2. Work experience as a practicing ergonomist/human factors engineer:
    4 years with a PhD
    5 years with a master's degree
    6 years with a bachelor's degree
3. Two or three work samples, which can include published books,
    research or technical reports, and inventions
4. Two letters of recommendation
5. Payment of fees

The application fee is $300, which includes $250 for certification and $50
for the first year. No written examination is required. An annual $60
renewal fee is required after certification. ORI can be contacted by mail at
10153 Vantage Point Court, New Market, MD 21744; by phone at (301)
865-4506; or by e-mail at bbanksori@aol.com.

Conclusion

Although certification by BCPE or ORI may help improve the quality and
cost-effectiveness of services, the reader is advised to keep abreast of certification issues through updates in *Work: A Journal of Prevention, Assessment and Rehabilitation* (e.g., Hart et al. 1993) and works by IOS Press
(the Netherlands).

References

BCPE (1994). Information on Certification Policies, Practices and Procedures (2nd
    ed). Bellingham, WA: BCPE.
BCPE (1998). http://www.bcpe.org. August 18.
Hart D. Isernhagen S, Matheson L (1993). Refining the practice of ergonomics.
    Work 3(3):69–72.
Rice VJB (1994a). Certification in ergonomics: an update and commentary. Work
    4(1):211–213.
Rice VJB (1994b). Ergonomics certification update. Work 4(1):71–72.

Appendix 14.1*

The following is a self-screening for Board Certification in Professional Ergonomics.

Directions

Assign a value between 0 and 5 to each item. After using subtotals to compute the total, review the interpretation of scores. Please note that *work* is defined as any purposive human activity requiring effort and skill.

Point Assignments

> 0 = Never exposed to this topic
> 1 = Learned from self-study or on-the-job experience
> 2 = Learned from seminars, short courses, or workshops
> 3 = Part of undergraduate program
> 4 = Part of graduate program in another field
> 5 = Part of graduate program in human factors/ergonomics

Self-Screening Form

A. Ergonomics
   1. Ergonomics approach to systems development   _____
   2. Ergonomics and society   _____
                                            Subtotal (10)   _____
B. Ergonomic approaches to people at work
   1. Work evaluation and investigation   _____
   2. Work activity or analysis   _____
   3. Introduction to ergonomic design   _____
   4. Design requirements and analysis and report   _____
   5. Instrumentation   _____
                                            Subtotal (25)   _____
C. Human characteristics and humans at work
   1. Anatomy   _____
   2. Physiology   _____
   3. Biomechanics and anthropometry   _____
   4. Human psychology   _____
   5. Organizational design and management   _____
   6. Physical environment of work   _____
                                            Subtotal (30)   _____

---

*Reprinted from Board for Certification in Professional Ergonomics (http://www.bcpe.org).

D. Supporting courses
    1. Quantitative and qualitative design and analysis _____
    2. Systems theory _____
    3. Technology or engineering _____
    4. Physics _____
    5. Business or economics _____
    6. Ethics and regulation _____
                                        Subtotal (30) _____

E. Application areas for ergonomics
    1. Workplace design _____
    2. Information design _____
    3. Work organization and design _____
    4. Health, safety, and well-being _____
    5. Training and instruction _____
    6. Occupational hygiene _____
    7. Architecture _____
    8. Participatory design processes _____
    9. Work-related musculoskeletal disorders _____
    10. Human-computer interaction _____
                                        Subtotal (50) _____

F. Field work (1 or 2 = reactive intervention to solve
    operational, safety, or health problems; 3–5 = proactive
    design to enhance productivity, safety, and well-being
    of the whole work system) _____
                                        Subtotal (5) _____
                                        TOTAL _____

Interpretation of Subtotals

A. Ergonomics (10 points possible)

> 0–3: Less than CEA preparation
> 4–6: CEA preparation
> 7–10: CPE preparation

B. Ergonomic approaches to people at work
(25 points possible)

> 0–8: Less than CEA preparation
> 9–15: CEA preparation
> 16–25: CPE preparation

C. Human characteristics and humans at work
(30 points possible)

> 0–8: Less than CEA preparation
> 9–15: CEA preparation
> 16–30: CPE preparation

D. Supporting courses (30 points possible)

>0–8: Less than CEA preparation
>9–15: CEA preparation
>16–30: CPE preparation

E. Application areas for ergonomics
(50 points possible)

>0–10: less than CEA
>11–20: CEA preparation
>21–50: CPE preparation

F. Field work (5 points possible)

>1 or 2: CEA preparation
>3–5: CPE preparation

Interpretation of Total Score

0–44

Having overall low scores in A–F (even if scores are high in any one lettered category) indicates that you may have an awareness of ergonomics, but you are unqualified to practice as an ergonomist.

45–75

If you scored points in all the categories in A–F and the total is within the range of 45 to 75 points, you may want to consider the CEA level of BCPE certification. You should keep in mind, however, that application fees are nonrefundable and that evaluation of all submitted materials will be in accordance with specific criteria developed by BCPE. A passing score on the CEA examination is also required.

76 and above

If most of your scored points in each of the six categories (A–F) are 4s and 5s (with very few score points of 0–3), you should apply for the CPE designation. You should keep in mind, however, that application fees are nonrefundable and that evaluation of all submitted materials will be in accordance with specific criteria developed by BCPE. A passing score on the CPA exam is also required.

What to Look for in the Self-Screening

Scoring points in each category is desirable. A balanced involvement of these topics is what makes ergonomics a unique field.

CHAPTER 15
Marketing

Karen Jacobs

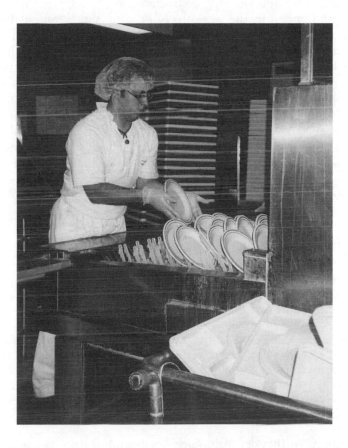

ABSTRACT

Marketing has an important role in the delivery of ergonomics. This chapter gives an overview of marketing with a focus on ergonomics consultation and provides a case study that illustrates the application of marketing strategies in the development of a new product.

Question: What do a microwave oven and consultation in ergonomics have in common?

Answer: They are both products that have been developed in response to consumers' needs.

The microwave oven was invented to meet the needs of two-career couples who had little time to spend on food preparation. Like the microwave oven, ergonomics developed out of a response to customer needs.

Ergonomics consultation in occupational and physical therapy responded to rising health care and workers' compensation costs by providing methods for preventing injuries in the workplace. Product development initiated in response to the changing needs of the public is part of a marketing approach. Since the early 1980s, marketing has become more common in health care. In fact, marketing has become necessary to survive in a competitive marketplace. All therapists should therefore have an understanding of marketing. Therapists should learn how to use marketing, just as they learned how to use the tools and techniques of their professions. Because little, if any, exposure to marketing is provided in the academic curriculum of occupational and physical therapy, therapists are encouraged to acquire a knowledge of marketing by attending workshops, taking continuing education courses, or pursuing degrees in business. In general, therapists need to become more business savvy.

Definition of *Marketing*

Marketing, a frequently misunderstood term, is most often used to identify a process involving public relations, selling, fund-raising, strategic planning, or development. According to Kotler (1975, p. 5),

> Marketing is the analysis, planning, implementation and control of carefully formulated programs designed to bring about voluntary exchanges of values with target markets for the purpose of achieving organizational objectives. It relies heavily on designing the organization's offering in terms of the target market's needs and desires, and on using effective pricing, communication, and distribution to inform, motivate and service the markets.

Paramount in this definition are needs and desires. Something that is identified as lacking in the market (an individual or group of individuals) reflects a *need*; a *desire* is a want or personal preference. The market is researched and analyzed to determine whether it reflects an absence of a good or service (need) or whether it prefers something in a different shape, form, time, or location (desire). According to Kiernan et al. (1989, p. 50),

> Once the need or want is established, the potential buyer must view the good or service being offered as satisfying a need or want better than any other available good or service. It is the packaging and support of a good or service that assure an ongoing relationship with the customer both for purposes of repurchase and for influencing initial purchases by other potential buyers.

Marketing should be considered a dynamic activity that includes the successful analysis of a need, the design of a good or service to meet the need, the uniting of that good or service with a potential user, and the use of a good or service by the customer. In an ideal situation, marketing is used before a product is developed. This has not always been the case. In particular, many industrial rehabilitation programs (e.g., work hardening) that may have begun with selling perspectives are now faced with the risk of becoming obsolete because they were developed as products for which no need currently exists at their cost, present locations, or format (Jacobs 1991).

Marketing Approach

Four components are involved in a marketing approach: (1) analyzing market opportunities, (2) researching and selecting target markets and market segments, (3) developing marketing strategies, and (4) executing and evaluating a marketing plan.

Analyzing Market Opportunities

The first step in a marketing approach is the analysis of various elements of the marketplace. The market itself needs to be defined and may be selected simply on the basis of geography. The market includes all actual or potential buyers of a product, service, or idea. In the case of ergonomics consultation, example markets are business and industry, occupational health or rehabilitation nurses, insurance companies, safety officers, lawyers, workers with injuries, and other health professionals. Identifying attractive target markets includes analyzing marketing opportunities, which entails a self-audit, consumer analysis, competition analysis, and environmental assessment (Jacobs 1989).

Self-Audit

A self-audit assesses strengths and weaknesses of, opportunities for, and threats to the individual therapist, service, or business (SWOT analysis). Factors to assess include the following:

1. Reputation of the organization or therapist in the community.
2. Therapists' qualifications: Does the therapist have a master's degree or specialized training in ergonomics, human factors, or biomechanics? Are any of the therapists certified as professional ergonomists or eligible for certification (see Chapter 14)?
3. Finances: Is advanced equipment available to perform work-site analysis, or can it be purchased if needed? Is the individual or company eligible to apply for grant funding (e.g., to develop "train the trainer" workshops at a designated work site)?

This self-audit assists in understanding how well or poorly prepared an individual or business is to meet the demands of the market. Ascertaining what an individual or business does well and maintaining that product or service at an optimal level is a critical aspect of marketing.

Consumer Analysis

Potential consumers must be identified for the provider to understand needs and desires for the product. Examples of consumers who might need or use ergonomics consultation are business and industry, occupational health or rehabilitation nurses, insurance companies, architects, attorneys, safety officers, workers with injuries, and health professionals.

Competition Analysis

Identifying other providers of similar services can give an overview of the kinds of services being offered in particular locations. Analyzing these services reduces the potential for overlap and helps identify areas that are not being served. Opportunities for collaboration or joint ventures can surface during a competition analysis.

Environmental Assessment

An environmental assessment predicts the effect demographics, political and regulatory systems, cultural and economic environments, psychographics, and technology may have on services. The following factors may have an impact on ergonomics.

Demographics

Because of economic necessity or preference, many older Americans continue to work after the traditional age of retirement. In the United States, 11% of the population, or 24 million people, have reached or passed the age of 65 years. By 2034, this percentage is expected to increase to 18%, and by 2050, one-fourth of the U.S. population will be over 65. To keep this working population active, occupational and physical therapists must become familiar with the aging process and learn to recognize the special needs of older workers. By becoming familiar with the physiologic effects of aging, therapists can develop intervention and prevention strategies that use ergonomics and, thus, assist in keeping this population actively engaged in the workforce (Coy and Davenport 1991).

Political and Regulatory Agencies
The Occupational Safety and Health Administration (OSHA) published guidelines for the meat-packing industry that are useful for an overall ergonomic program for most work sites (OSHA 1991). OSHA also proposed an industry-wide ergonomics standard called the "Ergonomics Protection Standard" (OSHA 1995). If these draft standards are approved, the need for qualified consultants to assist industry in compliance will increase. In addition, the Department of Labor has released a document called "Ergonomics and the Americans with Disabilities Act (ADA)," which states that people who suffer from ergonomic disorders are covered by the ADA if the physical or mental impairment substantially limits ability to perform essential functions of a job (cited in Smith 1993, p. 8).

A movement toward the establishment of state guidelines or standards in ergonomics has also been active. For example, on July 3, 1997, California OSHA introduced ergonomic standards to protect workers from work-related repetitive strain injuries (California Code of Regulations 1997). Therapists interested in consulting in industry should develop an understanding of guidelines and be aware of proposed standards. Up-to-date information can obtained from OSHA by phone (1-800-321-OSHA) and on the Internet (www.inquire@ergoweb.com).

Economic and Financial Factors
By the twenty-first century, 50% of the workforce is expected to suffer some type of occupational disorder. The cost to society will be billions of dollars each year (Sutherland and Counihan 1990). Low back pain alone accounts for millions of days lost from work and billions of dollars of lost productivity and workers' compensation claims. Clearly, injury prevention at the work site and health promotion are better alternatives to injury management (Jacobs 1992). The economic and financial benefits of injury prevention programs include less lost work time, increased safety and productivity, reduced errors, improved quality of service, and better employee relations (Sehnal and Christopher 1993). Good ergonomics can mean good economics (Bloswick 1993).

Researching and Selecting Target Markets

After marketing opportunities have been analyzed, the needs of the market can be determined through research, which might include observation, surveys, or even experimentation. After research is completed, the market is divided into target markets (i.e., groups of consumers with similar needs, wants, or interests). The groups are further segmented into distinct groups of consumers who might require separate products and promotions. For example, industry can be segmented into types of businesses (e.g., service industries and manufacturing industries). Service industries can be further segmented into businesses within certain geographic areas. Targeting a market is the act of evaluating and selecting one or more markets to enter.

Developing Marketing Strategies

A marketing approach develops a marketing mix to meet the needs, desires, or interests of a well-defined target market. Marketing involves influencing the demand for a product or service. A marketing mix consists of the four Ps: (1) product, (2) place, (3) price, and (4) promotion.

Product

The product is a marketing variable that needs to be designed for a specific target market. Ideally, a product line should be developed. For example, for ergonomics consultation to a hospital, products can include work-site analysis; audits for compliance with Titles II and III of the ADA; recommending intervention for workers with injury, such as splinting or redesigning a workstation; and implementing preventive programs, such as wellness and health promotion on the work site, including stress management or physical exercise.

Place

Where the product or service is provided is the place component of the marketing mix. Ergonomics consultation is usually provided at the work site; on occasion, therapists provide consultation in their own offices or provide expert testimony in court.

Price

The price or fee schedule for services should be based on cost, competitive factors, geography, and what the consumer is willing to pay. Four important methods for establishing a fee schedule are (1) unit value system, (2) cost-plus or overhead, (3) local survey or usual and customary fee, and (4) state code. Whatever method is selected, the price should be commensurate with perceived value.

Promotion

Promotion is the vehicle of communicating information to the consumer about the merits, place, and price of the product. According to Folts et al. (1993, p. 13),

[w]ork programs do not sell services; rather, they sell the benefits of those services. Clients do not want therapeutic modalities, exercises, or purposeful activities. Instead, clients desire the benefits treatment provides, such as pain reduction and the ability to return to work.

The value of ergonomics must be promoted. Instruments of promotion are advertising, sales promotion, publicity, and personal selling.

Advertising
Advertising involves the use of a paid message presented in a recognized medium by an identified sponsor with the purpose to inform, persuade, and remind. Some advertising vehicles include brochures, direct mail, or printed advertisement in the client company's monthly newsletter. Figure 15.1 provides an example of a national awareness campaign poster developed by American Occupational Therapy Association that was used to promote occupational therapy in ergonomics.

Sales Promotion
Sales promotion is the use of a wide variety of short-term incentives to encourage purchase of the product. This approach is optimized when used in conjunction with advertising. For example, at an open house for an industrial rehabilitation program, a successful sales promotion to increase new referrals is a business card drawing for a free ergonomic work-site analysis (Jacobs 1994, p. 40).

Publicity
An infrequently used marketing strategy, publicity is free promotion (Kotler 1983). Despite this positive feature, one has little control over placement, and thus directing the message at target markets becomes difficult. Examples of publicity for promoting ergonomics consultation are newspaper articles or radio public service announcements on topics such as stress management in the workplace and preventing cumulative trauma disorders. Figure 15.2 is a press release promoting occupational therapy's role in ergonomics. As of July 8, 1998, the release had been broadcast on 744 radio stations in all 50 states and generated 436 newspaper articles in 26 different states, reaching a total audience of 63,951,736 people in 1998.

Personal Selling
Personal selling, the most effective form of promotion, involves face-to-face communication between the therapist and the consumer. Some examples of personal selling are making presentations at meetings, providing continuing education workshops, and lecturing to professional organizations. In addition, word-of-mouth recommendations by recipients of ergonomics consultation are a powerful marketing tool.

It seems like such a simple thing, but every time you move the mouse or your hand a certain way the pain is so sharp it forces you to stop being the productive, hardworking, get-it-done-now person you've always been, and that's the most painful thing of all.

This year, millions of Americans in all lines of work will get a painful reminder of just how much they depend upon their hands. They'll develop job-related injuries that will interfere with their work performance and their quality of life. Fortunately, these people will be in good hands if they receive occupational therapy as part of their treatment program. Studies show that O.T. shortens recovery time. And since it teaches people healthy, efficient ways to perform job and everyday life tasks, occupational therapy reduces the chance of re-injury. If O.T. can do all that for a hand injury, just think how it can help people who have had strokes and sports injuries and those with developmental disabilities and chronic illnesses. For more information, call 1-800-668-8255 for a free brochure. Or email us at: praota@aota.org.

OCCUPATIONAL THERAPY
Skills for the job of living.

AOTA *The American Occupational Therapy Association, Inc.• 4720 Montgomery Lane • Bethesda MD • 20814-3425*

FIGURE 15.1 Advertisement developed by the American Occupational Therapy Association to promote occupational therapy's role in ergonomics. (Reprinted with permission from the American Occupational Therapy Association. Bethesda, MD.)

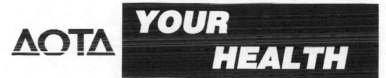

Facts From The American Occupational Therapy Association, Inc.

Preventing Carpal Tunnel Syndrome

by Karen Jacobs, EdD, OTR/L

(NAPS)—Here's some encouraging news: there are ways you may be able to help prevent repetitive motion injuries to your hands, wrists and fingers while on the job.

The American Occupational Therapy Association, Inc., offers the following advice:

Check your position

Keep shoulders erect, but relaxed, while sitting, place work close to you where it is easily accessible. Most work should be performed with elbows close to the body. Elbows should be bent to a 90 degree angle while working at your desk. Wrists should be only slightly bent, as they would look when you are holding a pencil.

If you use the telephone a lot, you may want to get a headset or speaker phone. Try not to cradle the telephone between your head and shoulder.

Check your equipment

The computer monitor should be placed about 26 inches from your eyes with the top of the screen at eye level.

You may be able to prevent shoulder, neck, and elbow problems by lowering the keyboard so its lowest point is positioned about an inch above your legs.

Give your body a break

Take a 10 minute break for every hour you spend at a computer terminal.

One of the better known workplace injuries is carpal tunnel syn-

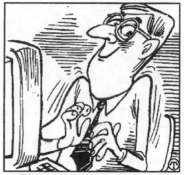

Some ways you may be able to help prevent repetitive motion injuries is by keeping shoulders erect, but relaxed, and taking 10 minute breaks every hour.

drome. It affects the hands, wrists and fingers. It is most often seen in keyboard operators and assembly line workers.

If you are experiencing any symptoms of carpal tunnel—such as numbness, weakness, pain and difficulty in moving your hands, wrists and fingers—you may want to see your doctor.

For more information about repetitive motion injuries, call The American Occupational Therapy Association, Inc., toll-free at 1-800-668-8255. Or you can visit www.aota.org on the Internet.

• *Dr. Jacobs is a faculty member at Boston University and currently president-elect of The American Occupational Therapy Association.*

FIGURE 15.2 Press release developed by the American Occupational Therapy Association to promote occupational therapy's role in ergonomics. (Reprinted with permission from the American Occupational Therapy Association. Bethesda, MD, 1998.)

Executing and Evaluating the Marketing Plan

After the target market has been selected and the marketing mix developed, the marketing plan should be initiated. Because marketing is a dynamic activity, a plan requires continual evaluation of its effectiveness. A time frame, such as a 12-month period, should be established to determine whether objectives and goals are being met. The marketing plan should be flexible to allow changes to be made as new opportunities and problems arise.

Case Study

The following case study demonstrates the use of marketing before the expansion of services.

A well-established, free-standing industrial rehabilitation center decided to start including ergonomics consultation as a service. The director of the center decided to perform a market analysis to determine the feasibility of such an expansion. In the first step, which involved identifying target markets, the director analyzed marketing opportunities; the analysis included a self-audit, a consumer analysis, a competitive analysis, and an environmental assessment.

Self-Audit

A SWOT analysis was performed to determine the strengths and weaknesses of, opportunities for, and threats to the center.

Strengths

- Three occupational and physical therapists with master's degrees; two of these therapists are CPEs.
- Excellent reputation in the community
- Located in an area with a high concentration of plastics and paper manufacturers

Weakness

- Limited financial resources for the purchase of equipment needed for work-site analysis

Opportunities

- The medical director of the center had been appointed medical director of a local plastics-manufacturing company.
- The center is eligible to apply for state funding provided by the Department of Industrial Accidents to develop a proposal for ergo-

nomics training for companies with workers at risk for cumulative trauma disorders.

Threat

- Two local physical therapists in private practice are expanding services to include ergonomics consultation.

Consumer Analysis

The consumer analysis revealed the following markets as potential users of ergonomics consultation:

- Local industry, in particular manufacturers whose employees perform repetitive upper-extremity tasks and material handling (e.g., paper manufacturers)
- Employees who work extensively with computers, such as insurance agency personnel

Competitive Analysis

A competitive analysis revealed two competitors within a 30-mile radius of the center. These competitors were identified in the self-audit under the "threat" category.

Environmental Assessment

An environmental assessment indicated that the center was located in an industrial community with an aging workforce. One manufacturer of plastics noted that over the last 2 years an increasing number of workers sustained cumulative trauma disorders. Concurrently, the number of lost work days per 100 workers increased steadily.

Market Segmentation

After the market analysis was completed in 2 weeks, a market segmentation was proposed. The potential consumers of ergonomics consultation were divided into distinct groups. For example, physicians were specified as orthopedic surgeons, occupational health practitioners, and neurologists. This market was further defined by the selection of only occupational health physicians as proposed primary referral sources for ergonomics consultation. Market segmentation was also performed for industrial sites.

The next step in the analysis involved developing marketing strategies specific to target markets by devising the optimal mix of product, place, price, and promotion. One of the target markets was a local plastics manufacturer. The center's product line for this manufacturer included baseline ergonomics screening surveys, work-site analyses, customized education and training programs, work-site modifications, and product design and evaluation (see Chapter 7 for more information on product design and evaluation). Ergonomics consultation would be provided at the work site, and the price of services would be based on cost-plus and consideration of what the competition was charging.

Promotion was aimed at the plastics industry. Personal selling was identified as the most effective sales mechanism: One of the center's therapists contacted the director of human resources of the plastics manufacturer to arrange for an appointment to promote ergonomics consultation. The development of a brochure was also suggested to delineate the center's expanded product line of ergonomics consultation. A time line was proposed to help determine whether the strategies resulted in contracts for ergonomics consultation.

When the market analysis was completed, expanding the center's product line to include ergonomics consultation on a trial basis (12 months) seemed feasible. The director evaluated the strategies after 6 months and again at the end of the year to determine whether the goals and objectives were being met.

Conclusion

The use of a marketing approach allows therapists to take a proactive approach in the health care environment and be ready to meet changing needs and wants of the marketplace. According to Schwartz (1991, p. 365),

> [o]ccupational therapy is strategically placed to assume a leadership role in work place injury prevention. . . . Prevention services offered by occupational therapists both minimize the incidence and severity of disability, for a far lower cost than occupational health physicians and other primary care providers have traditionally charged.

References

Bloswick D (1993). Developing Ergonomics Programs in Industry: A Practical Guide. Salt Lake City, UT: University of Utah Press.

California Code of Regulations. Title 8, Section 5110. The "Ergonomic" Regulation. Readopted April 17, 1997; effective July 3, 1997.

Coy J, Davenport M (1991). Age changes in the older adult worker: implications for injury prevention. Work 2:38–46.

Folts D, Jeremko J, Houk D (1993). Marketing's role in work programs. Work 3:13–18.

Jacobs K (1989). Work Hardening in the Health Care System. In L Ogden-Niemeyer, K Jacobs (eds), Work Hardening: State of the Art. Thorofare, NJ: Slack, 111–126.

Jacobs K (1991). A marketing approach to work practice. Work Programs Special Interest Section Newsletter 5:3–4.

Jacobs K (1992). From the Editor. Work 2:1.

Jacobs K (1994). Marketing Occupational Therapy Services. In K Jacobs, M Logigian (eds), Functions of a Manager in Occupational Therapy. Thorofare, NJ: Slack, 33–49.

Kiernan W, Carter A, Bronstein E (1989). Marketing and Marketing Management in Rehabilitation. In W Kiernan, R Schalock (eds), Economics, Industry, and Disability. Baltimore: Brookes, 49–56.

Kotler P (1975). Marketing for Non Profit Organizations. Englewood Cliffs, NJ: Prentice-Hall.

Kotler P (1983). Principles of Marketing: Instructor's Manual with Cases. Englewood Cliffs, NJ: Prentice-Hall.

OSHA (1995). Draft ergonomics protection standard. Federal Register 57(149): 34192–34200.

OSHA (1991). Ergonomic Program Management Guidelines for Meatpacking Plants. U.S. Department of Labor.

Schwartz R (1991). Prevention. In K Jacobs (ed), Occupational Therapy: Work Related Programs and Assessments. Boston: Little, Brown, 365–381.

Sehnal J, Christopher R (1993). Developing and marketing an ergonomics program in a corporate office environment. Work 3:22–30.

Smith M (1993). Ergonomic update: legislative, judicial, and other happenings. Prev Inj 2:8–9.

Sutherland R, Counihan W (1990). Functional restoration for the back-injured worker: a sports medicine approach. Occup Ther Prac 1:11–26.

Review Questions

(Answers are found in Appendix D.)

1. The four Ps of the marketing mix are
   (a) price, packaging, place, promotion
   (b) place, price, promotion, product
   (c) product, packaging, promotion, place
   (d) product, procedure, price, packaging

2. What are the components of a marketing approach?
   (a) Analyze market opportunities, research and select target markets and market segments, develop marketing strategies, and execute and evaluate the plan.
   (b) Develop a product, promote the product, and analyze the success of the product.
   (c) Market the product, research market segments, and evaluate the plan.
   (d) Analyze market opportunities, develop marketing strategies, and evaluate the plan.

3. A SWOT analysis, or self-audit, evaluates
    (a) strengths, weaknesses, organization, and treatment
    (b) support, weaknesses, opportunities, and treatment
    (c) strengths, weaknesses, opportunities, and threats
    (d) segments, weaknesses, organizations, and threats

4. Which is the most effective form of promotion?
    (a) Advertising
    (b) Publicity
    (c) Personal selling
    (d) Sales promotion

Appendices

APPENDIX A

Work-Site Job Analysis and Design Considerations

I. Job organization and structure
   A. Hours per shift
   B. Breaks
   C. Rest periods
   D. Job rotation
   E. Piece work
   F. Job-rate quotas
   G. Production incentives
   H. Work pace
   I. Work schedule
II. Tools and equipment
   A. Weight and size
   B. Mechanical aids for heavy tools and equipment
   C. Balances
   D. Sharpness
   E. Location
   F. Condition
   G. Temperature
   H. Power vs. manual
   I. Grasping surface, friction, and slip resistance
   J. Glove use and fit
   K. Sliding vs. lifting
   L. Torque
   M. Force requirements
   N. Handles
      1. Size and shape
      2. Thickness or diameter

      3. Grip or pinch design
      4. Serrations
      5. Friction with hand
      6. Length
      7. Surface material
      8. Compressibility of material (e.g., wood, metal, rubber)
      9. Heat or electrical conductivity
    10. Sharp edges
    11. Hand-tool position or resulting posture
    12. Ability to use in both hands
    13. Dampening material coating to minimize vibration
  O. Padding, bolsters, and cushions
  P. Curved vs. sharp edges and corners of tools and equipment
  Q. Use of tools vs. hands for pounding
  R. Foot pedal use, location, position, and number
III. Manual materials handling
  A. Force and weight of load
  B. Location of load in relation to the worker
     1. Horizontal distance
     2. Vertical distance
     3. Amount of twisting required to handle material
     4. Storage position for accessibility
  C. Size of load or container
  D. Load stability
  E. Location of coupling, handles, or cutouts
  F. Mechanical aid availability (e.g., carts, hoists, scissoring pallets or tables, two-wheelers)
  G. Availability of automation
  H. Lifting frequency
  I. Working surface (e.g., texture, level, and response to spills)
  J. Worker availability for two-person lifts
  K. Workplace layout and design
     1. Location and height of shelving, tables, and benches for positioning loads at easily accessible levels
     2. Presence of barriers or obstacles in work area
     3. Movement quality, symmetry, and balance during work
     4. Posture during work
  L. Environmental factors
     1. Lighting and illumination
     2. Vibration
     3. Temperature and humidity
     4. Noise level
     5. Air quality and circulation

M. Age and gender

N. National Institute of Occupational Safety and Health lifting equation

IV. Controls and display presentation

    A. Type of information

    B. Ease of reach for frequently used controls

    C. Feedback to indicate that control has been activated (e.g., tactile, auditory, visual)

    D. Information complexity (e.g., easy to read or identify)

    E. Size, shape, and color for control emphasis

    F. Placement of guards to prevent accidental activation

    G. Viewing distance, angle, and lighting

V. Seated work

    A. Chair

        1. Height adjustability

        2. Seat pan width and depth

        3. Backrest and lumbar support adjustability

        4. Armrests

        5. Footrests

        6. Caster base

        7. Maneuverability

        8. Ease of adjustment operation

        9. Size, appearance, and overall comfort

        10. Type of work performed during chair use

    B. Ease of job in seated position

    C. Location of objects to be lifted

    D. Location of objects to be handled

    E. Height of work surface

    F. Ability to alternate sitting and standing

    G. Dynamic vs. static work

    H. Posture

    I. Stretch breaks

VI. Standing work

    A. Standing surface

    B. Antifatigue mats

    C. Cushioned shoes or inserts

    D. Height of work surface

    E. Location of objects and equipment

    F. Rails, bars, and stools for footrest

    G. Ability to alternate standing and sitting

    H. Sit-stand chairs

    I. Dynamic vs. static work

    J. Posture

    K. Stretch breaks

VII. Psychosocial environment
   A. Job complexity
   B. Monotony and repetition
   C. Peer and social support
   D. Worker autonomy
   E. Accuracy requirements
   F. Excessive task speed or load
   G. Sensory deprivation and isolation

APPENDIX B

Americans with Disabilities Act Work-Site Assessment*

Company: _____   Areas evaluated: _____
Address: _____   Telephone: _____
Job title: _____
Primary function of company: _____
Contact person: _____
Reason for referral: _____
Date: _____   Evaluated by: _____

Method of evaluation:
_____ Observation of worker
_____ Simulation of job by worker
_____ Discussion of job with worker (identity)
_____ Review of company job description
_____ Review of *Dictionary of Occupational Titles*

Signature of company representative: _____

Terms:
Sedentary work: lift 10 lb maximum; occasionally carry small objects
Light work: lift 20 lb maximum; frequently lift or carry up to 10 lb
Medium work: lift 20 lb maximum; frequently lift or carry up to 25 lb
Heavy work: lift 100 lb maximum; frequently lift or carry up to 50 lb
Very heavy work: lift in excess of 100 lb; frequently lift or carry 50 lb
In terms of an 8-hour workday: Constantly   67–100%
                                  Frequently   34–66%
                                  Occasionally 1–33%

*Source: Modified from D Aja, K Jacobs, D Hermenau (1992). ADA Work Site Assessment.

Brief description of job:

_____

_____

_____

_____

Functional Body Positions of the Job

What is the maximum amount of sitting required?
_____ constant   _____ frequent   _____ occasional   _____ never
_____ essential   _____ marginal

What is the worker actually doing while sitting?

_____

_____

_____

What is the maximum amount of standing required?
_____ constant   _____ frequent   _____ occasional   _____ never
_____ essential   _____ marginal

What is the worker actually doing while standing?

_____

_____

_____

What is the maximum amount of walking required?
_____ constant   _____ frequent   _____ occasional   _____ never
_____ essential   _____ marginal

What is the worker actually doing while walking?

_____

_____

_____

What is the maximum amount of climbing required?
_____ constant   _____ frequent   _____ occasional   _____ never
_____ essential   _____ marginal

What is the worker actually doing while climbing?

_____

_____

_____

What is the maximum amount of balancing required?
_____ constant   _____ frequent   _____ occasional   _____ never
_____ essential   _____ marginal

What is the worker actually doing while balancing?

_____

_____

_____

What is the maximum amount of stooping required?
_____ constant   _____ frequent   _____ occasional   _____ never
_____ essential   _____ marginal

What is the worker actually doing while stooping?

_____

_____

_____

What is the maximum amount of kneeling required?
_____ constant   _____ frequent   _____ occasional   _____ never
_____ essential   _____ marginal

What is the worker actually doing while kneeling?

_____

_____

_____

What is the maximum amount of crouching required?
_____ constant   _____ frequent   _____ occasional   _____ never
_____ essential   _____ marginal

What is the worker actually doing while crouching?

_____

_____

_____

What is the maximum amount of crawling required?
_____ constant   _____ frequent   _____ occasional   _____ never
_____ essential   _____ marginal

What is the worker actually doing while crawling?

_____

_____

_____

What is the maximum amount of pulling required?
_____ constant   _____ frequent   _____ occasional   _____ never
_____ essential   _____ marginal

What is the worker actually doing while pulling?

_____
_____
_____

What is the maximum amount of pushing required?
_____ constant   _____ frequent   _____ occasional   _____ never
_____ essential   _____ marginal

What is the worker actually doing while pushing?

_____
_____
_____

What is the maximum amount of fingering required?
_____ constant   _____ frequent   _____ occasional   _____ never
_____ essential   _____ marginal

What is the worker actually doing while fingering?

_____
_____
_____

What is the maximum amount of feeling required?
_____ constant   _____ frequent   _____ occasional   _____ never
_____ essential   _____ marginal

What is the worker actually doing while feeling?

_____
_____
_____

What is the maximum amount of reaching at shoulder height or overhead required?
_____ constant   _____ frequent   _____ occasional   _____ never
_____ essential   _____ marginal

What is the worker actually doing while reaching at shoulder height or overhead? (Include reaching distance.)

_____
_____
_____

What is the maximum amount of reaching below shoulder height required?
_____ constant   _____ frequent   _____ occasional   _____ never
_____ essential   _____ marginal

What is the worker actually doing while reaching below shoulder height?
(Include reaching distance.)

_____

_____

_____

Environmental Conditions

What is the maximum amount of inside work required?
_____ constant   _____ frequent   _____ occasional   _____ never
_____ essential   _____ marginal

What is the worker actually doing when performing inside work?

_____

_____

_____

What is the maximum amount of outside work required?
_____ constant   _____ frequent   _____ occasional   _____ never
_____ essential   _____ marginal

What is the worker actually doing when performing outside work?

_____

_____

_____

Is the worker exposed to cold temperatures?
_____ constant   _____ frequent   _____ occasional   _____ never
_____ essential   _____ marginal

What is the worker actually doing when working in cold temperatures?

_____

_____

_____

Is the worker exposed to hot temperatures?
_____ constant   _____ frequent   _____ occasional   _____ never
_____ essential   _____ marginal

What is the worker actually doing when working in hot temperatures?

_____

_____

_____

Is the worker exposed to wet or humid conditions?
_____ constant _____ frequent _____ occasional _____ never
_____ essential _____ marginal

What is the worker actually doing when performing work in wet or humid conditions?

_____

_____

_____

Is the worker exposed to noise or vibration (circle whichever applies or both)?
_____ constant _____ frequent _____ occasional _____ never
_____ essential _____ marginal

What is the worker actually doing when performing work that exposes him or her to noise or vibration?

_____

_____

_____

Is the worker exposed to hazardous work?
_____ constant _____ frequent _____ occasional _____ never
_____ essential _____ marginal

What is the worker actually doing when performing hazardous work?

_____

_____

_____

Is the worker exposed to fumes, odors, dust, or toxic conditions?
_____ constant _____ frequent _____ occasional _____ never
_____ essential _____ marginal

What is the worker actually doing when exposed to fumes, odors, dust, or toxic conditions?

_____

_____

_____

Is the worker exposed to poor ventilation?
_____ constant   _____ frequent   _____ occasional   _____ never
_____ essential   _____ marginal

What is the worker actually doing when exposed to poor ventilation?

_____

_____

Intellectual Demands and Credentials

Is a specific educational degree, certificate, or license required by federal, state, or professional agencies to perform the job?
_____ yes   _____ no
_____ essential   _____ marginal

Credentials required:

_____

_____

Is previous experience required for the job?
_____ yes   _____ no
_____ essential   _____ marginal

Communication Demands

Is being able to read necessary to perform the job?
_____ yes   _____ no
_____ essential   _____ marginal

Nature of reading required:

_____

_____

Is being able to write necessary to perform the job?
_____ yes   _____ no
_____ essential   _____ marginal

Nature of writing required:

_____

_____

_____

Is being able to perform mathematical operations necessary for the job?
_____ yes _____ no
_____ essential _____ marginal

Nature of mathematical skills required:

_____
_____
_____

Is being able to see necessary to perform the job?
_____ yes _____ no
_____ essential _____ marginal

Visual skills required:

_____
_____
_____

Is being able to hear necessary to perform the job?
_____ yes _____ no
_____ essential _____ marginal

Auditory acuity required:

_____
_____
_____

Is being able to speak necessary to perform the job?
_____ yes _____ no
_____ essential _____ marginal

Command of language required:

_____
_____
_____

Equipment Use

During a work shift, is nonvehicular machinery or equipment used?
_____ yes _____ no

Name and function	Use						On the-job training?		Operator's license required?	
	Const.	Freq.	Occ.	Never	Essential	Marginal	Yes	No	Yes	No

Manual Lifting

Describe how objects are handled during a maximum-output day. Include height, weight, shape, frequency of movement, how the object is manipulated, and for what purpose (e.g., 60-lb rectangular boxes [13 in. × 10 in. × 5 in.] are lifted from the floor to a table 30 in. high at a rate of one lift per minute; the boxes are lifted to a table to be opened and the contents sorted).

Task	H origin	H dest.	V origin	V dest.	F	Asymmetric origin	Asymmetric dest.	Coupling	Weight

H = horizontal distance of the hands from the midpoint between the ankles; V = vertical distance of the hands from the floor; F = average frequency of lifting.

Recommended Weight Limit

Recommended weight limit (RWL) = LC × HM × VM × DM × AM × FM × CM

RWL = 51 lb × (10/H) × [1 − (0.0075 |V − 30|)] × [0.82 + (1.8/D)] × (1 − 0.0032A) × (FM from table) × (CM from table). *LC* stands for load constant, *HM* for horizontal multiplier, *VM* for vertical multiplier, *AM* for asymmetric multiplier, *CM* for coupling multiplier, *DM* for distance multiplier, and *FM* for frequency multiplier.

APPENDIX C

Job Analysis during Employer Site Visit*

Summary of Factors to Be Analyzed

Environmental conditions
Social conditions
Job tasks
Physical demands
Cognitive demands
Classification of work by amount of strength required
Physical barriers

Employer name: _____
Address: _____
Client name: _____
Job title: _____
Job location (include building name or number): _____
Date of visit: _____
Vocational rehabilitation specialist: _____

Instructions: Check any of the conditions listed in this analysis that are present in the work area.

Environmental Conditions

Condition	Definition
1. _____ Inside	Protected from weather conditions, as in factory or office work or long-distance truck driving.

---

*Source: Modified from a form created by MD Taber.

Condition	Definition
2. _____ Outside	No effective protection from the weather, such as postal work or outdoor labor.
3. _____ Extreme heat	Temperature sufficiently high to cause marked bodily discomfort, such as when working next to a hot stove or furnace or near a hot asphalt–spreading machine.
4. _____ Extreme cold	Temperature sufficiently low to cause marked bodily discomfort, such as when working in a cold storage room.
5. _____ Humid or wet	Atmospheric conditions in which moisture content is sufficiently high to cause marked bodily discomfort, such as when using a steam garment presser or being in contact with water or other liquids.
6. _____ Noise _____ (a) _____ (b)	(a) Sound loud enough to distract workers engaged in mental occupations, such as sounds greater than those made by a single typewriter or office machine; (b) sound loud enough to cause hearing damage, such as noise greater than 80 dB (approximately equal to the sound heard in a car in heavy traffic).
7. _____ Vibration	Oscillating movement or strain on the body or extremities from repeated motion or shock that may cause harm if endured day after day, such as operating a jackhammer.
8. _____ Mechanical hazards	Danger to fingers or limbs due to feeding animals or operating power-driven equipment.
9. _____ Electrical hazards	Danger due to possible electrical shock from electric wires, hazards transformers, or noninsulated electrical parts.
10. _____ (a) Fire _____ (b) Hot materials _____ (c) Chemical agents	Danger due to possible burns from any of these causes.

11. _____ Radiant energy   Exposure to radiant energy such as x-rays, radioactive material, or UV light.

12. _____ Poor ventilation   Insufficient or excessive movement of air or exposure to drafts.

13. _____ Moving objects   Exposure to moving equipment and objects in the immediate work area, such as automobiles, cranes, gurneys, and forklifts.

14. _____ Sharp tools   Exposure to tools or materials with sharp edges.

15. _____ Cluttered or slippery floors   Walking surfaces strewn with equipment, tools, or electrical wiring while work is being done, creating a risk of tripping or falling; wet, muddy, oily, or highly polished surfaces, which may cause worker to slip or lose footing.

16. _____ Elevated surfaces   Work occurs in places elevated above the ground, such as on catwalks, scaffolds, ladders, and roofs.

17. _____ Poor lighting   Nonadjustable lighting conditions that place excessive strain on vision during work; lighting conditions that are too dim or too bright.

18. Exposure to: Check specific condition if present.
_____ (a) Fumes
_____ (b) Odors
_____ (c) Dust
_____ (d) Mist
_____ (e) Gases

Social Conditions

Condition

Definition

19. ___ Working with others   Job duties that require communication and cooperation with other workers, customers, or the public; includes social skills and ability to tolerate frustration when dealing with others; workers who have such jobs include sales clerks, supervisors, and police officers.

Condition	Definition
20. _____ Working around others	Job duties that require the worker to work independently but near other workers, requiring only minimal verbal contact; examples include carpenters on construction crews or assembly line workers.
21. _____ Working alone	Job duties that require independent occupational effort and virtually no contact with fellow workers or the public, such as writers.
22. _____ Supervisor	Job duties that require direct supervision of other workers.
23. _____ Contact with violent or belligerent people	Job duties that require contact with people who may behave or speak in an aggressive, hostile, or threatening manner or with people who have a high probability of such behavior; workers who have such job duties are police officers, bouncers, and psychiatric aides.
24. _____ Working shifts that do not occur between 8:00 AM and 5:00 PM	Includes split shifts, rotating shifts, and mandatory overtime; does not include flex time (i.e., positions in which worker chooses to work earlier or later).
25. _____ Protective equipment	Equipment such as eye protection, canvas or rubber gloves, safety shoes, hard hats, and brightly colored vests worn regularly.

Job Tasks

Is the task critical? (circle one)	*Amount of time in one shift*	*Job tasks*
yes/no	_____	1. _____
		_____
		_____
		_____
		_____
		_____
		_____
yes/no	_____	2. _____
		_____
		_____
		_____
		_____
		_____
		_____
yes/no	_____	3. _____
		_____
		_____
		_____
		_____
		_____

Physical Demands

Physical requirements	Hours required in an 8-hour day	Minimum activity requirements	Distance	Job activity
Standing				
Sitting				
Walking				
Lifting				
Carrying				
Pushing				
Climbing				
Balancing				
Bending or squatting				
Twisting				
Rotating				
Crawling				
Kneeling				
Reaching above head				
Reaching at waist level				

Cognitive Demands

	Yes	No
1. Job requires complete independence of task.	____	____
2. Moderate amount of supervision is provided for this position.	____	____
3. Minimum supervision is given but is available on request.	____	____
4. Written directions are available to employee outlining the various steps of the job.	____	____
5. Verbal instructions are given initially during training, but constant cues are not available to employee concerning the job duties.	____	____

	Yes	No

6. The position is very structured.
7. The job is unstructured and requires much input from the employee regarding organization, planning, and sequence of task.
8. The following skills are required for the job:
   Short-term memory
   Long-term memory
   Organization
   Planning
   Sequencing
   Verbal fluency
   Reasoning
   Judgment
   Problem solving
   Safety awareness
   Visual-spatial skills
   Topographic orientation
   Fine-motor dexterity
   Gross-motor coordination
9. Work environment is distracting (e.g., abundance of noise, many people come in and out).
10. Employer appears willing to modify job (e.g., provides added supervision, structure, directions).

Classification of Work by Amount of Strength Required

Sedentary

Sedentary work involves lifting no more than 10 lb and occasionally lifting or carrying articles such as ledgers or hand tools. Although a *sedentary job* is defined as one that involves sitting, some walking and standing may be necessary to perform duties. Examples include the following: (1) A worker sits at a desk most of day, takes dictation, transcribes dictation on a typewriter, and occasionally walks to various departments (2) A worker sits at a drawing board, walks occasionally, and carries paper, instruments, and books.

Light

Light work involves lifting no more than 20 lb, with frequent lifting or carrying of objects up to 10 lb. Even though weight is negligible, a job fits into this category when it requires walking or standing to a considerable degree or when it requires sitting most of the time but entails pushing or pulling arm and or leg controls. Examples include the following: (1) A worker stands and walks behind a counter of a variety store all day to wrap and bag articles for customers. (2) A worker walks and stands constantly while arranging records in file cabinets and sits occasionally to sort paper. (3) A worker sits most of day and operates an industrial sewing machine.

Medium

Medium work involves lifting no more than 50 lb, with frequent lifting or carrying objects that weigh up to 25 lb. Examples include the following: (1) A worker assists in lifting patients, pushing gurneys, and pulling sheets from beds. (2) In the heaviest of several job duties, a worker lifts, pushes, and pulls to jack an automobile, remove a tire from a wheel, and remount the tire on the wheel.

Heavy

Heavy work involves lifting no more than 100 lb, with frequent lifting or carrying objects that weigh up to 50 lb. Examples include the following: (1) A worker pushes hand trucks up and down aisles of warehouse to fill orders and stoops to lift cartons of items with an average weight of 65 lb to place them on the truck. (2) A worker digs a trench to specified depth and width using a shovel.

Physical Barriers

	Yes	No
Parking		
1. Is parking that is adjacent or convenient to the work site provided?	____	____
2. Is the route from parking to work site barrier-free?	____	____
3. Are spaces indicated for handicapped individuals?	____	____
4. Are spaces at least 12 ft wide?	____	____
Ramp		
5. Is a ramp available for access to building?	____	____
6. Is the ramp at least 45 in. wide?	____	____
7. Is the slope no more than 1 in. in rise per 12 in. in length?	____	____
8. Does the ramp have at least one handrail?	____	____
9. Does the ramp have landings at top and bottom for 5 in. in direction of travel?	____	____
Building entrance		
10. Is at least one accessible building entrance a main entrance?	____	____
11. Does the door require less than 8 lb of force to open?	____	____

	Yes	No
12. Is at least 32 in. clearance provided?	___	___
13. Is an area of at least 5 in. × 5 ft provided in the direction of door swing?	___	___
14. Is the threshold flat, or does it have a maximum 0.5-in. slope?	___	___

Elevators

15. Are elevators directly accessible from a usable entrance?	___	___
16. Is the office or work site directly accessible from a usable main entrance or elevator?	___	___
17. Does the elevator car automatically come within 0.5 in. of building floor?	___	___
18. Are the highest controls within 54 in. of the floor?	___	___
19. Do elevator panels have braille and raised arabic symbols to the right of buttons?	___	___

Floors

20. Are floors made of a smooth, nonslip material or covered with low-nap carpet?	___	___

Doors

21. Do doors within work sites have 32-in. clear openings?	___	___
22. Are doors opened by lever handles instead of door knobs?	___	___
23. Are thresholds sloped and less than 0.5 in. high?	___	___
24. Are passageways at least 48 in. wide and free of tight turns?	___	___
25. Can existing obstructions within passageways or offices be easily moved?	___	___

Rest Room

26. Is a rest room convenient and accessible to work site?	___	___
27. Do entry doors have 32-in. clear openings?	___	___
28. Is passageway from rest room entrance to stall 43 in. wide at all points?	___	___
29. If a vestibule is between two doors, is it at least 5.5 ft long?	___	___
30. Is at least 29 in. of vertical clearance provided under sink?	___	___
31. Are the sink controls the single-lever type?	___	___
32. Does at least one rest-room stall have a 30-in. clear entrance?	___	___
33. Do stall doors open out?	___	___
34. Are stalls at least 36 in. wide?	___	___
35. Is the distance from the front of the seat to the closed door at least 48 in.?	___	___

	Yes	No
36. Is a handrail provided on each side of stall?	_____	_____
37. Are the handrails parallel to and 33 in. from the floor?	_____	_____

Water fountain

	Yes	No
38. Is at least one water fountain no more than 36 in. from floor, or has a cup dispenser been provided?	_____	_____
39. Has knee clearance of at least 27 in. been provided beneath fountain?	_____	_____
40. Are spout and controls in front?	_____	_____

Telephone

	Yes	No
41. Is a telephone available and accessible for use?	_____	_____
42. If not, is a public phone in an accessible area?	_____	_____
43. Is at least one telephone mounted so that the highest operable parts are no more than 54 in. above the floor?	_____	_____
44. Does the booth entrance provide 30 in. wide clearance?	_____	_____

Travel

	Yes	No
45. Does job require travel to noncompany sites that may not be accessible?	_____	_____

APPENDIX D

Answers to Review Questions

Chapter 1

1. Therapists must be aware of what is "normal" or expected to provide therapy that encourages regaining as much physical, emotional, and cognitive function as possible. The ergonomist must be aware of normal abilities to design items, products, environments, and so forth that match and do not exceed capabilities.
2. engineering, medicine, and psychology
3. "Honor thy user." Products and environments designed by ergonomists should match abilities, needs, and perceptions of the people who use them. The population for which an object or place is designed should be adequately considered. For example, an ergonomist should examine cultural differences such as language, physical size, and religious requirements or beliefs to determine whether a design can and will be used by the people for whom it is intended.
4. Assuming that a product matches human abilities, characteristics, and preferences based on a match to oneself or one's coworkers or on anecdotal evidence is not sufficient, as such a decision, made without scientific basis, can result in injury, illness, or inefficiency. Sample questions to be considered include the following: How much weight should be packed into boxes that have to be carried by men? By women? By men or women in teams? If the boxes must be lifted overhead for storage, should the amount of weight allowed in the box be changed? Does the box shape or the presence or absence of handles make a difference? Each task, environment, and product must be considered in terms of the entire system and series of requirements. Unless research is conducted and a systems approach used, solutions to design questions will be inaccurate and cause more problems or injuries than are solved.

5. Three factors that contribute to the paucity of ergonomics research for disabled populations are financial expense, lack of public support for spending, and lack of sufficient databases on which to base designs for special populations.

Chapter 2

1. d
2. c
3. d
4. d
5. b

Chapter 3

1. c
2. d
3. b
4. d
5. b

Chapter 4

1. b
2. a
3. c
4. a
5. a

Chapter 5

1. a and c
2. c
3. a, c, and d
4. d
5. a

Chapter 6

1. e
2. c
3. c
4. c

Chapter 7

1. b
2. d
3. d
4. b
5. d

Chapter 8

1. Usability testing involves evaluating a product to determine how easy (or hard) it is to use. Tests should be conducted with the people who will use the product. For example, if a hair dryer will be used by pre-teens, teenagers, and the elderly, all problems each group has with the product must be documented. The groups should also be asked about their likes and dislikes of the product and whether they think they would use it. Discovering problems people may have with a product before it goes on the market can help prevent injuries.
2. All patients, health care providers, and family or friends of a patient who might administer or use the equipment should be considered.
3. Errors are most often evidence of the failure of a system, rather than the failure of an individual. This philosophy has been more effective in reducing medically related human errors than blaming the individual (whether the individual is a patient or a health care worker). If someone must be trained to use or is incorrectly using a product, a problem exists with the design of the product. When possible, the best idea is to design the product so the mistake cannot be made.
4. *Context* refers to the necessary circumstances in which the item will be used or the task will be conducted. *Ecologic validity* refers to how closely the testing environment resembles the actual environment (i.e., how closely it resembles the context). The context can affect the user's ability to use a product. For example, the design of a warning label and instructions on a package of sleep suppressants (e.g., Vivarin, No-Doz) should take into consideration the user's sleepiness, which can impair concentration and the ability to read.
5. A design must be proposed, tested, rejected (or accepted), and revised repeatedly to obtain the best possible design. A minimum of three iterations are recommended: (1) product development (prototype or pilot testing), (2) efficacy testing (performance testing in a controlled setting), and (3) field testing (evaluation in a setting similar to the environment in which the product will be used). Even when a product is on the market, it should be evaluated and redesigned if problems are identified or new procedures or pertinent products are developed.
6. (1) Identify subject-matter experts.

   (2) Define the project and raise questions about the product through discussion between the investigators, subject-matter experts, and representatives from the user groups.

   (3) Identify design objectives.

   (4) Analyze tasks and functions.

   (5) Develop performance criteria.

   (6) Select measurement techniques to quantify objective and subjective performance.

   (7) Recruit and train subjects.

   (8) Conduct formal or informal testing.

   (9) Initiate re-evaluation or redesign.

Chapter 9

1. e
2. c
3. a and c
4. b
5. all except e

Chapter 10

1. c
2. c
3. b
4. e
5. b

Chapter 11

1. e
2. a
3. e
4. e
5. a
6. b
7. d
8. e
9. d
10. e

Chapter 12

1. c
2. a
3. a
4. c
5. e

Chapter 13

1. d
2. c
3. d
4. a
5. d

Chapter 14

Review questions not provided.

Chapter 15

1. b
2. a
3. c
4. c

Index

Note: Page numbers followed by *f* indicate figures; page numbers followed by *t* indicate tables.